Medical Intelligence Unit

Strategies in Vaccine Design

Medical Intelligence Unit

Strategies in Vaccine Design

Gordon L. Ada

Australian National University
Canberra

R.G. Landes Company
Austin

MEDICAL INTELLIGENCE UNIT

STRATEGIES IN VACCINE DESIGN

R.G. LANDES COMPANY
Austin

CRC Press is the exclusive worldwide distributor of publications of the Medical Intelligence Unit.
CRC Press, 2000 Corporate Blvd., NW, Boca Raton, FL 33431. Phone: 407/994-0555.

Submitted: November 1993
Published: February 1994

Production Manager: Elinda McKenna
Copy Editor: Francine Daniel

Printed on recycled paper by Walsworth Publishing Co., Marceline, Missouri, U.S.A.

Please address all inquiries to the Publisher:
R.G. Landes Company, 909 Pine Street, Georgetown, TX 78626
or
P.O. Box 4858, Austin, TX 78765
Phone: 512/ 863 7762; FAX: 512/ 863 0081

ISBN 1-57059-094-X
CATALOG # LN9094

While the authors, editors and publisher believe that drug selection and dosage and the specifications and usage of equipment and devices, as set forth in this book, are in accord with current recommendations and practice at the time of publication, they make no warranty, expressed or implied, with respect to material described in this book. In view of the ongoing research, equipment development, changes in governmental regulations and the rapid accumulation of information relating to the biomedical sciences, the reader is urged to carefully review and evaluate the information provided herein.

Library of Congress Cataloging-in-Publication Data

Strategies in vaccine design / [edited by] Gordon L. Ada.
p. cm.—(Medical intelligence unit)
Includes bibliographical references and index.
ISBN 1-57059-094-X (hard cover) : $89.95
1. Synthetic vaccines. 2. Vaccines—Design. I. Ada, G. L., 1922- . II. Series.
[DLNM: 1. Vaccines, Synthetic—immunology. 2. Immunity, Cellular—immunology.
QW 805 S898 1994]
QR189.2.S77 1994
615'.37—dc20
DNLM/DLC
for Library of Congress

93-46422
CIP

CONTENTS

CONTRIBUTORS

Gordon L. Ada
Division of Cell Biology
John Curtin School of Medical Research
The Australian National University
Canberra, ACT, Australia
Chapter 1

Nancy J. Alexander
Contraceptive Development Branch
National Institute of Child Health and Human Development
National Institutes of Health
Chapter 12

Jörg Arnoldi
Department of Immunology
University of Ulm
Albert-Einstein-Allee 11
Ulm, Germany
Chapter 6

Robert Blanden
Division of Cell Biology
John Curtin School of Medical Research
Australian National University
Canberra, ACT, Australia
Chapter 5

Peter A. Bretscher
Department of Microbiology
University of Saskatchewan
Saskatoon, Saskatchewan
Canada
Chapter 7

R. Mark L. Buller
Laboratory of Viral Diseases
National Institute of Allergy and Infectious Diseases
National Institutes of Health
Bethesda, MD
Chapter 10

Gregory F. Burton
Departments of Microbiology, Immunology and Anatomy
Medical College of Virginia
Virginia Commonwealth University
Richmond, VA
Chapter 3

Mario Clerici
Accociato di Immunologia
Nell Unitersita' di Milano
Via Abamono
MIlano, Italy
Chapter 8

Peter D. Cooper
Division of Cell Biology
John Curtin School of Medical Research
Australian National University
Canberra, ACT, Australia
Chapter 9

CONTRIBUTORS
Continued

Peter C. Doherty
Department of Immunology
St. Jude Children's Research Hospital
332 North Lauderdale
Memphis, TN and
Departments of Pathology and
Pediatrics
University of Tennessee
Memphis, TN
Chapter 4

Hikmat Hayder
Division of Cell Biology
John Curtin School of Medical Research
Australian National University
Canberra, ACT, Australia
Chapter 5

Sam Hou
Department of Immunology
St. Jude Children's Research Hospital
332 North Lauderdale
Memphis, TN
Chapter 4

Zoher F. Kapasi
Departments of Microbiology,
Immunology and Anatomy
Medical College of Virginia
Virginia Commonwealth University
Richmond, VA
Chapter 3

Stefan H. E. Kaufmann
Department of Immunology
University of Ulm
Albert-Einstein-Allee 11
Ulm, Germany
Chapter 6

Michael B. McChesney
California Regional Primate
Research Center
School of Veterinary Medicine and
Department of Medical Pathology
School of Medicine
University of California, Davis
Davis, CA
Chapter 12

Christopher J. Miller
California Regional Primate
Research Center
Department of Veterinary Pathology
Microbiology and Immunology
School of Veterinary Medicine

Department of Medical Pathology
School of Medicine
University of California, Davis
Davis, CA
Chapter 12

CONTRIBUTORS
Continued

Alistair J. Ramsay
Viral Engineering and Cytokine Research Group
Division of Cell Biology
John Curtin School of Medical Research
The Australian National University
Canberra, ACT, Australia
Chapter 11

Ian A. Ramshaw
Viral Engineering and Cytokine Research Group
Division of Cell Biology
John Curtin School of Medical Research
The Australian National University
Canberra, ACT, Australia
Chapter 11

Janet C. Ruby
Viral Engineering and Cytokine Research Group
Division of Cell Biology
John Curtin School of Medical Research
The Australian National University
Canberra, ACT, Australia
Chapter 11

Sally R. Sarawar
Department of Immunology
St. Jude Children's Research Hospital
332 North Lauderdale
Memphis, TN
Chapter 4

Gene M. Shearer
National Institutes of Health
National Cancer Institute/DCBDC
Experimental Immunology Branch
1000 Rockville Pike
Bethesda, MD
Chapter 8

Andras K. Szakal
Departments of Microbiology, Immunology and Anatomy
Division of Immunobiology
Medical College of Virginia
Virginia Commonwealth University
Richmond, VA
Chapter 3

Geraldine Taylor
AFRC Institute for Animal Health
Compton Laboratory
Compton, Berkshire, England
Chapter 2

John G. Tew
Departments of Microbiology, Immunology and Anatomy
Medical College of Virginia
Virginia Commonwealth University
Richmond, VA
Chapter 3

Ralph Tripp
Department of Immunology
St. Jude Children's Research Hospital
332 North Lauderdale
Memphis, TN
Chapter 4

PREFACE

About 50 vaccines are in use for medical purposes. Some are more efficacious than others. Most are to control agents which cause acute infections, that is, infections from which most people recover in a matter of one or a few weeks provided the challenge dose is not too high. Following recovery from the infection, most people possess immunity to the infectious agent (provided its antigenic specificity does not markedly change). The most successful of these vaccines include the live attenuated viruses—vaccinia, yellow fever, polio, and so on. Most of these were developed in an empirical fashion, such as prolonged tissue culture and a balance between attenuation and immunogenicity so that the preparation provides long-lasting immunity without causing significant disease. Immunologists made little contribution to the development of these vaccines. The guideline was to find something that works and use it!

When of necessity attention had to be turned to persistent infections such as malaria and with the arrival of HIV, AIDS, it became increasingly clear that this approach to vaccine development was unlikely to be successful. As the efficacy of a vaccine depends very largely on the nature and persistence of the immune response, there was a need to establish the immunological correlates of protection, the antigens important in this respect and the most effective methods to induce those protective responses. For years, it had seemed that immunologists, to be regarded as true exponents of the discipline, had to work with preparations such as DNP and/or KLH. But in the last decade or so, the challenge of these persisting infectious diseases has drawn an increasing number of talented immunologists into the arena of infectious diseases.

The infectious process can be divided into four stages—infection, replication, prevention of replication, and clearance of the infection. The adaptive immune response may prevent the infection (pre-formed antibody) and control and clear the infection (antibody and cell-mediated responses). Probably few vaccines induce 'sterilizing immunity', i.e., antibody completely prevents infection from occurring, so increasing attention has been paid to the later stages—control and clearance of the infection.

In this volume, after a general overview of the immune response, eleven essays review current knowledge and concepts mainly in these two areas. Antibody has an important role in controlling infections but until recently was thought unlikely to clear an intracellular infection. That this can occur, perhaps in unusual circumstances, is shown very clearly with respiratory syncytial viral infections in an animal model (Chapter 2). Efficacious vaccines generally provide long-term production of antibody. From discussions at vaccine meetings, I believe that the complex mechanism involved and the implications for successful vaccine development are not appreciated by many vaccinologists, so the remarkable series of events leading to memory B cell production and the recruitment of these cells to form antibody-secreting cells are outlined in Chapter 3.

The events leading to memory T cell development are not so well understood. In contrast to B cell memory, it is controversial whether there is a requirement for antigen persistence in order to have long-lived T cell memory. Some of the properties of T memory cells in this respect are reviewed in Chapter 4, which serves as an introduction to the exciting recent developments concerning the properties and roles of different T cell subsets. Four of the leading groups in these areas discuss the roles of $CD8^+$ CTLs and $CD4^+$ TH1 and TH2 cell populations (Chapters 5-8). The importance of $CD8^+$ CTLs was first recognized in viral infections, but it has now become very clear that they are also important in both some bacterial and parasitic infections. On the other hand, the question of susceptibility versus resistance to different infections in model systems and in a few human infections is increasingly being attributed to the balance between TH1 and TH2 cellular activity. Altogether, these four chapters present the latest information - and opinions - in this very important area. One offshoot of these studies has been a recognition of the importance of antigen dose in determining the characteristics of the subsequent immune response. Adjuvants are also increasingly being viewed in terms of the preferential induction of one or other (or both!) of these different responses and recent findings in this area are presented in Chapter 9.

In contrast to subunit and peptide-based preparations, infectious agents have their own (in-built as it were) adjuvanticity which contributes to the success of the live attenuated viral vaccines. Molecular biology is making it possible to replace the traditional approaches to attenuation with a much more specific technology: the deletion of specific nucleic acid segments from the viral genome leading to a controlled and hence reproducible level of attenuation while retaining immunogenicity. This is most clearly seen with some poxviruses and these developments are reviewed in Chapter 10. The net result is to add to the attractiveness of these preparations as vectors of DNA coding for antigens of other disease agents. An additional approach is to include also in the genome of the vector DNA coding for different lymphokines. This may not only contribute to the attenuation of the virus but also may influence the type of immune response generated (Chapter 11).

Globally, sexually-transmitted diseases are a major cause of morbidity. Many of the agents also show great antigenic variation. The advent of AIDS with its very high mortality rate has served to focus more attention on mucosal immunity, particularly of the female reproductive tract. It is fitting that the final chapter (Chapter 12) should report current progress on the mechanism of infection by SIV in monkeys at this site and approaches to obtaining persisting immunity. Substantial success would not only increase the chances of a vaccine greatly decreasing via secretory IgA the infectious HIV load, but also open the way to effectively combating other STDs, which are the major cause of human infertility.

I would like to thank the many colleagues who contributed so effectively to this volume.

Gordon Ada

CHAPTER 1

Vaccination Strategies to Control Infections: An Overview

Gordon L. Ada

INTRODUCTION

The mammalian body is enveloped in a sea of microorganisms, the great majority of which are harmless to the host; colonization of body cavities by some of these is in fact necessary for the health of the mammalian host. For example, the female vagina is normally colonized by several bacterial species which secrete products that contribute to the maintenance of a healthy environment.[1] Disease situations can develop when other bacteria or certain viruses or parasites become established at this site.

The greatest contribution to community welfare in industrialized countries was the introduction, particularly in the 19th century, of public health measures such as the provision of clean water supplies and adequate sanitary arrangements. This was followed in industrial countries by the development of a variety of vaccines against a number of viral and bacterial infections which, by the late 20th century, had reduced previously killer diseases such as measles and polio to minor public health problems. This was not the case in developing countries where a variety of parasitic, viral and bacterial infections were a major cause of morbidity and mortality. The challenge of malaria and the advent of HIV leading to the global AIDS pandemic drew the world's attention to the need for a greater effort in vaccine research.

Most human vaccines currently in use were developed empirically with the primary aims of safety and ability to protect the vaccinated host from disease when subsequently exposed to the wild-type agent. Although the efficacy of a vaccine depends upon the type and persistence of the immune

Strategies in Vaccine Design, edited by Gordon L. Ada, D.Sc.

response it generates, such knowledge was widely considered to be superfluous until comparatively recently. It is now acknowledged by most in this field that the development of effective vaccines to protect against chronic persistent infections such as malaria and HIV will be greatly assisted by a detailed knowledge of the desirable immune responses and how best to achieve them.

TYPES OF INFECTIONS

A wide variety of situations can exist, but some categorization can be made.

ACUTE VERSUS PERSISTENT INFECTIONS

The former apply to those infections which, in the great majority of those infected, either overwhelm the immune system and the infected host dies, or the host can mount a sufficiently strong immune response to limit and finally clear the infection. In the case of persistent infections, though the host may mount a strong immune response, it does not result in the clearance of the infection. There is a variety of reasons why this failure occurs and they mainly involve evasion of the cell-mediated immune responses (see below).

INTRACELLULAR VERSUS EXTRACELLULAR GROWTH PATTERNS

Some microorganisms, particularly certain bacteria (e.g., the pneumococcus) and certain parasites (e.g., schistosomes) live and replicate in the body outside cells. Other microorganisms such as all viruses, some bacteria (e.g., mycobacteria) and parasites (e.g., malaria) grow and replicate inside cells (obligate intracellular parasites). Because of these differences, the type of immune response required to control these infections also differs.

TYPES OF IMMUNE RESPONSES

There are two main types of immune responses: nonadaptive, nonspecific responses and adaptive, specific responses.

NONADAPTIVE, NONSPECIFIC RESPONSES

This type of response includes the actions of different classes of cells such as eosinophils, PMN cells, NK cells and others and of factors such as complement and interferons which can have an important role in the limitation of replication of some microorganisms, especially viruses. They act early in an infection so that in the absence of specific antibody, they may form the first line of defense. Thus complement may directly lyse viruses which have a lipid envelope, and NK cells can recognise and destroy some infected cells. In this way, their action may have a degree of selectivity, but not specificity. Their second most important characteristic is that there is no evidence that they may display memory; that is, as a result of a first experience with an infectious agent, there is no enhancement of activity upon exposure a second time to the same agent at a later time, say months.

It is particularly these two properties – specificity and memory – which distinguish the nonadaptive from the adaptive immune responses.

Adaptive, specific responses

These responses are the hallmark of one class of cell, the lymphocyte, which shows both specificity and memory. There are two main classes–B cells and T cells. B cells make antibody (immunoglobulin, Ig), a humoral effector response. As competent but naive cells (able to respond upon exposure at a future time to specific antigen), they express two types of Ig receptors (IgM, IgD) on their surface. Following recognition of an antigen and subsequent activation (see below), they secrete different isotypes of Igs – initially IgM followed by IgG, IgE or IgA. There are a number of subclasses of IgG each of which has particular characteristics.

The situation with T cells is more complicated. Upon activation they may have regulatory roles via helper (TH) or suppressor (TS) activities as well as effector roles, mediating delayed type sensitivity (DTH, TD) or cytotoxic (CTL, TC) activities. Most T cells express antigen receptors composed of α, β chains, but recently a smaller population of cells has been detected which expresses receptors composed of γ, δ chains. The latter cells are found mainly in special sites such as those adjacent to mucosal surfaces and often recognize certain types of antigens, such as heat shock proteins. T cell responses are generally referred to as cell-mediated (CMI) in contrast to the soluble product, antibody, secreted by activated B cells. This terminology was originally used following the finding that whereas the effect of antibody could be directly demonstrated by transfer of immune serum to another host, transfer of cells was required to demonstrate an effect such as delayed type hypersensitivity (DTH). It is now realized that many of the effects of T cells are also manifested by secreted factors (variously called interleukins, lymphokines or cytokines) which are inter-cell messengers and generally act only in the close proximity of the donor cell.

(i) Specificity

Following the declaration of the Clonal Selection Theory by F. M. Burnet[2] in 1957, it was soon established that individual B lymphocytes had receptors of a single specificity as Burnet had predicted, thus accounting for the exquisite specificity of the immune system. A similar situation was later found to apply to T cells.

(ii) Memory

A. Glenny[3] was the first to demonstrate the different kinetics which distinguish a primary versus a secondary immune response. In 1949, Burnet pointed out that the hypothesis of antibody formation current at that time, the Instruction Theory, could not provide an explanation for this effect.[4] The more rapid and earlier production of antibody which characterizes a secondary response could only be explained on the basis of an increased number of specific cells producing antibody. Thus, it appeared likely that one factor in immunologic memory would be an increased number of cells of a given specificity.

Antigen presentation and recognition

The receptors on B cells and free antibody recognize mainly amino acid or sugar sequences (called epitopes). These may form a linear or continuous sequence in an antigen molecule or a discontinuous sequence formed by adjacent peptide sequences in individual molecule or even by adjacent protein molecules, present for example, as a mosaic on the surface of a virus or in the flagella of some bacteria. All epitopes have a preferred conformation, and presentation in this form is important for the generation of antibodies of high affinity to the antigen itself.

In direct contrast to the above situation, T cell receptors recognize a complex of a peptide, derived from degraded protein antigens, with a major histocompatibility (MHC) antigen.[5] As the receptor sees an epitope composed of the foreign peptide and part of the MHC molecule, the peptide itself is called a determinant. Th cells recognize peptides derived from the processing in lysozymes of exogenous antigens The peptides complex with class II MHC molecules which are then expressed at the cell surface; such responses are called class II MHC restricted. The peptide bound may vary in length from about 12 to 20 amino acids. The three dimensional structure of the complex has recently been resolved.[6] The responding T cell is characterized by a membrane marker, the CD4 molecule.

In the case of proteins synthesized in the cytoplasm of the cell, such as self antigens or newly synthesized antigens of an infectious agent, some molecules may be degraded in the cytoplasm to form peptides which then may complex with class I MHC molecules. These complexes, expressed at the cell surface, are recognized by CTL (or their precursors), so that these responses are called class I MHC-retricted responses; the membrane marker on these T cells is the CD8 molecule. The three dimensional structure of the class I MHC/peptide complexes was the first to be resolved.[7] It was subsequently found that the peptide was generally nine amino acids long and required a motif (possessing certain amino acids at certain positions) in order to fit into a groove at the tip of the MHC molecule.

Consequently, there are two requirements for T cell recognition–the antigen-presenting cell (APC) must produce appropriate peptides, and secondly, the host must have T cells possessing receptors with the requisite specificity to recognize the epitope composed of the peptide and MHC molecule. There are thus two levels at which the genetic makeup of the host can substantially influence the T cell response and hence the overall immune response.

ACTIVATION OF LYMPHOCYTE

T CELLS

Activation of naive Th cells and CTLs may involve three different components[8,9] – recognition of the peptide:MHC antigen complex by the T cell receptor, recognition of other ligands on the APC plasma membrane (such as the murine molecular complex, B7) by other receptors (CD28) on the T cell membrane and perhaps the secretion of one or more cytokines by the APC. In the case of Th cells, the biochemical pathway leading to activation is known in some detail. The cell begins to produce IL-2, an interleukin of central importance; this is followed by the expression of a cellular receptor for the molecule which initiates an autocrine pathway of activation with the result that cellular differentiation occurs and a range of other interleukins is produced. The action of activated T cells is mediated to a large extent by these factors acting on other cells, such as B cells.

The ability to clone activated lymphocytes led to the finding first in mice[10] and later in humans that at least two classes of Th cells, Th1 and Th2, might exist during an immune response. Recent findings[11] suggest for example that IL-12 produced by macrophages induces precursor or naive T cell to differentiate into Th1 cells. IL-4 seems to be the cytokine which causes naive T cells to differentiate into Th2 cells. These two T cell types could be distinguished by the pattern of lymphokines they produced, as will be discussed shortly

The initial requirements for activation of naive CTLs are basically similar to the above. Though it may be likely that normally Th cells (Th1 cells?) may have a role in the differentiation and maturation of CTLs via the provision of cytokines, it has been shown that mice treated with anti-CD4 antibody and hence lacking $CD4^+$ T cells generate levels of $CD8^+$ CTLs[12] within the 'normal' range. Thus, Th cells seem not to be mandatory for CTL induction and maturation.

B CELLS

Polysaccharides which are poorly processed by T cells, especially those of the very young, bind specifically to a B cell receptor and activate the cell to the extent that it will produce and secrete IgM antibody of that specificity. Sometimes, a particular IgG subclass, IgG2a, may be produced (in mice) following IgM production.

Antigens which are predominantly protein in nature will not only be taken up and processed by APCs but also bind to B cells expressing a receptor specific for an epitope on the antigen. The binding and subsequent endocytosis of the antigen:B cell receptor complex will be more efficient in the case of polymeric antigens. It has been shown that this process of antigen attachment and endocytosis may result in a concentration of antigen within the B cell of up to 1000-fold higher than is present in the external medium. The subsequent processing of the Ag:Ab complex within the cell contributes to cell activation. This, together with factors from the APCs (e.g., dendritic cells) processing the same antigen results in an upregulation of class II MHC antigens in the B cell. This allows the expression of (foreign antigen) peptide:MHC antigen complexes at the surface of the cell. It may be that this partially-activated B cell may sometimes act as a 'professional' APC and stimulate naive T cells. To do this it would need in addition to express the 'co-stimulatory' factors outlined above and this may not be a regular occurrence. The more general situation is that B cells at this stage of activation would be recognized by already activated Th cells which, upon interaction with the B cell, would then secrete those interleukins (IL-4, 5, 6) which cause the B cells to differentiate further. This involves a switch in the Ig synthetic machinery from IgM/IgD to IgG, IgE or IgA and finally to become the plasma cell whose sole task is to produce Ig of a specificity either the same as or similar to (allowing for somatic hypermutation) that of the original IgM receptor.

It is important to realize that the form of the antigen binding via epitopes of a single specificity to the naive B cell can vary greatly in complexity, from say a peptide to a particle possibly as complex as a virus. The different antigens in such a particle do not necessarily need to be bound covalently to the antigen containing the particular epitope recognized by the

B cell receptor, in order to be endocytosed by the cell and processed. The benefit of such a situation is that the greater the variety of antigens processed by a given B cell, the greater the variety of peptides produced that may bind to class II MHC molecules. In turn, this increases the opportunity for Th cells of a variety of different receptor specificities to interact with the B cell. The net result is a great facilitation of B cell differentiation. (This assumes of course that the APC which originally activated the naive Th cells had also processed antigens of a similar range of complexity).

Subclasses of T cells

As indicated above, there is increasing awareness of the complexity of T cell populations. There is in general insufficient information about the role of γ, δ receptor chain T cells vis-a-vis α, β receptor chain T cells, and not enough to be able to specify the extent to which a vaccine should aim to and/or be able to activate that population. This information may only come when transfer experiments involving such cells (in the absence of classical CTL populations) are carried out.

In addition, there are reports of $CD4^+$ or $CD8^+$ T cells which have suppressor activity, but in general, their mode of action has not been accurately defined. A vaccine should aim not to induce such responses, and there is little indication to date that such responses do occur following standard vaccination procedures. They are not discussed further in this chapter.

Currently, the three classes of T cells which are of main concern to vaccine designers are Th1, Th2 and CTLs. As explained above, T cells work very largely through the production and secretion of cytokines, and these factors greatly influence the differentiation pattern of other cells such as B cells. Table 1 shows some of the characteristics of these three cell types.[3] Several points are worth noting.

(i) To date, Th1 and Th2 cells have mainly been demonstrated in persistent infections,[13,14] suggesting that chronic stimulation favors the emergence of these two dominant T cell types. It has been thought that short-term stimulation may produce predominantly a 'precursor' cell-type (TH0) which might have a 'common' or broader range pattern of cytokines[3] but the recent findings (mentioned above) regarding the effect of IL-12 throws some doubt on this possibility. Another difficulty with such a proposal is that some cytokines, at least in in vitro experiments, are antagonists. Thus, IL-4 and IFN–γ are mutually inhibitory, and IL-10 inhibits the production of IFN–γ . Nevertheless, two later chapters in this volume describe examples where both types of T cells are found simultaneously.

(ii) Th1 and CTLs have in part a common pattern of cytokines so that one can predict what their role would be to control the replication of intracellular pathogens, either by activating phagocytic cells via cytokines such as INF–γ, by inhibiting replication of the infectious agent such as viruses (Th1, CTLs) or by direct lysis of infected cells (CTLs). However, Th1 cells are the main if not the only cell-type mediating DTH responses and as this response is also cytokine mediated, there must be some differences in the cytokine profiles of these two cell types.

(iii) Initially in the murine system, but also now in the human system, different cytokines have been shown to influence Ig isotype production.

(iv) It has also been suggested that Th1 cells may provide help for the generation of CTLs, but at least in the case of several viral infections ablation of $CD4^+$ T cells did not influence either the production of primary or secondary CTL activity.[15]

The question of vaccine design for stimulation of these subsets is discussed later in this chapter.

THE TIME SEQUENCE OF RESPONSES DURING AN ACUTE INFECTION

Figure 1 summarizes experiments designed to follow two main responses during a non-lethal influenza virus infection in mice.[16,17] After intranasal inoculation, virus (curve A) replicates in the lung (3-4 $\log_{10}$ ID_{50}), reaches maximum titers by days 3-6 (depending upon the size of the inoculum) and then decreases so that infectious virus is no longer detectable after days 9-12. This disappearance of infectious virus has been confirmed in a murine influenza virus system using PCR analysis to look for viral RNA.[18] Curve B represents CTL activity, which peaks a few days after the viral titer peaks and then activity declines, disappearing some days after infectious virus can no longer be detected. As infectious virus is required for CTL generation, this disappearance of CTL activity has been interpreted to reflect the short half-life of these effector cells.[4] However, a recent finding has described the effect of IL-4 in cell culture in causing the conversion of CTLs into non-cytolytic $CD8^-CD4^-$ cells that make Th2-type cytokines.[19] As IgA and IgG producing antibody-secreting cells (ASCs) have just begun to appear at

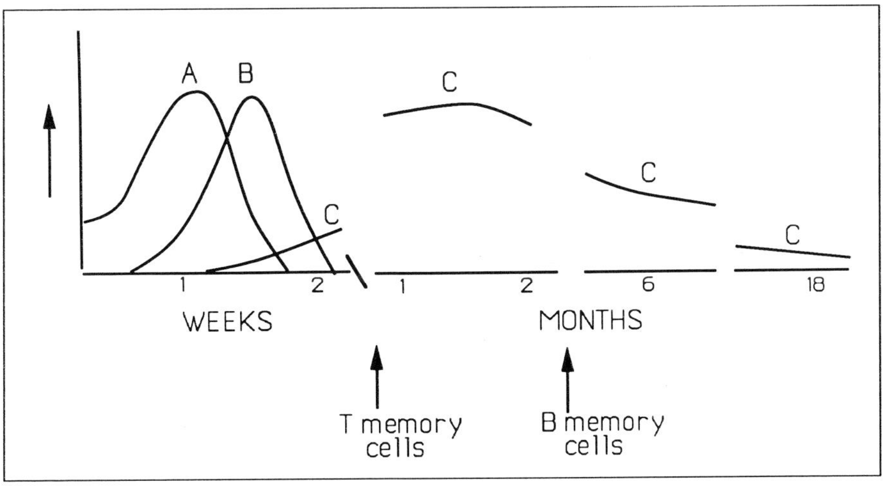

Fig. 1. Time sequence of infectious process and subsequent immune responses in a murine influenza virus infection.
Ordinate. Increase in infectivity/effector cell numbers.
Abscissa. Time after initiation of infection.
Curves. A. Growth and disappearance of infectious virus.
B. Appearance and disappearance of effector CTLs.
C. Appearance and continuing presence of antibody-secreting cells.
Arrows. Time of presence of maximum numbers of memory T or B cells.
Reproduced with kind permission from ref. 16.

about the time CTL activity disappears, the possibility of such an effect occurring under 'natural' conditions in vivo needs to be examined. However, memory CTLs reach maximum levels of frequency by about two weeks, at about the same time that CTL activity is no longer detectable. They survive for a long period, with a half-life of possibly a year or more in mice.[20]

ASCs (IgM) first appear between days 5-10 and IgA and IgG producing cells some days later. The highest frequency of ASCs (IgA, IgG) occurs at about 3 months and then levels slowly decrease, but some (IgG producers) are still found 20 months after the initial infection. Memory B cells also peak at about 3 months, and in number vary from 100-1000 times the frequency of precursor cells in uninfected lungs. Although not shown in the figure, Th cells are the first specific response, being detected within 2-3 days after the infection. They are found for some considerable time (months at least) from then on.

THE ROLE OF DIFFERENT IMMUNE RESPONSES

Prevention of infection

Though there may be a number of nonspecific factors which limit an infectious process, e.g., a thick layer of mucin at a mucosal surface or carriage of virus by cilia away from susceptible cells in the respiratory tract, specific antibody is the only efficient effector mechanism for either completely or very largely preventing infection by any infectious agent. The protection against a variety of infectious agents afforded to human infants by maternal antibody acquired at birth is the best evidence for this role of specific antibody. There are many examples in model systems where transfer of specific antibody to a host has protected the host from at least frank disease when challenged by the agent. For example, transfer of specific anti-influenza virus IgG to mice prevented infection of the lower respiratory tract following intranasal inoculation of the virus, but did not prevent infection of the cells lining the mucosal surface of the respiratory tract.[21] In contrast, transfer of a hybridoma expressing anti-hemagglutinin poly IgA, which is converted into s.IgA on passage to the mucosal lumen, completely prevented infection of the mucosa in most mice.[22] This may be one of the few documented occasions where s.IgA, in the absence of other effector mechanisms, has completely prevented infection, a situation sometimes called "sterilizing immunity". Furthermore, in mice convalescent from a respiratory influenza virus infection, anti-α, but not anti-μ or anti-γ, destroyed the resistance to a second infection of mucosal cells with the homologous virus.[23] The wide relevance of these observations becomes apparent when it is realized that, other than vector-borne agents, the great majority of infectious agents infect via a mucosal surface.

Limitation of replication

As previously outlined, nonadaptive responses are the main mechanism for limiting replication of the agent before the adaptive response is generated. Though there is no evidence in any system that nonadaptive responses can clear an infection, the recent availability of a wide range of 'doctored' mice, which lack the ability to produce different products such as B_2-microglobulin and hence class I MHC molecules, may produce such evidence. The use of such mice to date has indicated both the extent to which different systems are linked, usually through cytokine effects, and hence the extent to which other mechanisms may compensate for the deficiency.

Recovery from Infection

Most of the evidence indicating the extent to which the different immune responses can control and clear an infection comes from 'experiments of nature', and by transfer experiments mainly in model systems. Thus, agammaglobulinemic people can survive infections by viruses such as measles or influenza, and this earlier led to the belief that cell-mediated immune responses were important in this respect. For many years, nude (nu+/nu+) mice were useful models in assessing the roles of different components. Intranasal infection of these mice with influenza led to a persisting lung infection,[24] even though such mice are known to have 'activated' macrophages and a high level of NK cell activity.

In the case of extracellular pathogens, antibody must remain the main mechanism for clearing the infection though activation of phagocytic cells such as macrophages by cytokines such as INF–γ would help in the disposal of the antibody-coated organism. Even with intracellular pathogens, specific antibody can help to control an infection by neutralizing the infectivity of newly-produced infectious progeny or by lysing infected cells expressing antigens either by antibody-dependent cellular cytotoxicity (ADCC) or by a complement dependent mechanism. Transfer of high titer anti-influenza antibody to influenza-infected nude mice greatly reduced infectious viral titers but as time passed and the antibody titer waned higher viral titers returned.[25] In the early 1960s, transfer of immune sera to children with malaria relieved the symptoms of, but did not cure, the disease[26] and it has been claimed that the transfer of immune sera to HIV-infected children may have some benefit.[27] In the last two cases, it is possible that greater effects might have been seen if the infectious agent had not been subject to great antigenic variation, leading possibly to immune selection of mutant organisms.

For intracellular pathogens, accumulated evidence strongly indicates that CMI responses are mainly responsible for clearing infections of any type and some of the later chapters in this monograph deal specifically with this aspect. There are ostensibly three related mechanisms–particular cytokines with anti-infectious agent activity, cells with cytolytic activity and cells mediating delayed-type hypersensitivity (DTH). The two cell types are $CD8^+$ CTLs and $CD4^+$Th1. Both cell types secrete certain cytokines (Table 1). Primary $CD8^+$CTLs generated during viral, some bacterial and parasitic infections are strongly cytolytic. That is, they do not require further stimulation by exposure to antigen in in vitro culture to show this activity. In a murine influenza viral infection, such preparations may show relatively weak DTH reactivity[28] but this has not been observed in a herpes infection. In contrast, primary $CD4^+$Th1 cells may show strong DTH but are rarely if ever cytolytic, at least in normal, i.e., not doctored, mice.[29] When restimulated and cultured in vitro or especially after cloning, $CD4^+$ T cell preparations are frequently cytolytic. Such a preparation having cytolytic activity was shown to clear a murine influenza virus infection.[30]

Table 1. Some characteristics of $CD8^+$ cytotoxic T cells (CTLs) and of $CD4^+$ T helper 1 cells (Th1) and T helper 2 cells (Th2)

$CD8^+$CTLs:

- Class I MHC restricted,
- *Secrete IL-2, IFN-γ, TNF_B*
- Primary cells, i.e. cells from infected hosts (and without further activation by antigen in vitro) lyse virus-infected cells in vitro
- Mediate little, sometimes no, DTH reactivity

$CD4^+$ TH1 cells:

- Class II MHC restricted
- *Secrete IL-2, IFN-γ, TNF_B*
- Primary cells taken directly from infected tissues generally do not lyse virus-infected cells in vitro
- Major mediator of DTH reactivity
- Provide help for IgG_{2a} (mice) or IgG_1 (human) antibody production
- Provide help for CTL production? Not mandatory

$CD4^+$ TH2 cells:

- Class II MHC restricted
- Secrete IL-4,-5, -6,-10
- Provide help for antibody production (IgM, IgA, IgE, some IgG isotypes)

The contribution each may make to clearance of an infection may vary. A recent experiment in which nude mice were infected with a recombinant vaccinia virus expressing the gene for INF–γ, showed that in the complete absence of effector T cells having receptors, expression of the gene for this cytokine resulted in the clearance of the infection.[31] Though it may be doubted whether infection of normal mice with vaccinia virus would induce similar levels of INF–γ, this experiment shows the potential importance of this cytokine response. Though it is difficult to obtain direct proof that CTLs lyse infected cells in vivo as they clearly do in vitro, the available indirect evidence is entirely consistent with this interpretation. Therefore, these cells currently are seen as having at least two separate functional activities.

There are eight (possibly more) different classes of virus where in model systems, it has been shown that transfer of $CD8^+$CTLs can protect from a lethal infection and/or clear the infection.[32] In transfer experiments showing the protective effect of ($CD8^+$) class I MHC-restricted effector T cells, the controls frequently involved transfer of the corresponding class II MHC-restricted ($CD4^+$) effector T cells; such controls rarely showed a protective effect. In the murine influenza virus model system, $CD4^+$ preparations were frequently shown to express DTH activity.[33] In one set of experiments, transfer of cells to mice, previously given a lethal dose of influenza virus intranasally induced a strong infiltration of mononuclear cells into the lungs and shortened the time to death. In contrast, transfer of cells showing strong CTL activity resulted in survival of the mice.[34] Transfer of virus-specific Th cell clones gave variable results: influenza virus HA-specific clones either did not reduce viral titers or resulted in higher viral titers which the authors also attributed to DTH reactions.[35] Other than work with herpes infection in mice showing that at an early stage of the infection transfer of $CD4^+$ T cells possessing DTH activity is protective,[36] I am unaware of any consistent evidence in other viral systems that $CD4^+$ T cell preparations expressing DTH reactivity contribute in a major way to the clearance of a viral infection.

A recent publication on antiviral protection by $CD8^+$ versus $CD4^+$ T cells concludes that $CD4^+$ T cells may mediate antiviral protection, but their efficiency is rather weak compared to $CD8^+$ T cell-mediated protection correlating with cytotoxic activity in vitro.[37] At the same time, I am unaware of any case where specific antibody, if present in sufficient concentration in vivo, does not at least substantially limit a viral infection, though there are well documented cases, e.g., dengue virus infections, where infection may be enhanced. Currently, the bulk of the available evidence suggests that antiviral vaccines for prophylaxis should preferentially aim to induce Th2 and CTL responses. This is especially so in the case of mucosal infections if it can be shown that specific s.IgA can neutralize viral infectivity.

The situation might well be quite different with many intracellular bacterial and parasitic infections. Particularly where there is little evidence that antibody is relatively important in preventing infection, the case for vaccines inducing Th1 cells would be strong. For example, the findings with *Leishmania major* infections in mice are particularly striking.[38] Th1 responses were the dominant response in resistant mice whereas Th2 responses were dominant in susceptible mice. In another murine model, *B. pertussis* respiratory infection, Th1 cells but not $CD8^+$ T cells were shown to be an important protective response[39] at a time when antibody levels were very low or non-detectable. The extent to which DTH activity may have contributed to this protective effect is unclear. Other reports give some idea of the complexity which may exist. On the one hand, using β_2-microglobulin deficient mice (unable to make class I MHC T cell responses), the findings indicated that functional $CD8^+$ cells and possibly T cells bearing the γ, β antigen receptor, were a necessary component of a protective immune response to *M. tuberculosis.*[40] In apparent contrast, T cell clones derived from patients with tuberculoid leprosy were found to have a lymphokine secretion pattern similar to Th1 cells, suggesting that "mycobacteria selectively induce human T cells with a Th1-like cytokine secretion profile".[41]

In a murine model of plasmodia infection (malaria), it was earlier found that both antibody and CTLs can protect against a sporozoite infection.[42] Using cloned Th1 and Th2 T cell preparations to investigate the protective mechanisms at the blood-stage parasitemia, it has been recently found[43] that the former could protect via a nitric oxide dependent mechanism in the primary parasitemia, whereas Th2 cells protected in the later stages by enhancement and accelerated production of specific IgG_1 antibody. As one approach to developing a malaria vaccine may involve the induction of protective mechanisms operating at different stages of the infection, these results provide something of a challenge to the vaccine developer.

The Need for Immunological Memory

As the evidence suggests that both effector T cells and ASCs have a short half-life, of the order of some days or a week, it is deduced that the constant presence of antibody after an infection only occurs because of the generation and activation of memory B cells. Both T and B memory cells are formed during an immune response to protein antigens and they may differ from naive cells in several ways.

(i) Either qualitatively or quantitatively in the expression of different markers;[44,45]

(ii) Following an acute infection, there may be increases (10-1000 fold) in the frequency of cells with a specificity similar to that of their precursors;[17]

(iii) Both T and B memory cells are generally more easily activated by antigen than are naive cells.[46,47]

Whereas naive B cells express only IgM and IgD antigen receptors, memory B cells may express other Ig isotypes. Following stimulation, B cells follow one of two paths. One group matures and secretes mainly IgM antibodies in a primary response. The other group migrates to the lymphoid follicles and, with T cell help, undergoes clonal expansion with somatic hypermutation of the receptors to become memory cells expressing other Ig isotypes.

The events leading to the generation of memory T cells is less well understood.

Long-lived antibody production

Particularly after immunization with a live attenuated viral vaccine, specific antibody may exist for many years even in the known absence of specific re-stimulation. Possible explanations for this may include

(i) The infectious agent may persist, providing a continuous supply of antigen. It has earlier been shown[18] that this cannot be a general explanation;

(ii) There could be re-stimulation by cross-reacting antigens. This also cannot be a general explanation. Volunteers for HIV vaccine trials were recently found to have anti-vaccinia antibodies though they had been vaccinated at least 15 years previously. The only other pox virus known to replicate in humans is monkey pox and human monkey pox virus infections are known to occur very rarely.

(iii) Idiotype:anti-idiotype interactions might provide an explanation. Such interactions are known to occur in the short term but there is little evidence for long-term (years) effects. Nevertheless, they might contribute to the phenomenon.

(iv) Persistence of non-infectious antigens. This is now well documented and accounts for the main findings as outlined next.

Antigen persistence and affinity maturation of antibody.

(i) Antigen:antibody complexes attach to the surface of follicular dendritic cells (FDCs) via complement and possibly Fc receptors.

(ii) Particularly for surface antigens, such as viral glycoproteins, localization in their native (protease-resistant) conformation favors long-term persistance. Localization of antigen in the form of polymers, and even as infectious virus[48] has been observed. This helps to account for the observation that many protective high-affinity viral antibodies recognize highly conformational epitopes.

(iii) Memory B cell formation requires antigen localization at this site.
(iv) Antigen:antibody complexes bud off the FDCs to form iccosomes (immune complex coated bodies) and are processed within memory B cells. With T cell help, these become antibody-secreting cells.
(v) As time passes and in the absence of a second infection or vaccination, decreasing levels of antigen on the FDCs results in the selection of memory cells expressing receptors of higher affinity, thus leading over time to the production of antibody of increasingly higher affinity, a critically important feature of the immune response. A later Chapter provides details of these processes.

General Immunological Requirements for an Optimally Successful Vaccine

The above considerations lead to the formulation of four general requirements.[16]

(i) Activation of APCs, involving the processing of antigens by either the lysosomal or cytoplasmic route, expression of co-stimulatory factors at the cell surface and possibly also secretion of cytokines. Such cells are sometimes referred to as 'professional' APCs. Dendritic cells are highly competent in this respect.
(ii) Activation, replication and differentiation of T and B cells, leading to the generation of a large pool of memory cells of both types.
(iii) Generation of effector T cells to sufficient peptide determinants and epitopes, preferably from conserved regions of antigens, both to limit the effects of antigenic variation of protective antigens and to minimize the effects of MHC antigen polymorphism in an outbred population.
(iv) Long-term persistence of conformationally intact antigen (as antigen:antibody complexes), and preferably as antigenic aggregates, to allow the continuing formation of, followed by the recruitment of, B memory cells to form ASCs, thus ensuring the continuing formation of antibody of increasingly higher affinity.

CONCLUDING REMARKS

The purpose of this first chapter has been to serve as an introduction, mainly in immunological terms, to the remaining chapters, each of which discusses in more detail particular aspects and/or ways of modifying the immune response. It is inevitable that the more we learn about the immune response, the more complicated it appears. New information is now appearing at a very fast rate, and some of it is sufficiently novel to make one query the correctness of some cherished beliefs. Because of this, it becomes increasingly difficult to write a relatively short but basically correct summary. There are many aspects barely mentioned in this chapter, and only some of these are discussed in later chapters. Hopefully, the short and sometimes simplified presentations in this chapter provide a useful stepping stone to appreciating the more detailed presentations in the following chapters.

References

1. Cohen MS, Heine RP. Mucosal defenses and microbial pathogens of the genital tract. In: Quinn DC, ed. Advances in Host Defense Mechanisms. Sexually Transmitted Diseases. Raven Press, New York. 1992; 8: 39-56.
2. Burnet FM. A modification of Jerne's theory of antibody production using the concept of clonal selection. Aust J Sci 1957;20: 67-69.
3. Ada GL. Vaccines. In: Paul WE, ed. Fundamental Immunology. 3rd ed. Raven Press, New York.1993: 1309-1352.
4. Ada GL, Nossal GJV. The clonal-selection theory. Sci. Amer.1987; 255:62-9.
5. Neefjes JJ, Schumacher TNM, Ploegh HL. Assembly and intracellular transport of major histocompatibility complex molecules. Curr Opin Cell Biol 1991; 3: 601-9.
6. Bjorkman PJ, Saper MA, Samraoir B et al. Structure of the human class I histocompatibility antigen, HLA-A2. Nature 1987; 329: 506-12.
7. Brown JH, Jardezky TS, Gorge JC et al. Three-dimensional structure of the human class II histocompatibility antigen HLA-DR1. Nature 1993; 364: 33-39.
8. Schwartz R H. Costimulation of T lymphocytes: The role of CD28, CTLA-4, and B7/BB1 in interleukin-2 production and immunotherapy. Cell 1992; 71: 1065-8.
9. Lanzavecchia A. Identifying strategies for immune intervention. Science 1991; 260: 937-43.
10. Mossman TR, Schumacher JH, Street NF et al. Diversity of cytokine synthesis and function of mouse $CD4^+$ T cells. Immunol Rev 1991; 123: 209-29.
11. Hsieh C-S, Macatonia SE, Tripp CS et al. Development of Th1 $CD4^+$ T cells through IL-12 produced by Listeria-induced macrophages. Science 193; 260: 547-9.
12. Buller RM, Holmes KL, Hugin A et al. Induction of cytotoxic T cell responses in vivo in the absence of $CD4^+$ helper cell. Nature 1987; 328: 77-9.
13. Finkelman FD, Katoma IM, Urban JF et al. Suppression of in vivo polyclonal IgE responses by monoclonal antibody to the lymphokine B-cell stimulatory factor. Proc Nat Acad Sci 1986; 83: 9675-9.
14. Sher FA, Fiorentino DF, Casper P et al. Production of IL-10 by CD4+ lymphocytes correlates with downregulation of Th1 cytokine synthesis in helminth infections. J Immunol 1991; 147: 2713-6.
15. Liu Y, Mullbacher A. The generation and activation of memory class I MHC restricted cytotoxic T cell responses to influenza A virus in vivo do not require $CD4^+$ T cells. Immunol Cell Biol 1989; 67: 413-20.
16. Ada GL. The immune response to antigens: the immunological principles of vaccination. Lancet 1990; 335: 523-6.
17. Ada GL, Jones PD. The immune response to influenza infection. Curr Top Microbiol Immunol 1986; 128: 1-54.
18. Eichelberger MC, Wang M, Rowlands DJ et al. Influenza virus RNA in the lung and lymphoid tissues of immunologically intact and CD4-depleted mice. J Gen Virol 1991;72: 1695-8.
19. Erard F, Wild M-T, Garcia-Sanz JA, Le Gros G. Switch of CD8 T cells to noncytolytic $CD8^-$ $CD4^-$ cells that make Th2 cytokines and help B cells. Science 1993; 260: 1802-5.
20. Ashman RB. Persistence of cell-mediated immunity to influenza A virus in mice. Immunology 1982; 47: 165-8.

21. Ramphal R, Cogliano RE, Shands JW, Small PA. Serum antibody prevents lethal murine influenza pneumonitis but not tracheitis. Infect. Immun. 1979; 25: 992-6.
22. Renegar KB, Small PA. Passive transfer of local immunity to influenza virus infection by IgA antibody. J Immunol 1991; 146: 1972-8.
23. Renegar KB, Small PA. Immunoglobulin A mediates murine anti-influenza virus immunity. J Virol 1992; 65: 2146-8.
24. Yap KL, Braciale TJ, Ada GL. Role of T cell function in recovery from murine influenza infection. Cell Immunol 1979; 43: 341-51.
25. Askonas BA, McMichael AJ, Webster RG. The immune response to influenza viruses and the problem of protection against infection. In: Beare H. ed. Basic and Applied Influenza Research. CRC Press, Boca Raton, Fl. 1982; pp. 159-188.
26. Cohen S, McGregor IA, Carrington S. Gamma-globulin and acquired immunity to human malaria. Nature 1961; 192: 733-7.
27. Dwyer JM. Manipulating the system with immune globulin. New Eng J Med 1992; 326: 107-113.
28. Leung K-N, Ada GL. Two T cell populations mediate delayed type hypersensitivity to murine influenza virus infection. Scand J Immunol 1980; 12: 129-139.
29. Muller D, Koller BH, Whitton JL et al. LCM-specific class II-restricted cytotoxic T cells in B_2-microglobulin deficient mice. Science 1992; 255: 1576-1577.
30. Luchacher AE, Morrison LA, Braciale VL, BracialeTJ. In: Steinman RM, North RJ, eds. Mechanisms of host resistance to infectious agents, tumors and allografts. Rockefeller Press, New York. 1986; pp. 223 -254.
31. Ramshaw I, Ruby J, Ramsey A et al. Expression of cytokines by recombinant vaccinia viruses: a model for studying cytokines in virus infections in vivo. Immunol Rev 1992; 127; 157-182.
32. Ada GL. Vaccines and the immune response. In: Webster RG, Granoff A, eds. Encyclopedia Virol. Academic Press, New York. 1993; In press.
33. Leung K-N, Ada GL, McKenzie IFC. Specificity, Ly phenotype and H-2 compatibility requirements of effector cells in delayed-type hypersensitivity responses to murine influenza virus infection. J Exp Med 1980; 151: 815-26.
34. Leung K-N, Ada GL. Different functions and immunopathological effects of subsets of effector T cells in murine influenza virus infection. Cell Immunol 1982; 67: 312-24.
35. Askonas BA, Wraith DC, Taylor PM. Cytotoxic T cells in influenza: their role and specificities. Prog Immunol 1986; VI: 770-8.
36. Nash AA, Gell PGH. Membrane phenotype of murine effector and suppressor T cells involved in delayed hypersensitivity and protective immunity to herpes simplex virus. Cell Immunol 1983 75:348-55.
37. Binder D, Kundig TM. Antiviral protection by CD8+ versus CD4+ T cells. Cells correlating with cytotoxic activity in vitro are more efficient in anti-vaccinia virus protection than CD4-dependent IL. J Immunol 1993; 146: 4301-4307.
38. Coffman RL, Chatelain R, Leal LMC et al. Leishmania major infection in mice - a model system for the study of CD4+ T cell subset differentiation. Rev Immunol 1991; 142: 36

39. Mills KHG, Barnard A,Watkins J et al. Cell-mediated immunity to *Bordetella pertussis* : Role of Th1 cells in bacterial clearance in a murine respiratory infection model. Infect Immunity 1993; 61: 399-410.
40. Flynn J L, Goldstein MM, Triebold K J et al. Major histocompatibility complex class I-restricted T cells are required for resistance to Mycobacterium tuberculosis infection. Proc Nat Acad Sci. 1992; 89: 12013-7.
41. Haanen BAG, de Waal Malefijt R, Res PCM et al. Selection of a human T helper type 1-like T cell subset by Mycobacteria. J Exp Med 1991; 174: 583-92.
42. Weiss WR, Sedegah M, Beaudoin RL et al. $CD8^{+}$T cells (cytotoxic/suppressors) are required for protection in mice immunized with malaria sporozoites. Proc Nat Acad Sci 1988; 85: 573-8.
43. Taylor-Robinson AW, Phillips RS, Severn A et al. The role of Th1 and Th2 cells in a rodent malaria infection. Science 1993; 260: 1931-3.
44. Schittek B, Rajewsky K. Maintenance of B cell memory by long-lived cells generated from proliferating precursors. Nature 1990; 346: 749-51.
45. Vitetta ES, Berton MT, Burget C et al. Memory B and T cells. Ann Rev Immunol 1991; 9: 193-217..
46. Hill AB, Blanden RV, Parrish CR et al. Restimulated Tc cells have a higher apparent avidity of interaction with targets than primary virus-immune Tc cells as indicated by anti-CD8 blocking. Immunol Cell Biol 1992; 70: 259-65.
47. Hilbert DM, Cancro MP, Scherle PA et al. T-cell derived IL-6 is differentially required for antigen-specific antibody secretion by primary and secondary B cells. J Immunol 1989; 143: 4019-24.
48. Pantaleo G, Graziosi C, Demarest JF et al. HIV infection is active and progressive in lymphoid tissues during the clinically latent stage of disease. Nature 1993: 362: 355-8.

CHAPTER 2

The Role of Antibody in Controlling and/or Clearing Virus Infections

Geraldine Taylor

It is well established that pre-existing antibodies can prevent infection and the efficacy of vaccines has traditionally been assessed by measuring the neutralizing antibody response. However, there is often a poor correlation between the ability of sera to neutralize virus infectivity in vitro, and protection in vivo. Cell-mediated immune mechanisms, in particular lysis of virus-infected cells by $CD8^+$ T cells and the anti-viral action of cytokines, appear to be the main effectors of recovery from virus infection, however, antibody can play a role in virus clearance. Little is known about how antibodies act at defined stages of virus infection to protect the host. Studies on the ability of monoclonal antibodies (mAb) specific for virus-coded proteins to passively immunize naive animals have led to the identification of viral antigenic determinants that are important in immunity and have defined the mechanisms by which these antibodies exert their protective effects in vivo. It is clear from such studies that the relationship between in vivo and in vitro effects of mAbs on virus growth and pathogenesis is complex, and differs from virus to virus and perhaps even from host to host. In this chapter, studies using mAbs to respiratory syncytial virus (RSV) will be described to illustrate how antigens which are related to in vivo protection have been determined for this virus, how the properties of the antibodies that determine protection were identified and how this knowledge may be exploited for therapy and vaccine design.

Strategies in Vaccine Design, edited by Gordon L. Ada, D.Sc.

RESPIRATORY SYNCYTIAL VIRUS

RSV is a pneumovirus within the paramyxovirus family and is a major cause of lower respiratory tract disease in children and calves.[1] The virus encodes 10 proteins, 2 of which are non-structural (1B and 1C) and 8 structural.[2] The large surface glycoprotein (G) mediates attachment of the virus to cells and the fusion (F) surface glycoprotein mediates penetration of the virus into cells and fusion between infected cells and adjacent cells; M1 and M2 (or 22K) are associated with the viral envelope; the N, P and L proteins are associated with the nucleocapsid; the SH protein is expressed on the cell surface and appears to play a critical role in the formation of syncytia induced by the F protein.[3] Human (H) and bovine (B) strains of RSV are antigenically related to 80-84% amino acid homology in the F protein between human and bovine strains of virus.[4] In contrast, the G glycoprotein of RSV is not well conserved and human and bovine strains can both be divided into at least 2 subgroups based on their reactivity with monoclonal antibodies to the G protein.[5,6]

The greatest morbidity in both infants and calves occurs during the first 6 months of life, when maternal antibody is still present and epidemiological evidence for the role of maternal antibody in protection is conflicting (see ref. 1). Reinfection with RSV is common and frequently accompanied by severe disease, indicating that immunity following natural infection is incomplete. However, there is a pattern of increasing levels of serum antibody with successive infections which parallels an accumulative acquisition of resistance to severe disease (see ref. 1). Problems have been encountered with the use of both live and inactivated virus vaccines in children and calves.[1] Live vaccines, given intramuscularly (i.m.) were poorly effective in infants and calves with maternal antibodies and exacerbation of disease has been observed in calves given live RSV vaccine i.m.[7] A formalin-inactivated RSV vaccine not only failed to protect infants and young children against infection but also resulted in an exacerbated respiratory disease.[8,9] The reasons for the failure of the vaccine to confer protection are not clear. However, a high ratio of ELISA-binding to neutralizing antibodies was observed in sera of immunized children, suggesting that epitopes of the F or G proteins were altered after formalin treatment.[10] The occurrence of severe disease in the presence of maternal antibodies and the exacerbated disease seen in vaccine recipients have led to the suggestion that antibody may not be protective and could contribute to the pathogenesis of RSV infections. These observations highlight the need to identify the protective epitopes on RSV proteins and the immune effector mechanisms that protect against infection, in order to develop safe and effective vaccines against RSV.

PASSIVE PROTECTION WITH ANTIBODY TO RSV

Studies in cotton rats, ferrets and owl monkeys have demonstrated that passive immunization with convalescent sera or human immune globulin, containing high levels of neutralizing antibodies to RSV, protected the lower respiratory tract against RSV infection.[11] Furthermore, histopathological examination of the lungs of passively immunized animals showed no evidence of potentiation of disease. Passively transferred human serum was more effective against virus in the lung than in the nose[12] and was effective when given therapeutically;[12,13] the therapeutic dose was over 100x less when administered intranasally when compared with parenteral inoculation.[14]

Studies with monoclonal antibodies to RSV have also shown that antibody can protect against infection. A comparison of the ability of 41 murine and 12 bovine monoclonal antibodies (produced from heterohybridoma cells) specific for individual proteins of RSV to passively immunize mice showed that mAbs to the F or G proteins can protect the lung against infection with HRSV when the Mabs were given intraperitoneally (i.p.) or intravenously (i.v.) 24h prior to intranasal (i.n.) challenge (Table 1[15,16]). Similar results were obtained with murine mAbs in cotton rats.[17] These findings are similar to those for other paramyxovirus infections where antibodies to the HN/G and F envelope proteins can protect against infection and/or disease.[18-26] As seen with polyclonal sera, there was no increase in the severity of lung lesions, even after passive transfer of non-protective mAbs[15] and the protective dose was up to 40-fold more effective if given by the i.n. route when compared with parenteral inoculation (unpublished observations). The possibility that the reduction in virus titer was an in vitro artifact caused by the interaction of virus and antibody after homogenization of the lung was excluded by showing that lung homogenates from passively immunized mice mixed with virus did not reduce virus titer.[15]

mAbs to the F protein that completely protected against RSV infection when given 24h prior to virus challenge were also highly effective in clearing an established RSV infection. Thus, mAbs to the F protein given i.p. 4 or 5 days after infection, at the time of maximum titers of virus in the lungs, eliminated the virus from the lungs within 6h. Furthermore, virus did not reappear in the lungs of nude mice persistently infected with RSV, when the mAb was administered on day 4 of infection, even when the antibody had declined below levels previously shown to be protective (Table 2). These findings contrast with those in nude mice infected with influenza virus, where there was only a transient decrease in virus in the lungs and tracheas

Table 1. Passive protection of mice against infection with the A2 strain of RSV with monoclonal antibodies

Protein specificity	No. mAbs	No. giving reduction in virus titer of $\log_{10}$[a]			
		>2.0	1.0-2.0	<1.0	None
F	12 Bov[b]	4	0	4	4
	23 Mu[c]	6	4	10	3
G	13 Mu	6	3	1	3
N	3 Mu	0	0	1	2
P	1 Mu	0	0	0	1
22K	1 Mu	0	0	0	1

[a] Reduction in virus titer in lungs of mice given mAbs intraperitoneally 24h prior to intranasal challenge with RSV compared with control animals.

[b] Bov = bovine monoclonal antibodies.

[c] Mu = murine monoclonal antibodies.

Table 2. Comparison of the therapeutic effects of a mAb to the G protein and an mAb to the F protein against RSV infection in nude mice

mAb[a]	Specificity	RSV titer in lungs (log_{10} PFU/g)			
		D5	D14	D21	D28
11	F	<1.7	<1.7	<1.7	ND
None		4.9 ± 0.1	4.4 ± 0.2	4.2 ± 0.2	ND
29	G	3.7 ± 0.7	1.7 ± 0.2	ND	<1.7
None		5.0 ± 0.3	4.5 ± 0.2	ND	3.7 ± 0.2

[a] Nude mice inoculated intranasally with approx. 104 PFU of HRSV were given 200µl mAbs in ascitic fluid intraperitoneally on D4 of infection.

(These experiments were done in collaboration with Jim Stott and Julie Furze, IAH Compton).

when high titer antibody was administered i.p. 5 days after infection with influenza virus.[27] mAbs to the G protein, which prevented infection when given 24h prior to RSV challenge, had little immediate impact on virus replication when administered to nude mice on day 4 of infection. Virus was not cleared from the lungs until 2 to 3 weeks after infection (Table 2). Thus mAbs to the F protein were more effective against RSV infection than those to the G protein, when given therapeutically. Furthermore, the 8 highly protective mAbs to the F protein recognized all strains of human and bovine RSV studied[6]. In contrast, protective mAbs to the G protein are either subgroup or strain-specific.[5,28]

Since mAbs to the F and G protein of RSV are effective against experimental RSV infection in mice and cotton rats, it is important to determine if such antibodies are effective against RSV infection in a natural host for the virus. Hence, bovine mAbs, which were effective against RSV infection in mice, have been examined for their ability to protect calves against RSV infection. Gnotobiotic calves were given 0.3 mg/kg body weight of bovine mAb B4, B13 or B1 by the intratracheal (i.t.) route 24h prior to i.n. and i.t. challenge with BRSV. RSV infection was significantly reduced in the lungs of the calves given B4 and B13 when compared with animals given B1 or PBS (Table 3). Furthermore, the development of lung lesions was suppressed in calves given B4 or B13 when compared with control animals or animals given B1 (unpublished observations). There was no increase in the severity of lung lesions even after passive transfer of a non-neutralizing but complement-fixing antibody (B1).

These studies highlight the importance of antibodies to the F and G protein in protection against RSV infection and failed to implicate antibody in the pathogenesis of disease.

IDENTIFICATION OF THE MECHANISMS BY WHICH MABS PROTECT

A number of virus-antibody interactions have been demonstrated in vitro, which could act to control virus infections in vivo. Neutralization of free virus would be expected to be of major importance both in preventing infection and in limiting the spread of infection in extracellular fluids. The variety of different

Table 3. Prophylactic effects of bovine mAbs to the F protein on RSV infection in calves

Treatment[a]	No. calves	No. lung samples infected/total[b]
B4	3	1/9 (11%)
B13	4	1/12 (8%)
B1	4	11/12 (92%)
PBS	9	26/27 (96%)

[a] Calves were given 15mg bovine mAb intratracheally 24h prior to intranasal and intratracheal challenge with bovine RSV.

[b] Three lung homogenate samples were assayed for virus from each calf 7 days after challenge with RSV.

(These experiments were done in collaboration with Lewis Thomas, Sara Wyld and Julie Furze, IAH Compton).

mechanisms by which viruses can be neutralized, such as aggregation of virions, inhibition of attachment of virus to the cell, inhibition of virus penetration, inhibition of virus uncoating have been reviewed extensively by Dimmock.[29] The spread of infection could also be limited by antibody which prevents the direct cell-to-cell transmission of virus, such as antibodies to the F protein of paramyxoviruses[30] or inhibits the release of progeny virus from infected cells, such as antibodies to the neuraminidase of influenza virus.[31] Antibody may also contribute to recovery from an established infection by lysis of virus-infected cells. This may be mediated by antibody-dependent cell-mediated cytotoxicity (ADCC) or complement-dependent lysis (CDL) involving the classical or alternative complement pathways.[32] The isotype of the antibody may have implications for protection in vivo, since the isotype can affect the tissue distribution of the antibody, play a role in the interaction of antibody with cells bearing the appropriate Fc receptor, in the activation of complement and in aggregation of virions (see Dimmock[29]). Thus, human IgG1 and IgG3 are good activators of the classical complement pathway, and only human IgG1 and to a lesser extent IgG3 mediate ADCC.[33,34] The importance of IgG isotype in protection against LCMV infection of mice was suggested by the observation that all protective mAbs were IgG2a, while IgG1 mAbs mapping to the same epitopes were not protective.[35] The finding that $F(ab')_2$ fragments, which retained neutralizing activity in vitro, were not protective against LCM in vivo, despite daily administration, together with the observation that the mAbs were protective in C5-deficient mice suggested that protection may involve ADCC. Furthermore, other studies indicate that murine IgG2a antibody is more effective than IgG1 at mediating ADCC.[36] There is evidence, based on studies to examine the ability of $F(ab')_2$ fragments to protect, that cells with Fc receptors are involved in viral clearance or ADCC for several other viruses, e.g., foot-and-mouth disease virus,[37] Semliki forest virus,[38,39] Venezuelan equine encephalomyelitis virus,[40] herpes simplex virus.[41] However, since F(ab')2 fragments have a short half-life in vivo, their inability to protect in some studies may be related to insufficient serum concentrations of antibody. Although a correlation between CDCL and the ability of antibody to protect has been demonstrated in some virus infections,[42,43] there is little definitive evidence for a role for complement in antibody-mediated protection in vivo. Furthermore, complement does not appear to be of major importance in virus infections of man as complement deficiencies appear to be associated with increased susceptibility to certain bacterial rather than viral infections.[44,45]

Identification of the Mechanisms by which mAbs to the G Protein Protect Against RSV Infection

In order to identify the mechanisms by which mAbs to G protein protect against infection, the biological properties of the antibodies were examined. As shown in Table 4. all the mAbs, except an IgM antibody, which may be unable to gain access to the lungs, protected against infection, indicating that there was no correlation between IgG isotype and protection. Of the 10 mAbs shown in Table 4, only one neutralized virus (mAb 29), and the protective effect of this mAb was no greater than those of the non-neutralizing antibodies. There are other examples of protection mediated by non-neutralizing antibodies, e.g., HSV,[46,47] Yellow fever virus.[48,49] Only five mAbs to the G protein lysed virus-infected cells in the presence of rabbit complement, indicating that there was no

Table 4. Biological properties of mAbs to the G protein of HRSV

mAb	Isotype	ELISA titer[a]			Neut.[b]	CDCL[c]	Mouse
		A2	8/60	127	(log_{10})		protection[d]
29	G2a	7.1	7.4	<2.5	>2.0	5.7	2.7
30	G1	7.0	<3.0	<2.5	<1.0	<2.5	1.7
31	G2a	6.3	<3.0	<2.5	<1.0	4.7	>2.8
37	M	5.4	<3.0	<2.5	<1.0	2.2	0
38	G2a	5.9	<3.0	<2.5	<1.0	2.2	2.4
22	G2a	<1.5	3.9	<1.5	<1.0	>2.0	>2.1
25	G1	<1.5	3.5	<1.5	<1.0	0	>2.1
26	G1	<1.5	3.6	<1.5	<1.0	0	>2.1
27	G1	<1.5	2.9	<1.5	<1.0	0	>2.1
32	G1	<1.5	3.8	<1.5	<1.0	0	>2.1

[a] Log_{10} antibody titer against HRSV strain A2 (subtype A), 8/60 (subtype B) and BRSV strain 127.

[b] Log_{10} titer antibody giving 50% plaque reduction titer.

[c] % specific ^{51}Cr release from CV-1 cells infected with recombinant vaccinia virus expressing the G protein of the A2 strain of HRSV (for mAbs 29 to 38) or CV-1 cells infected with the 8/60 strain of HRSV (for mAbs 22 to 32) in the presence of rabbit complement.

[d] Log_{10} reduction in virus titer in the lungs of passively immunized mice compared with controls 5 days after challenge with the A2 strain (for mAbs 29 to 38) or 8/60 strain (for mAbs 22 to 32) of HRSV.

(These experiments were done in collaboration with Jim Stott and Julie Furze).

correlation between complement-lysis and protection. Furthermore, there were no differences in the ability of these mAbs either to prevent RSV infection or to clear an established infection in mice deficient in the C5 component of complement when compared with controls (unpublished observations). Further studies in mice treated with cobra venom factor, to deplete the C3 component of complement, will help to resolve the importance of complement in the protection mediated by these mAbs. Studies comparing the efficacy of $F(ab')_2$ or Fab fragments of antibody should help to determine the importance of ADCC in the protection mediated by mAbs to the G protein.

Identification of the mechanisms by which mAbs to the F protein protect against RSV infection

In order to identify the mechanisms by which mAbs to the F protein protect against RSV infection, the biological properties of the mAbs[15,50] were compared. As shown in Table 5, there was no correlation between either the IgG isotype, virus-neutralization titer in vitro, or the ability of the mAbs to lyse virus-infected cells in the presence of complement and protection against RSV

Table 5. Correlation of in vitro properties of mAbs to the F protein with protection in vivo

mAb	Isotype	$\log_{10}$ Neut. titer[a]	% CDCL[b]	Fusion inhibition[c]	Protection[d]
14	G1	3.8	0	-	0.9
16	G1	2.0	0	-	0.6
17	G2b	<1.0	59	-	0.6
18	G2b	3.4	43	-	1.6
21	G2a	<1.0	68	-	1.0
B1	BG1	<1.0	40	-	0
11	G2b	3.3	57	+	>3.5
13	G2b	2.5	43	+	>3.5
19	G2a	3.4	2	+	>3.5
20	G2a	4.3	76	+	>3.5
B4	BG1[e]	4.5	62	+	>3.5
B5	BG1	3.9	65	+	3.1
B13	BG1	5.3	0	+	>3.5
B14	BG13	5.5	0	+	>3.5

[a] 50% plaque reduction titer.

[b] Complement-dependent cell lysis expressed as % specific ^{51}Cr release from RSV-infected cells by rabbit complement and 1/100 dilution of mAb.

[c] Inhibition of the formation of multinucleated giant cells in MA104 cells infected with RSV 24h prior to the addition of mAb.

[d] $\log_{10}$ reduction in virus titer in the lungs of passively immunized mice compared with controls 5 days after RSV challenge.

[e] BG1 is bovine IgG1.

infection. Thus, although all neutralizing mAbs reduced virus titers in the lung, the neutralizing titers of the highly protective mAbs (11,13,19,20,B4, B5, B13 and B14) were similar to those of Mabs (14 and 18) that gave only partial protection. Further, some non-neutralizing antibodies (mAbs 17 and 21) could reduce virus titers. Three of the highly protective mAbs (19, B13 and B14) failed to lyse virus-infected cells in the presence of rabbit complement (CDCL), and three of the mAbs (17, 18 and 21) giving only partial protection and one mAb (B1) giving no protection were effective in CDCL. The only property of the mAbs to the F protein that correlated with high levels of protection was the ability of the antibodies to inhibit the formation of multinucleated giant cells.[50] Such antibodies would be effective in preventing the cell-to-cell transmission of RSV, but it is not clear how they could mediate clearance of intracellular virus.

In order to determine the role of different isotypes in protection, it is important to compare antibodies with the same paratope but with different isotypes. This can be done by selection of heavy chain gene switch variants which occur spontaneously in hybridomas secreting mAbs[51] or through genetic engineering.[33] An Ig class-switch variant was isolated from an IgG1-secreting hybridoma (mAb 16) by sequential sub-lining. After 10 weeks in culture, a variant secreting an IgG2b antibody (mAb 43) was isolated that on the basis of competitive binding studies, appeared to recognize the same epitope as that recognized by mAb 16. Despite the ability of mAb 43 to lyse virus-infected cells in the presence of complement, the prophylactic properties of these two mAbs were identical (Table 6). However, in contrast to the IgG1 antibody (mAb 16) which was ineffective against RSV infection when given on day 4 of infection, the IgG2b antibody (mAb 43) was able to reduce the virus titer in the lung by $\log_{10}$ 0.7 PFU/g. This slightly increased therapeutic potential of the IgG2b mAb when compared with the IgG1 antibody could be due to CDCL activity or increased ADCC activity of the IgG2b antibody.

Further studies showed that Fab fragments, produced by papain digestion, of two of the protective mAbs were highly effective against RSV infection in mice when given either prophylactically or therapeutically by the intranasal route. The fractions were examined for anti-RSV activity by ELISA using antisera specific for the Fab or Fc regions of mouse immunoglobulin

Table 6. Comparison of the prophylactic and therapeutic properties of an Ig switch variant and the original mAb against RSV infection

mAb	Isotype	RSV titer in lungs ($\log_{10}$ PFU/g)	
		mAb d-1	mAb d4
16	IgG1	3.8 ± 0.2	4.8 ± 0.1
43[a]	IgG2b	3.7 ± 0.3	4.0 ± 0.2
Control		4.7 ± 0.3	

[a] mAb 43 is an immunoglobulin switch variant of mAb 16 specific for the F protein of RSV.

(These experiments were done in collaboration with Lynne Harrison and Julie Furze).

and by a plaque reduction assay. The ELISA indicated that the Fab fragments of the mAbs were not contaminated with significant amounts of undigested IgG (Table 7) and that they neutralized RSV in vitro (unpublished observations). The Fab fragments were administered by the intranasal route to overcome problems associated with the rapid half-life of Fab fragments in serum, access to tissues in vivo and also because less antibody is required to protect when it is given by the intranasal route compared with the parenteral route as described above. The Fab fragments were highly effective both prophylactically and therapeutically against RSV infection in mice. Further studies showed that there was only a four-fold difference in efficacy between Fab fragments of mAb 19 and intact immunoglobulin. Thus, these antibodies mediated their prophylactic and therapeutic effects through a mechanism that is independent of complement fixation, complement receptors or Fc receptors. These results are similar to those reported by Prince et al[52] in cotton rats passively immunized with human IgG containing high titers of antibody to RSV. The latter studies showed that antibody-clearance of RSV from the lungs occurred in the absence of complement and that $F(ab')_2$ fragments prepared from human IgG cleared virus to a similar extent as intact IgG in complement-depleted cotton rats.

Since RSV is cell-associated and can spread through cellular fusion it is not clear how intracellular virus can be eliminated following the binding of Fab fragments to the F protein expressed on the surface of infected cells. There are several other viruses that appear to be cleared by mechanisms which do not involve complement or ADCC but affect the intracellular level of viral gene expression.[53-56] Bivalent antibody binding to viral antigens expressed on the cell surface may transduce a signal across the plasma membrane to internal proteins which affect viral gene expression as has been suggested for measles virus infected cells.[57,58] Alternatively, antibody-mediated inhibition of viral gene transcription may result from endocytosis of antibody bound to virus-infected cells as has been demonstrated in rabies

Table 7. Prophylactic and therapeutic effects of Fab fragments of mAbs to the F protein on RSV infection in mice

Antibody[a]	ELISA titer		RSV titer in lungs on D5	
	Anti-Fc	Anti-Fab	mAb d-1	mAb d4
19	4.4	4.3	<1.7	<1.7
19 Fab	<2.0	4.6	<1.7	<1.7
None			4.5 ± 0.1	4.6 ± 0.1
20	5.1	5.1	<1.7	<1.7
20 Fab	<2.0	4.8	<1.7	<1.7
None			4.5 ± 0.1	4.5 ± 0.1

[a] Mice inoculated intranasally with approx. 25μg of intact Ig or Fab fragments 24h prior to or 4 days after intranasal challenge with approx. 10^4 PFU RSV.

(These experiments were done with Julie Furze).

virus-infected cells.[56] It will be important to determine if the fusion-inhibiting mAbs to the F protein exert their anti-viral effects by influencing viral gene expression and unraveling the molecular mechanisms by which antibodies mediate these effects.

THE RELATIVE IMPORTANCE OF ANTIBODY AND T CELLS IN PROTECTION AGAINST RSV INFECTION

Studies in mice depleted of T cell subsets using mAbs to $CD4^+$ and $CD8^+$ T cells showed that clearance of RSV required both T cell subsets.[59] In addition, both T cell subsets appeared to contribute to illness. The enhanced illness and alveolitis observed in previously infected mice rechallenged with virus were mediated by $CD8^+$ T cells, and the peribronchovascular accumulations of lymphocytes in such animals were mediated by $CD4^+$ T cells. Mice depleted of B cells by treatment with anti-μ antibody cleared RSV with the same kinetics as control animals.[60] Whereas in mice prolonged RSV shedding only occurred in animals depleted of both $CD4^+$ and $CD8^+$ T cells, depletion of $CD8^+$ T cells in cattle was sufficient to delay clearance of virus from the respiratory tract.[61] In contrast, there were no significant differences in virus clearance in control calves and those depleted of $CD4^+$ T cells, despite a suppression of the antibody response. These studies highlight the importance of T cells in recovery from RSV infection.

Studies on the effects of passive transfer of $CD4^+$ or $CD8^+$ T cells into mice infected with RSV have shown that both T cell subsets can mediate virus clearance in the absence of antibody. However, passively immunized mice developed more severe lung lesions than control animals.[62,63] As mentioned previously, a formalin-inactivated RSV vaccine not only failed to confer protection against RSV infection but resulted in exacerbated disease after subsequent natural infection. Exacerbation of disease may have been related to the cellular immune response since amelioration of the enhanced disease in mice vaccinated with formalin-inactivated virus was achieved by treatment with antibody to $CD4^+$.[64] These findings of disease-enhancing functions of T cells in RSV infection contrast with the findings for antibodies, which appear to either protect against lung lesions or have no effect on their development. Hence knowledge of the epitopes recognized by protective mAbs to the F and G proteins may aid the design of a vaccine that will induce protective antibodies without stimulating potentially pathogenic T cell responses.

Linear epitopes that are recognized by neutralizing mAbs have been identified for a number of viruses and synthetic peptides corresponding to these epitopes can induce neutralizing antibodies in immunized animals (see ref. 29). Although the proportion of anti-peptide antibodies that recognize native virus is often low, there has been some limited success in inducing protection against virus challenge with peptide-based vaccines.[65-67]

CHARACTERIZATION OF THE ANTIGENIC SITES ON THE G PROTEIN RECOGNIZED BY PROTECTIVE MABS

Norrby et al[68] using overlapping peptides, identified a peptide corresponding to amino acid residues 174-188 of the G protein of subgroup A HRSV which binds to human convalescent sera, rabbit hyperimmune sera and murine mAbs. Among our G protein-specific mAbs, this peptide reacted with mAbs 30 and 31, both of which protected mice from RSV infection (Table 4). Immunization of mice with a peptide corresponding to 174-187, coupled to keyhole limpet hemocyanin induced high levels of antibody to RSV as detected by ELISA and although these antibodies were not neutralizing, mice were protected against challenge with RSV.[69] Furthermore, studies by Olmstead et al,[70] using recombinant vaccinia viruses expressing carboxy terminally truncated mutants of the G protein showed that the region from amino acids 180 to 230 was critical for protection. However, if the protection induced by peptide G174-187 is mediated by antibody, it would not be expected to protect against heterologous subgroup HRS viruses, as mAbs which react with this epitope only recognize subgroup A HRS viruses. Furthermore, recombinant vaccinia viruses expressing the G protein of either subgroup of HRSV are poorly protective against heterologous challenge.[71]

CHARACTERIZATION OF THE ANTIGENIC SITES ON THE F PROTEIN RECOGNIZED BY PROTECTIVE MABS

The epitopes on the F protein recognized by protective mAbs have been mapped by a variety of methods, including competitive inhibition of binding, analysis of antibody-escape mutants, binding to proteolytic fragments of the F protein and binding to synthetic peptides. Several laboratories have identified at least three antigenic areas on the F protein which are involved in neutralization, two of which are also fusion-inhibiting.[72,28,50] We have located the two areas (II and IV[73]) on the F protein which contain overlapping epitopes recognized by fusion-inhibiting mAbs of both murine and bovine origin and also partially protective or nonprotective mAbs. Thus, protective murine mAbs 11 and 13 and bovine mAbs B4 and B5 map to site II and murine mAbs 19 and 20 and bovine mAbs B13 and B14 map to site IV. Sequence analysis of the F protein of antibody-escape mutants indicated that amino acid changes that modified epitopes of antigenic area II clustered in the region 258 to 275; changes at amino acid 429 altered the reactivity of mAbs mapping to antigenic area IV.[73] A synthetic peptide corresponding to the region 255 to 275 of the F protein reacted with protective mAbs B4 and B5 and another corresponding to the region 417 to 435 reacted with protective mAbs 19 73, B13 and B14 (unpublished observations). Trudel et al,[74] mapped the epitope recognized by a neutralizing mAb to amino acid residues 221-237, and other neutralizing mAbs have been mapped to amino acid residues 283-327[75] and 200-225 of the F protein.[76] By analogy with other paramyxoviruses, it is assumed that the fusion activity RSV depends upon the proteolytic processing of the F protein precursor.[2] This modification generates the new N terminus of the F1 subunit, proposed to interact with lipid membranes through a short hydrophobic peptide. However, the areas of the F protein which are recognized by fusion-inhibiting mAbs are located distant from the fusion sequence in a linear map. These findings indicate that binding of antibodies to other regions of the F protein can influence the biological activity of the fusion peptide.

Identification of epitopes recognized by fusion-inhibiting, protective mAbs provides the opportunity to determine if a synthetic or recombinant vaccine containing only these epitopes can be produced which will induce protective antibodies in animals. Fusion-inhibiting antibodies have been induced by a peptide from the V3 region of HIV-1 gp120 expressed in Ty virus-like particles.[77] However, most synthetic peptides representing regions of the F protein of RSV and which bind to protective mAbs induce antibodies that recognize the peptide but not the native F protein.[78,79] A low level of anti-viral antibody was induced in mice by a peptide corresponding to amino acid residues 215-255.[79]

PROSPECTS FOR THE CONTROL OF RSV INFECTIONS WITH MABS

The prophylactic and therapeutic effects of human immune globulin (IVIG) containing high levels of neutralizing antibody to RSV in cotton rats and owl monkeys[12,13] stimulated a small trial to examine the effects of IVIG on RSV infection in infants and young children hospitalized for RSV infection. This study showed that treatment with IVIG resulted in significant reductions in nasal shedding of RSV and improvement in oxygenation when compared with placebo controls.[80] The studies described above with mAbs suggest that highly protective, fusion-inhibiting mAbs have great potential for the prevention or treatment of RSV infections in infants and calves. The dose of fusion-inhibiting mAb required to prevent or clear RSV infection in the lungs of mice was 2-5 mg/kg body weight when given i.v. or i.p.[81] This is 10 to 100x less than the dose of IVIG required to protect against RSV infection when given prophylactically and 4,000x less than the dose required to clear virus when given therapeutically to cotton rats.[11] Thus one of the major advantages of mAbs as opposed to polyclonal sera is that the higher concentration of specific antibody that can be obtained with mAbs should decrease the amount of globulin required for prophylaxis or therapy to levels that could be administered i.m. rather than i.v. Human mAbs are difficult to produce by conventional hybridoma techniques and the application of mouse mAbs is limited in man by the immune response against mouse protein and recognition of mouse antibody effector domains by the human immune system. However, the latter does not appear to be critical for the protection mediated by fusion-inhibiting mAbs to RSV. As an alternative, it is possible to use genetic engineering to transfer the antigen-binding regions from a mouse antibody to a human immunoglobulin.[82] This technique of CDR grafting has been used to produce a human mAb to RSV which contains the antigen-binding sites from a highly protective murine mAb.[81] The reshaped human mAb recognized all clinical isolates of RSV examined and was as effective as the original murine antibody both in the prevention and clearance of RSV infection in mice. These findings raise the hope that the reshaped antibody will be clinically effective against RSV infection in infants.

A human Fab fragment specific for the F protein of RSV has been produced from a combinatorial antibody library expressed on the surface of phage.[83] The Fab fragment has a neutralizing titer of 0.1-1.0 μg/ml, which is similar to that described for the humanized mAb described above.[81] The ability of intranasally administered Fab fragments, obtained from papain-digests of protective mAbs, to protect against and clear an established RSV infection in mice (Table 7), raises the possibility that human or bovine Fab fragments derived from combinatorial antibody libraries could be administered to children or calves by aerosol. Alternatively, Fab fragments could be incorporated into full-length IgG molecules for administration systemically.

CONCLUSIONS

As seen in other virus infections, there is a discrepancy between in vivo and in vitro protective activities of mAbs specific for the F and G proteins of RSV. Neutralizing mAbs to the F protein that also inhibited the formation of multinucleated giant cells were the most potent protective component so far identified. These antibodies mediated their protective effects in the absence of secondary effector mechanisms such as complement-mediated lysis or ADCC of virus-infected cells. Antibody did not appear to contribute to the development of lung lesions. In contrast T cells, which are also able to clear RSV infection, can contribute to severe lung pathology. Thus an effective vaccine may be one that induces high levels of fusion-inhibiting antibody without stimulating an adverse T cell response.

It has been suggested that it may not be possible to actively immunize very young or high-risk infants to prevent RSV disease given that natural RSV infection does not provide adequate or durable immunity. However it has been possible to vaccinate young calves and protect against RSV disease.[84,85] Since there is an accumulative acquisition of resistance to severe disease with successive infections, it may be that protective epitopes on the F protein are poorly immunogenic and are only recognized after several infections.

There is a correlation between levels of maternal IgG antibodies to RSV and the resistance of infants to infection during the first months of life.[86] Therefore, vaccination of mothers in the last trimester of pregnancy in order to boost the maternal gift of fusion-inhibiting antibody may provide a better means of protecting the infant than vaccination in the first few months of life when maternal antibody may interfere with vaccine efficacy. Vaccination of the mother would also remove a major source of infection for the infant.

Because of the adverse reactions associated with the formalin-inactivated RSV vaccine, and the problems of developing a live vaccine that is safe, stable and immunogenic in young infants with maternal antibody, it is unlikely that a vaccine suitable for use in infants will be available in the near future. At present, passive immunization with IVIG is most likely to offer protection against RSV infection. Prophylactic administration of fusion-inhibiting mAbs to infants with underlying cardiopulmonary disease or with immunodefficiency, or to immunosuppressed adults may protect those individuals at most risk of severe disease. Such mAbs could also help to eliminate virus from the lungs of those with severe lower respiratory tract disease or even of those with early mild disease and so prevent hospitalization. mAbs have also been used successfully to clear virus infections in the CNS.[55,56,87] For example, mAbs to rabies virus have been identified that can abrogate virus infection even after CNS invasion by inhibiting virus spread from cell to cell and by blocking RNA transcription and replication.[56]

In conclusion, the identification of mAbs which are highly protective in vivo, and the delineation of their mechanism of action has important practical implications both in the design of effective vaccines and in the selection of potential antibodies for prophylaxis and therapy of viral infections.

References

1. Stott EJ, Taylor G. Immunity to respiratory syncytial virus. In: Dimmock NJ, Minor PD ed. Immune Responses, Virus Infections and Disease. Oxford, IRL Press, 1989:85-104.
2. Collins PL. The molecular biology of human respiratory syncytial virus (RSV) of the genus Pneumovirus. In: Kingsbury DW, ed. The Paramyxoviruses. New York, Plenum Press, 1991:103-62.
3. Heminway BR, Yang Y, Tanaka Y et al. Role of the human respiratory syncytial virus small hydrophobic protein in membrane fusion. Abstracts IXth Int Cong Virol 1993; P17-2:167.
4. Lerch RA, Anderson K, Amann VL et al. Nucleotide sequence analysis of the bovine respiratory syncytial virus fusion protein mRNA and expression from a recombinant vaccinia virus. Virol 1991; 181:118-31.
5. Anderson LJ, Hierholzer JC, Tsou C et al. Antigenic characterisation of respiratory syncytial virus strains with monoclonal antibodies. J Inf Dis 1985; 151:626-33.
6. Furze J, Wertz G, Lerch R et al. Antigenic heterogeneity of the attachment protein of bovine respiratory syncytial virus. J Gen Virol 1993; in press.
7. Kimman TG, Sol J, Westenbrink F et al. A severe outbreak of respiratory tract disease associated with bovine respiratory syncytial virus probably enhanced by vaccination with modified virus. Vet Quart 1989; 11:250-3.
8. Kapikian AZ, Mitchel RH, Chanock RM et al. An epidemiological study of altered clinical reactivity to respiratory syncytial (RS) virus infection in children previously vaccinated with an inactivated RS virus vaccine. Amer J Epid 1969; 89:405-21.
9. Kim HW, Canchola JG, Brandt CD et al. Respiratory syncytial virus disease in infants despite prior administration of antigenic inactivated vaccine. Amer J Epid 1969; 89:422-34.
10. Murphy BR, Prince GA, Walsh EE, et al. Dissociation between serum neutralising and glycoprotein antibody responses of infants and children who received inactivated respiratory syncytial virus vaccine. J Clin Microbiol 1986; 24:197-202.
11. Hemming VG, Prince GA. Respiratory syncytial virus: Babies and antibodies. Infect Agents Dis 1992; 1:24-32.
12. Prince GA, Hemming VG, Horswood RL et al. Immunoprophylaxis and immunotherapy of respiratory syncytial virus infection in the cotton rat. Virus Res 1985; 3:193-206.
13. Hemming VG, Prince GA, Horswood RL et al. Studies of passive immunotherapy for infections of respiratory syncytial virus in the respiratory tract of a primate model. J Inf Dis 1985; 152:1083-7.
14. Prince GA, Hemming VG, Horswood RL et al. Effectiveness of topically administered neutralizing antibodies in experimental immunotherapy of respiratory syncytial virus infection in cotton rats. J Virol 1987; 61:1851-4.
15. Taylor G, Stott EJ, Bew M et al. Monoclonal antibodies protect against respiratory syncytial virus infection in mice. Immunol 1984; 52:137-42.
16. Kennedy HE, Jones BV, Tucker EM et al. Production and characterisation of bovine monoclonal antibodies to respiratory syncytial virus. J Gen Virol 1988; 69:3023-32.
17. Walsh EE, Schlesinger JJ, Brandriss MW. Protection from respiratory syncytial virus infection in cotton rats by passive transfer of monoclonal antibodies. Infect

Immun 1984; 43:756-58.
18. Giraudon P, Wild TF. Correlation between epitopes on hemagglutinin of measles virus and biological activities: passive protection by monoclonal antibodies is related to their hemagglutination inhibiting activity. Virol 1985; 144:46-58.
19. Malvoisin E, Wild F. Contribution of measles virus fusion protein in protectiveimmunity: anti-F monoclonal antibodies neutralise virus infectivity and protect mice against challenge. J Virol 1990; 64:5160-62.
20. Rydbeck R, Love A, Norrby E. Protective effects of monoclonal antibodies against parainfluenza virus type 3-induced brain infection in hamsters. J Gen Virol 1988; 69:1019-24.
21. Orvell C, Grandien M. The effects of monoclonal antibodies on biologic activities of structural proteins of sendai virus. J Immunol 1982; 129:2779-87.
22. Wolinsky JS, Waxham MN, Server AC. Protective effects of glycoprotein-specific monoclonal antibodies on the course of experimental mumps virus meningoencephalitis. J Virol 1985; 53:727-34.
23. Love A, Rydbeck R, Utter G et al. Monoclonal antibodies against the fusion protein are protective in necrotizing mumps encephalitis. J Virol 1986; 58:220-22.
24. Meulemans G, Gonze M, Carlier MC et al. Protective effects of HN and F glycoprotein-specific monoclonal antibodies on experimental Newcastle disease. Avian Pathol 1986; 15:761-8.
25. Umimo Y, Sato TA, Suguira A. Protective effect of monoclonal antibodies to Newcastle disease virus in passive immunization. J Gen Virol 1990; 71:1199-1203.
26. Hirayama N, Senda M, Nakashima N et al. Protective effects of monoclonal antibodies against lethal canine distemper virus infection in mice. J Gen Virol 1991; 72:2827-30.
27. Kris RM, Yetter RA, Cogliano R et al. Passive serum antibody causes temporary recovery from influenza virus infection of the nose, trachea and lung of nude mice. Immunol 1988; 63:349-53.
28. Garcia-Barreno B, Palomo C, Penas C et al. Marked differences in the antigenic structure of human respiratory syncytial virus F and G glycoproteins. J Virol 1989; 63:925-32.
29. Dimmock NJ. Neutralisation of animal viruses. Curr Topics Microbiol Immunol 1993; 183:1-150.
30. Merz DC, Scheid A, Choppin PW. Importance of antibodies to the fusion glycoprotein of paramyxoviruses in the prevention of infection. J Exp Med 1980; 151:275-88.
31. Becht H, Hammerling U, Rott R. Undisturbed release of influenza virus in the presence of univalent antineuraminidase antibodies. Virol 1971; 46:337-43.
32. Sissons JG, Oldstone MBA. Antibody-mediated destruction of virus-infected cells. Adv Immunol 1980; 29:209-60.
33. Bruggemann M, Williams GT, Bindon CI et al. Comparison of the effector functions of human immunoglobulins using a matched set of chimeric antibodies. J Exp Med 1987; 166:1351-61.
34. Lucisano Valim YM, Lachman PJ. The effect of antibody isotype and antigenic epitope density on the complement-fixing activity of immune complexes: a systematic study using chimaeric anti-NP antibodies with human Fc regions. Clin Exp Immunol 1991; 84:1-8.
35. Baldridge JR & Buchmeier MJ. Mechanisms of antibody-mediated protection against lymphocytic choriomeningitis virus infection: mother-to-baby transfer of humoral protection. J Virol 1992; 66:4252-57.

36. Kaminski MS, Kitamura K, Maloney G, et al. Importance of antibody isotype in monoclonal anti-idiotype therapy of a murine B cell lymphoma. A study of hybridoma class switch variants. J Immunol 1986; 136:1123-30.
37. McCullough KC, Crowther JR, Butcher RN, et al. Immune protection against foot-and-mouth disease virus studied using virus-neutralising and non-neutralising concentrations of monoclonal antibodies. Immunol 1986; 58:421-28.
38. Boere WAM, Benaissa-Trouw BJ, Harmsen T, et al. Mechanisms of monoclonal antibody-mediated protection against virulent Semliki Forest virus. J Virol 1985; 54:546-51.
39. Wust CJ, Crombie R, Brown A. Passive protection across subgroups of alphaviruses by hyperimmune non-cross-neutralizing anti-Sindbis serum. Proc Soc Exp Biol Med 1987; 184:56-63.
40. Mathews JH, Roehrig JT, Trent DW. Role of complement and the Fc portion of immunoglobulin G in immunity to Venezuelan equine encephalomyelitis virus infection with glycoprotein-specific monoclonal antibodies. J Virol 1985; 55:594-600.
41. McKendall RR. IgG-mediated viral clearance in experimental infection with herpes simplex virus type 1: Role for neutralisation and Fc-dependent functions but not C' cytolysis and C5 chemotaxis. J Inf Dis 1985; 151:464-70.
42. Schlesinger JJ, Brandriss MW, Walsh EE. Protection against 17D Yellow fever encephalitis in mice by passive transfer of monoclonal antibodies to the nonstructural glycoprotein gp48 and by active immunization with gp48. J Immunol 1985; 135:2805-9.
43. Schmaljohn AL, Kokubun KM, Cole GA. Protective monoclonal antibodies define maturational and pH-dependent antigenic changes in Sindbis virus E1 glycoprotein. Virol 1983; 130:144-54.
44. Hirsch RL. The complement system: its importance in the host response to viral infection. Microbiol Rev 1982; 46:71-85.
45. Morgan BP, Walport MJ. Complement deficiency and disease. Immunol Today 1991; 12:301-6.
46. Rector JT, Lausch RL, Oakes JE. Use of monoclonal antibodies for analysis of antibody-dependent immunity to ocular herpes simplex virus type 1 infection. Infect Immun 1982; 38:168-74.
47. Balachandran N, Bacchetti S, Rawls WE. Protection against lethal challenge of BALB/c mice by passive protection of monoclonal antibodies to five glycoproteins of herpes simplex virus type 2. Infect Immun 1982; 37:1132-7.
48. Gould EA. Neutralizing (54k) and non-neutralizing (54 and 48k) monoclonal antibodies against structural and non-structural yellow fever virus proteins confer immunity in mice. J Gen Virol 1986; 67:590-5.
49. Brandriss MW, Schlesinger JJ, Walsh EE et al. Lethal 17D yellow fever encephalitis in mice. I. Passive protection by monoclonal antibodies to the envelope proteins of 17D yellow fever and Dengue 2 viruses. J Gen Virol 1986; 67:229-34.
50. Taylor G, Stott EJ, Furze J et al. Protective epitopes on the fusion protein of respiratory syncytial virus recognised by murine and bovine monoclonal antibodies. J Gen Virol 1992; 73:2217-23.
51. Hale G, Cobbold SP, Waldman H et al. Isolation of low-frequency class-switch variants from rat hybrid myelomas. J Immunol Methods 1987; 103:59-67.
52. Prince GA, Hemming VG, Horswood RL et al. Mechanism of antibody-

mediated viral clearance in immunotherapy of respiratory syncytial virus infection in cotton rats. J Virol 1990; 64:3091-92.
53. Alexanderson S, Larsen S, Cohn A, et al. Passive transfer of antiviral antibodies restricts replication of Aleutian mink disease parvovirus in vivo. J Virol 1989; 63:9-17.
54. Liebert UG, Schneider-Schaulies S, Baczko K et al. Antibody-induced restriction of viral gene expression in measles encephalitis in rats. J Virol 1990; 64:706-713.
55. Levine B, Hardwick JM, Trapp BD et al. Antibody-mediated clearance of alphavirus infection from neurons. Science 1991; 254:856-60.
56. Dietzschold B, Kao M, Zheng YM et al. Delineation of putative mechanisms involved in antibody-mediated clearance of rabies virus from the central nervous system. Proc natl Acad Sci USA 1992; 89:7252-56.
57. Fujinami RS, Oldstone MBA. Alterations in expression of measles virus polypeptides by antibody: molecular events in antibody-induced antigenic modulation. J Immunol 1980; 125:78-85.
58. Weinmann-Dorsch C, Koschel K. Coupling of viral membrane proteins to phosphatidylinositide signalling system. FEBS Lett 1989; 247:185-88.
59. Graham BS, Bunton LA, Wright PF et al. Role of T lymphocyte subsets in the pathogenesis of primary infection and rechallenge with respiratory syncytial virus in mice. J Clin Invest 1991; 88:1026-33.
60. Graham BS, Bunton LA, Rowland J et al. Respiratory syncytial virus infection in anti-μ-treated mice. J Virol 1991; 65:4936-42.
61. Taylor G, Thomas LH, Howard CJ et al. Effect of T cell depletion on respiratory syncytial virus infection in calves. Abstracts IXth Int Cong Virol 1993; P31-20:236.
62. Cannon MJ, Openshaw PJM, Askonas BA. Cyt otoxic T cells clear virus but augmentlung pathology in mice infected with respiratory syncytial virus. J Exp Med 1988; 168:1163-8.
63. Alwan WH, Record FM, Openshaw PJM. $CD4^+$ T cells clear virus but augment disease in mice infected with respiratory syncytial virus. Comparison with the effects of $CD8^+$ T cells. Clin Exp Immunol 1992; 88:527-36.
64. Connors M, Kulkarni AB, Firestone C-Y, et al. Pulmonary histopathology induced by respiratory syncytial virus (RSV) challenge of formalin-inactivated RSV-immunized BALB/c mice is abrogated by depletion of $CD4^+$ T cells. J Virol 1992; 66:7444-51.
65. Bittle JL, Houghten RA, Alexander H et al. Protection against foot and mouth disease by immunization with a chemically synthesized peptide predicted from the viral nucleotide sequence. Nature 1982; 298:30-3.
66. DiMarchi R, Brooke G, Gale C et al. Protection of cattle against foot-and-mouth disease by a synthetic peptide. Science 1986; 232:639-41.
67. Dietzschold B, Gore M, Marchadier D et al. Structural and immunological characterization of a linear virus-neutralizing epitope of the rabies virus glycoprotein and its possible use in a synthetic vaccine. J Virol 1990; 64:3804-9.
68. Norrby E, Mufson MA, Alexander H, et al. Site directed serology with synthetic peptides representing the large glycoprotein G of respiratory syncytial virus. Proc Natl Acad Sci 1987; 84:6572-76.
69. Trudel M, Nadon F, Seguin C, et al. Protection of BALB/c mice from respiratory syncytial virus infection by immunization with a synthetic peptide derived from the G glycoprotein. Virology 1991; 185:749-57.

70. Olmstead RA, Murphy BR, Lawrence LA et al. Processing, surface expression, and immunogenicity of carboxy-terminally truncated mutants of the G protein of human respiratory syncytial virus. J Virol 1989; 63:411-20.
71. Sullender WM, Anderson K, Wertz GW. The respiratory syncytial virus subgroup B attachment glycoprotein: Analysis of sequence, expression from a recombinant vector, and evaluation as an immunogen against homologous and heterologous subgroup virus challenge. Virol 1990; 178:195-203.
72. Beeler JA, Van Wyke Coelingh K. Neutralisation epitopes on the F glycoprotein of respiratory syncytial virus: effect of mutation upon fusion function. J Virol 1989; 63:2941-50.
73. Arbiza J, Taylor G, Lopez JA et al. Characterization of two antigenic sites recognized by neutralizing monoclonal antibodies directed against the fusion glycoprotein of human respiratory syncytial virus. J Gen Virol 1992; 73:2225-34.
74. Trudel MF, Nadon C, Seguin G et al. Identification of a synthetic peptide as part of a major neutralization epitope of respiratory syncytial virus. J Gen Virol 1987; 68:2273- 80.
75. Paradiso PR, Hu BT, Arumugham R et al. Mapping of a fusion related epitope of the respiratory syncytial virus fusion protein. Vaccine 1991; 9:231-7.
76. Bourgeois C, Corvaisier C, Bour JB, et al. Use of synthetic peptides to locate neutralising antigenic domains on the fusion protein of respiratory syncytial virus. J Gen Virol 1991; 72:1051-8.
77. Griffiths JC, Berrie EL, Holdsworth LN et al. Induction of high titer neutralizing antibodies, using hybrid human immunodefficiency virus V3-Ty-virus-like particles in a clinically relevant adjuvant. J Virol 1991; 65:450-6.
78. Trudel M, Stott EJ, Taylor G et al. Synthetic peptides corresponding to the F protein of RSV stimulates murine B and T cells but fail to confer protection. Arch Virol 1991; 117:59-71.
79. Lopez JA, Andreu D, Carreno C et al. Conformational constraints of conserved neutralizing epitopes from a major antigenic area of human respiratory syncytial virus fusion (F) glycoprotein. J Gen Virol 1993; 74:2567-77
80. Hemming VG, Rodriguez W, Kim HW et al. Intravenous immunoglobulin treatment of respiratory syncytial virus infections in infants and young children. Antimicrob Agents Chemother 1987; 31:1882-6.
81. Tempest PR, Bremner P, Lambert M et al. Reshaping a human monoclonal antibody to inhibit human respiratory syncytial virus infection in vivo. Bio/ Technol 1991; 9:266-71.
82. Jones PT, Dear PH, Foote J et al. Replacing the complementarity determining regions in human antibody with those from a mouse. Nature 1986; 321:522-5.
83. Barbas CF, Crowe JE, Cababa D et al. Human monovalent Fab fragments derived from a combinatorial library bind to respiratory syncytial virus F glycoprotein and neutralize infectivity. Proc Natl Acad Sci 1992; 89:10164-8.
84. Stott EJ, Thomas LH, Taylor G et al. A comparison of three vaccines against respiratory syncytial virus in calves. J Hyg Camb 1984; 93:251-61.
85. Howard CJ, Stott EJ, Thomas LH et al. Protection against respiratory disease in calves induced by vaccines containing respiratory syncytial virus, parainfluenza type 3 virus, Mycoplasma bovis and M. dispar. Vet Rec 1987; 121:372-6.
86. Ogilvie MM, Vathenen AS, Radford M et al. Maternal antibody and respiratory syncytial virus infection in infancy. J Med Virol 1981; 7:263-71.
87. Wright KE, Buchmeier MJ. Antiviral antibodies attenuate T-cell-mediated immunopathology following acute lymphocytic choriomeningitis virus infection. J Virol 1991; 65:3001-6.

CHAPTER 3

The Generation and Maintenance of Antibody and B Cell Memory: The Role of Retained Antigen and Follicular Dendritic Cells

Gregory F. Burton
Andras K. Szakal
Zoher F. Kapasi
John G. Tew

INTRODUCTION

Successful immunizations typically result in potent immune responses which are maintained for long periods of time. Studies of long-term immune responses have shown that immunogens used for induction are retained for many months to years in secondary lymphoid tissues. We believe that this retained immunogen plays a vital role in the induction of potent antibody (Ab) responses, their affinity maturation and long term maintenance. This chapter will focus on the role of retained antigen (Ag) in generating and maintaining long-term humoral responses in vivo. The contributions of lymphocytes, macrophages and Ag-retaining follicular dendritic cells (FDC) to the long-term maintenance of these responses will be discussed. Furthermore experimental approaches will be described that have the potential to render Ag more immunogenic in vivo. These techniques may result in immunization protocols which require fewer injections of immunogen than conventional protocols yet still provide equivalent or greater responses. Studies examining features which contribute to high-affinity long-term Ab responses are frequently conducted outside of the body where cells, Ags and cytokines

---

Strategies in Vaccine Design, edited by Gordon L. Ada, D.Sc.

may be mixed together and the response monitored. Although these studies have contributed much to our understanding of interactions that can occur between cells, the implicit assumption is that the same cells and factors will associate in the same manner in vivo. However, lymphoid tissues have a highly organized architecture and cells do not randomly associate. When cells are isolated from these tissues for study in vitro, the complex architecture is destroyed and therefore only a part of the system is examined. Thus the in vitro environment may not represent events as they occur in vivo. In order to optimally manipulate the immune system to facilitate vaccinations, its in vivo operation must be understood.

Most vaccination protocols rely on an initial priming injection followed by one or more "booster" immunizations to get high titers of high-affinity Ab that is maintained for a long period. With this in mind, the secondary or anamnestic response will be the major focus in this discussion. We think it is significant that Ag can be used in secondary responses in a highly efficient manner–a few picograms of Ag are adequate to induce microgram levels of specific Ab in spite of feedback inhibition mediated by Ab produced during the primary response.[1-3] The presence of specific Ab represents a fundamental difference between primary and secondary Ab responses. In secondary responses, specific Ab rapidly converts the immunogen into immune complexes which are then transported into draining secondary lymphoid tissues. The vast majority of these immune complexes are eliminated by phagocytic cells in the classical macrophage mediated pathway.[4,5] However, a small portion of complexes are trapped on the surface of follicular dendritic cells (FDC) which are able to retain them for many months to years.[6] This FDC-mediated pathway of Ag handling is referred to as the "alternate Ag pathway"[4,5] and will be discussed here in the context of its importance to the induction and maintenance of long-term Ab responses.

LONG-TERM RETENTION OF AG IN LYMPHOID FOLLICLES

Soluble Ag injected into immunologically naive hosts rapidly appears in the lymph and equilibrates throughout the blood. In the absence of specific Ab, soluble Ag is able to freely diffuse through draining lymphoid tissues and interact with immune cells having appropriate receptors. If the Ag is radiolabeled, clearance may be studied and in naive animals yields a biphasic curve. The first phase, resulting from catabolism, begins almost immediately after Ag injection and continues slowly for the first few days. By about the fourth day, sufficient Ab is generated to begin the much more rapid second phase of immune clearance.[6,7] Ag complexed with specific Ab is eliminated effectively by macrophages in the afferent and efferent sinuses of lymph nodes, the sinusoids of the liver and the marginal sinuses of the spleen. In addition, FDC also trap some immune complexes but in contrast to macrophages which endocytose and destroy immune complexes, FDC trap and retain picogram amounts of Ag on their surfaces for long periods of time. The mechanism for this Ag trapping on FDC appears to differ based on the tissue that is being examined. In the spleen, the Ag trapping and retention mechanism requires the presence of complement[9-11] and is sensitive to low dose γ-irradiation.[12-14] In lymph nodes, non-phagocytic cells with dendritic morphology trap immune complexes.[15] These cells, which may be "pre-FDC", are referred to as Ag transport cells (ATC) because they transport Ag onto FDC in the lymphoid follicle. Although Ag complexed with Ab will localize in follicles of either the spleen or lymph nodes, the lymph node pathway does not require the presence of complement [11] and is not sensitive to doses of γ-irradiation up to 1800 rads[12,13] (Burton, unpublished). Ag transport and subsequent localization in lymphoid follicles appear to be rapid events. In primary responses, retained Ag may be present in the spleen as early as four days after initial injection.[8] The kinetics are even more rapid in anamnestic responses where radiolabeled Ag can be detected on ATC in draining lymph nodes 1-2 minutes after injection.[15]

Ag trapping and retention in lymphoid follicles is exquisitely localized to draining lymphoid tissues. Ag injected into a single hind foot of an immune mouse will be initially localized in the draining lymph nodes and to a small extent in the spleen.[6,16] Within four months of Ag challenge, it is no longer detectable in the spleen but is confined to the draining lymph nodes. With increasing time, Ag becomes more and more focused to the lymphoid follicles nearest the site of Ag injection and by one year after Ag challenge specific antibody forming cells (AFC) are almost exclusively confined to the most proximal draining lymph node.[16]

THE ROLE OF FDC-DERIVED AG IN GENERATION AND MAINTENANCE OF AB RESPONSES

Ag retained in lymphoid follicles on FDC is believed to play a vital role in maintaining specific humoral immunity.[6,17] Data supporting this concept come from mice immunized in either a fore or hind foot with human serum albumin (HSA).[17] Regardless of the site of injected Ag the mice responded with an average HSA specific Ab level of 800mg/ml. Surgical removal of non-draining lymph nodes or sham surgery had no significant effect on anti-HSA levels. However, removal of draining lymph nodes with their FDC-retained Ag resulted in almost a 50% decrease in serum anti-HSA levels and this was not restored throughout an 18 week period.[17] Experiments performed by Gray and Skarvall[18] also support the importance of retained Ag in long-term B cell memory. Memory B and T cells from the thoracic ducts of immune rats were transferred into irradiated congenic recipients which did not have retained Ag. Twelve weeks after transfer, the ability to elicit specific memory responses was almost absent. However, responses from animals receiving a small amount of Ag at the time of cell transfer showed normal memory. In work done in our laboratories, transfer of memory cells followed by Ag leads to rapid follicular localization (Burton, Lu and Tew, unpublished).

Further data supporting the role of FDC-retained Ag in induction and maintenance of anamnestic Ab responses have come from in vitro studies of the "spontaneous Ab response".[7] A "spontaneous Ab response" is defined as an anamnestic response (IgG response) that occurs spontaneously (no Ag added). For example, spontaneous responses may be demonstrated in organ fragment cultures prepared from draining lymph nodes removed from hyperimmune mice. Culture fluid obtained after six day culture showed that organ fragments with picogram amounts of retained Ag spontaneously (in the absence of added Ag) produced μg quantities of specific Ab and the amount of Ab produced was directly correlated to the amount of Ag retained. In contrast lymph nodes without retained Ag (i.e., non-draining) produced little Ab spontaneously, but could be induced by adding Ag, indicating that memory cells are present but that Ag is required for Ab production. Interestingly, 10 μg of exogenous Ag was required to induce an optimal Ab response using cells from non-draining lymph nodes whereas only picogram quantities of FDC-retained Ag were required for draining lymph nodes suggesting that FDC-retained Ag is very immunogenic.

The finding that Ag retained on FDC was able to elicit a spontaneous Ab response suggested it must be retained in its native configuration since surface immunoglobulin receptors on B cells generally do not recognize degraded or "processed" Ag. This was confirmed when FDC-retained Ag was recovered and found to be precipitable by specific Ab and capable of co-migration with native Ag on a sizing column.[19] Another tenant of the hypothesis that FDC-retained Ag is important for long-term Ab maintenance is that Ag must be present for long periods. Experiments have shown that the half-life of HSA retained on FDC is in the order of 5.1 to 20 weeks.[20] Studies using the histochemically detectable Ag, horseradish peroxidase (HRP) showed Ag present on FDC even after one year.[16] Furthermore, cells producing anti-HRP could only be observed in draining lymph nodes where FDCs were present with retained HRP.[16] These data indicate that FDC-retained Ag is present for long periods of time and support the concept that retained Ag is functioning in the maintenance of specific Ab responses.

Since there was only a few hundred picograms of Ag retained in lymphoid follicles,[7] we sought to determine how such small quantities were capable of inducing and maintaining Ab responses. In 1988, Szakal et al[21] discovered that small quantities of FDC-retained Ag were released and made available to specific B cells in the microenvironment of the follicle in a novel manner (as microscopic immune complex coated bodies or iccosomes). These structures form in a relatively complex manner through the interaction of subpopulations of FDCs. Iccosomes were first recognized in isolated preparations of FDCs by scanning electron microscopy.[22] Latter transmission electron microscopic studies revealed some of the complicated details of iccosome formation and dispersion. Iccosomes begin their development on the dendrites of a subpopulation of FDCs and form small 0.3-0.5 μm "beads." We referred to these FDCs as "beaded" FDC in contrast to FDCs with filamentous or "filiform" dendrites.[22] Short-term cell culturing has shown that FDCs with filiform dendrites can transform into FDCs with "beaded" dendrites in vitro.

In addition to these two populations of FDCs, a third population was observed to contribute to the formation of iccosomes. These FDCs had veils and irregular or pleiomorphic dendrites. The irregular, less differentiated appearance of the dendrites of these FDCs suggests a younger FDC population than the filiform and the beaded populations of FDCs.[5,22] These pleiomorphic FDCs are also distinguished by the heavy layering of immune complexes present on distinct areas of their dendrites (or veils). These FDCs closely resemble the more mature forms of ATCs. The importance of these ATC-like FDCs to iccosome formation is their close interaction with the dendrites of "beaded" FDCs. This interaction may be described as "Ag or immune complex loading." In this process immune complexes are transferred onto the surface of the "beads" by a mechanism thought to involve interaction between Fc receptors on the beads and the immune complexes of pleiomorphic FDCs and the simultaneous enveloping of the beads by the immune complex carrying dendrite.[5] Once the enveloping dendritic processes are shed, the "beads" with their thick, even coat of periodically arranged immune complexes are released from the dendrites and become dispersed among the B cells of the follicle. Subsequently, these fully formed iccosomes were seen in different stages of endocytosis by B cells.[5,21]

High resolution electron microscopy revealed a spiraling periodicity (440-490 Å) of immune complexes on filiform dendrites of FDC[22] and on the surface of free iccosomes. This periodicity may facilitate interaction between B cells and immune complexes since it has been reported that optimal stimulation of B cells occurs when epitopes are spaced 120-670 Å apart.[5,23]

Iccosomes first appeared within 24 hours of injection of immune mice with Ag[21] and were dispersed in the developing germinal center and endocytosed by B cells by day three. By day five after Ag challenge, iccosomes were rarely seen in germinal centers but the majority of germinal center lymphocytes contained endocytosed Ag-Ab complexes.[5,21] Endocytosed iccosomal Ag (HRP) could be followed to the Golgi apparatus where the Ag appeared to be processed as judged by the apparent decrease in the peroxidatic activity of the Ag. Germinal center B cell presentation of this processed iccosomal Ag to T helper cells was subsequently shown by in vitro experiments.[24] Germinal center B cells were isolated at successive time points after antigenic challenge and assayed for their ability to present the in vivo-obtained Ag to T cells in vitro. Antigen presentation was assayed as the function of IL-2 production by T cells. The results of this study closely correlated with the kinetics of iccosome formation and endocytosis, and showed that germinal center B cells efficiently processed and presented the iccosomal Ag obtained from FDCs to T helper cells.[24]

The significance of iccosomes may be better appreciated if one considers the microenvironment of follicular B cells. Memory B cells localized in follicles bind to Ag on the convoluted dendritic processes of FDCs.[15] However, due to the relatively large size of these processes, B cells do not readily endocytose them. Thus, Ag has to be made available for endocytosis in an appropriate size and form. The iccosome's small size, the periodic disposition of immune complexes on its surface for B cell binding and the presence of Ag within the core of the iccosome provides the Ag in small packets to B cells in a readily palatable form.

Since iccosomes were only detected in vivo between one to three days after Ag challenge, we reasoned that Ag availability must be highly regulated. One likely candidate for regulating the availability of Ag on FDC was the level of specific Ab present. Low levels of Ab would induce Ag release and subsequent Ab synthesis whereas high Ab concentrations would inhibit the release of Ag and therefore turn off Ab production. We reasoned that Ab might act at the level of the FDC. High concentrations of Ab could interact with Ag on FDC processes and crosslink them so that Ag would not be available to surrounding cells. This hypothesis was supported by ultrastructural observation of FDC after Ag challenge.[4,5,21] Initially Ag was freely available to surrounding cells but by day 14 after Ag challenge, FDC-Ag was found in tightly coiled "ball of yarn" configurations that would shield Ag from other cells. To assess the role of Ab feedback on Ag availability two types of experiment were performed. The first was done in vitro using the spontaneous Ab response model where specific Ab was added during various times of culture.[25,26] When Ab was added during the first three days of culture, a marked (>90%) suppression of the specific response was observed whereas addition of Ab on the fourth day had little effect. The addition of Ab in the form of Fab'$_2$ fragments did not inhibit the spontaneous response[26] supporting the hypothesis that crosslinking of Ag on FDC may play a role in Ag availability. Thus the crosslinking through Fab to Ag on one dendrite and Fc on another dendrite may serve as the mechanism for the formation of the "ball of yarn" like convolutions of FDC dendrites shown by electron microscopy that hide the Ag from follicular B cells.[21]

Experiments have also been performed in vivo by Bystryn, Graf and Uhr.[27,28] Rabbits (and in other experiments mice) were immunized with two Ag and then exchange transfused with blood from rabbits immune to only one of the Ag thus mimicking a memory response with retained Ag when Ab levels were low. These rabbits responded to the loss of a single Ab specificity by production of Ab of only the specificity that had been removed. This would be predicted if the infused Ab interacted with FDC-retained Ag (as would occur naturally when Ab levels were high) to protect it from immunocompetent cells while the other Ag would be available since only low levels of Ab would be present. Taken together these experiments indicate that specific Ab serves as a feedback regulator of Ab responses and that Ag availability may play a role in this regulation.

IMMUNOGENICITY OF FDC-RETAINED AG

Following the discovery that FDC could form and release iccosomes, we sought to determine the relative immunogenicity of FDC-retained (iccosomal) Ag in comparison to free Ag. Increasing doses of OVA-bearing FDC or of free OVA were incubated with T and B memory cells obtained from OVA immune mice and adoptively transferred to irradiated syngeneic mice and the amount of anti-OVA produced determined.[29] Mice receiving FDC-retained OVA produced significantly greater quantities of anti-OVA than mice receiving free OVA. It took 1000 pg of free OVA to elicit Ab responses that were equivalent to those obtained from only 100 pg of FDC-retained OVA.[29] FDC were also shown to provide augmentation of Ab responses in an Ag-independent manner suggesting an adjuvant-like effect. In other studies looking at the immunogenicity of FDC-retained Ag and iccosomes, we found that aged mice (>24 months of age) could trap and localize Ag on FDC, but that this function was aberrant and iccosome release could not be observed.[30] We reasoned that this inability to form iccosomes might contribute to the inability of aged mice to mount and maintain normal primary and anamnestic responses. To test this, identical amounts of Ag from normal or aged mice were mixed with T and B memory cells from normal young mice and transfered into other young mice. Some FDC were also sonicated to release pre-formed iccosomes and create in vitro iccosome-like structures. These preparations were also incubated with memory cells and adoptively transferred as above. Mice receiving Ag on FDC from normal mice responded with predicted levels of Ab while those receiving the same amount of Ag on FDC from old mice did not. In contrast, Ab levels were equivalent in mice given iccosome-like Ag (sonicated FDC) regardless of the source of Ag (aged FDC or young). Furthermore, Ag in the form of iccosome constructs gave higher responses than those obtained using Ag on intact FDC suggesting that the iccosome is a particularly palatable form of Ag. We feel that these findings are important in light of the observation that many aged humans also have impaired responses. Administration of Ag on iccosomes or iccosome-like liposomes to these individuals might prove efficacious.

SIGNIFICANCE OF GERMINAL CENTER FORMATION IN THE GENERATION AND MAINTENANCE OF AB AND B CELL MEMORY

INTRODUCTION

One important consequence of Ag challenge is the formation of germinal centers in secondary lymphoid tissues. Germinal centers are recognized as foci of rapidly proliferating B cells around sites where FDC have trapped Ag. These structures are associated with the development of B cell memory,[10,31,32] the induction of a population of AFC,[4,5,33,34] hypermutation of immunoglobulin genes,[35-38] and selection of appropriately mutated B cells.[39]

Germinal centers are comprised of some 80-85% B cells, ~5% $CD4^+$ T cells and a small population of FDC. A specialized macrophage, called a "tingible body" macrophage can also be found associated with germinal centers and is believed to play a role in removing apoptotic B cells.[39] These macrophages were so named because of the tingible bodies (stainable nuclear material) that are seen in phagocytic vacuoles. Examination of the events associated with the development of a germinal center (referred to as the germinal center reaction) has shown that it can be functionally divided into two stages (early and late) which have different functions as explained below.[16,33,37,38,40-42]

EVENTS IN THE EARLY STAGE OF THE GERMINAL CENTER REACTION: AB PRODUCTION

Early in the germinal center reaction (days 1-5), Ag-specific cells interact with FDC-retained Ag and iccosomes and some cells begin to develop into AFC.[40] These plasma cell precursors (which have the germinal center B cell phenotype) migrate out of the follicles and home to the bone marrow and certain other sites where they mature into plasma cells.[40,41] The major events leading to AFC in follicles are as follows: As soon as Ag can be seen on FDC, germinal centers begin to form around the FDC and there is a one-to-one correlation between the number of FDC-Ag retaining sites and germinal centers in a lymph node.[43] Shortly after secondary Ag challenge, germinal centers become edematous and iccosomes are released and endocytosed[5,24] by Ag-specific B cells.[44] The interaction of B cells with FDC results in B cells acquiring the activation state and costimulatory molecules (MHC class II and B7) necessary to successfully present Ag.[45] Germinal center B cells then process and present iccosomal Ag to T cells which respond by releasing interleukins thought to be associated with the induction of a population of AFC. We and others have found that AFC are present in the germinal centers by day three after Ag challenge and have largely disappeared by day seven.[5,33,34] Cytologically, the vast majority of these cells appear as immature plasma cells (pre-plasmablasts). Isolation and culture of germinal center cells three days after Ag challenge results in spontaneous production of specific Ab. If cells are isolated at earlier or later times, they must be further induced with cytokines to produce Ab suggesting that Ag-specific cells are present in the germinal centers but that needed secondary signals are not. This development of AFC appears to be linked to iccosome release and when iccosome release is not observed, induction of AFC in the germinal centers is delayed and Ab responses are impaired.[40]

Shortly after Ag challenge, cells having the phenotype of germinal center B cells (PNA^{Hi}, IgD^-, IgM^{Lo}) appear to be migrating out of follicles. We reasoned that FDC might provide signals that allow B cells to increase their mobility and at the same time respond to chemoattractive signals. We found that FDC could provide a potent primary signal to B cells which made the cells responsive to chemoattractants such as those found in bone marrow cultures.[46] Thus it appears that during the early stage of the germinal center reaction when iccosome release is occurring and when AFCs are found in the germinal center, FDCs can provide signals which could facilitate B cell emigration from the germinal center and contribute to the ability of these cells to migrate toward factors present in bone marrow and other sites of plasma cell accumulation.

To determine if AFC induced in the follicle migrated through the lymph and blood to distal locations (e.g., bone marrow), thoracic duct lymph and peripheral blood were examined for the presence of cells having the phenotype of germinal center B cells (i.e., blasting cells which were highly reactive with the lectin peanut agglutinin PNA^{Hi}).[41] Cells isolated three days following Ag challenge—when iccosomes are released—included numerous cells with the germinal center phenotype whereas cells isolated at other times did not.[41] Furthermore, culture of these cells showed spontaneous production of Ab specific for the Ag retained on FDC in germinal centers. Lastly, cells from germinal centers of immune mice were isolated three days after Ag challenge and found to home to bone marrow.[41,42]

The mechanism for homing to bone marrow is not known but it appears that B cells receive signals prompting them to leave the germinal centers. After entering the blood via the efferent lymph, these cells circulate and home to bone marrow (and certain other sites) which support terminal maturation. Culture of day-3 germinal center B cells with bone marrow cells or supernatant fluids results in at least a two-fold increase in Ab production indicating the importance of bone marrow factors in terminal differentiation.[41] Furthermore, bone marrow has a factor or factors present which can attract day-3 germinal center B cells but not those isolated before day 3 or after day 6 indicating that there is a narrow window during which this unique population of B cells is responsive to migratory signals.[42,47] This pathway from the lymphoid follicles to bone marrow early after secondary immunization is consistent with data showing that the majority of Ab production occurs in bone marrow.[48,49]

Events in the Late Stage of the Germinal Center Reaction: B Cell Memory

The latter stage of the germinal center reaction appears to be directed toward generating the B memory cell pool. It is during this stage when the majority of germinal center growth occurs[5,43] and somatic hypermutation of B cell immunoglobulin genes takes place.[37,38] When iccosome release is completed, the associated edema disappears and the B cells begin a marked proliferative state which continues for about 10 days at which time the germinal center has reached peak size.[5,32,43] Since germinal center B cells are in close proximity to FDC, we sought to determine if the FDC could contribute to the B cell proliferative response. Earlier Schnizlein et al[50] reported that FDC appeared to promote proliferation of LPS-activated B cells. To determine if FDC could augment B cells which had been stimulated in a more physiological manner (Ag as opposed to the mitogen LPS), we isolated resting B cells and cultured them in the presence of anti-mu (Ag surrogate), IL-4 (T cell surrogate) and FDC.[51] We found that FDC caused a consistent two-to-three-fold augmentation of the proliferative capacity of the B cells and that this was a costimulatory signal which first required the activation of the cells either with the Ag and T cell surrogates or with mitogen. Furthermore, this costimulatory signaling was independent of MHC haplotype (i.e., B cells and FDC could be MHC disparate).

In recent experiments we tried to further characterize the FDC-mediated costimulatory activity and determine if iccosomes or iccosome-like fragments could also provide this activity. Preliminary studies suggest that although iccosomes can provide potent augmentation of Ab production, they appear to inhibit B cell proliferation (Qin and Tew, unpublished). We think that this apparent difference in signaling between FDC and their product (iccosomes) may contribute to the differential focus of the two stages of the germinal center reaction: when iccosomes are released, Ab formation is the focus and when iccosome release is completed, expansion of the B cell population and selection of high-affinity clones is favored.

High-affinity clones begin to appear at about day 10 of a primary response and around day 6 of an anamnestic response.[36-38,52] It appears that the germinal center B cell population is oligoclonal[35,36,53,54] and thus a rapid expansion of the small number of B cells clones prior to the beginning of somatic hypermutation would allow a larger number of B cells to undergo mutation and thus a higher chance of mutant clones emerging with a higher affinity for Ag.[55] It has been suggested that B cell blasts in the dark zone (area of greatest proliferation) of the germinal center will undergo apoptosis if not selected by Ag and that interaction with Ag-FDC would rescue the cell from this fate. Since Ag is present in limiting quantity on FDC, cells which had high-affinity immunoglobulin receptors (as a consequence of mutation) would be able to more efficiently compete for the Ag and thus be preferentially selected and spared from programmed cell death.[35,53] In contrast, cells with low affinity receptors would not effectively compete for limited Ag and therefore undergo apoptosis and be removed by tingible body macrophages (TBM) in the germinal centers. As the number of B cells in the germinal center increases, so does the number of TBM and this appears to peak during the time when somatic hypermutation is ongoing.

CHARACTERISTICS OF AB RESPONSES THAT ARE NOT MAINTAINED LONG-TERM

Unlike most proteins, carbohydrate Ags often elicit poor anamnestic Ab responses which suggests that functional populations of memory cells are lacking.[56] Interestingly, carbohydrate Ags do not readily induce germinal center reactions.[57] If germinal centers are not formed properly, it does not seem surprising to us that immune responses to carbohydrate Ags are characterized as being of low affinity (suggesting a lack of somatic mutation) and are of limited heterogeneity.[58] Furthermore, responses to carbohydrate Ags are often predominated by Ab of the IgG_2 isotype,[59,60] which in the system we have studied[60] is not maintained for long periods of time in the absence of a continuous source of the Ag.[61] Our studies have been carried out in juvenile periodontitis patients which frequently respond to *Actinobacillus actinomycetemcomitans* serotype b by making high titers of Ab (10-1000 μg/ml) against the serotype specific carbohydrate.[59,60] This serotype specific carbohydrate Ag of *A. actinomycetemcomitans* is the immunodominant Ag and virtually all of the Ab is reactive with this Ag[62] and is IgG_2.[59,60] Interestingly, this Ab is of very low avidity compared to high avidity protein Ags from the same organism when studied using ammonium isothiocyanate as a dissociating agent.[63] It required about 3M ammonium isothiocyanate to dissociate half the Ab reactive with an *A. actinomycetemcomitans* protein Ag as opposed to less than 1M to dissociate half the IgG_2 Ab from the serotype specific carbohydrate Ag (Califano and Tew, Unpublished). Interestingly, when juvenile periodontitis patients are given periodontal treatment, including antibiotics which are known to eliminate *A. actinomycetemcomitans*, the serum Ab reactive with this organism rapidly declines.[61] The implications are that not only is memory short lived but that the immune system lacks the ability to maintain the Ab response for long periods in the absence of the organism.

We suspect that the lack of germinal center formation, memory cell production, somatic mutation, and long term maintenance of Ab production is related to a lack of FDC function. We reason that it may be possible to engineer Ags to be trapped and maintained on FDC and this may lead to Ab responses to carbohydrates with high levels of memory and the long term maintenance of significant levels of high-affinity Ab. Thus the recognition of the role of FDC and persisting Ag in these processes could lead to improved vaccines for certain carbohydrate Ags.

DIRECTING AG TO FDC

Targeting Ags to FDC might be advantageous, since the Ag-FDC complex plays a vital role in germinal center formation, memory cell production, somatic mutation, and long term maintenance of Ab production. This approach might reduce the amount of Ag required and lead to vaccination protocols using fewer immunizations with lower doses of Ag. Targeting Ag to specific cells in vivo has been accomplished by conjugating Ags or haptens to Ab specific for molecules present on the target cells. Some of the molecules targeted include surface immunoglobulin,[64,65] class II major histocompatibility molecules,[66-68] T cell markers (e.g., Thy-1)[69] and Fcγ receptors.[70] Some of these procedures have resulted in augmented immune responses using only nanogram amounts of Ag in the absence of adjuvants.[70]

Recently Mjaaland and Fossum[69] immunized animals with haptens conjugated to FDC-specific monoclonal Ab and found that some animals responded with primary responses having the characteristics of anamnestic responses. Hapten specific IgG was rapidly produced and appeared to be maintained. This seems significant and deserves further study. Targeting Ag to more than one cell type may result in further augmentation of responses including production of more Ab and longer memory. Two likely candidates for targeting of Ag are FDC—which present Ag to B cells and T cell-associated dendritic cells (e.g., interdigitating cells, Langerhans cells)—which present Ag to T cells. In this fashion we would predict that both T and B cells would be stimulated and would result in rapid germinal center formation. Thus by coupling Ag to monoclonal antibodies that bind to FDC, Ag could be engineered to go to FDC where germinal centers and strong anamnestic Ab responses would be elicited. For example, this approach might allow high-affinity responses to be elicited and maintained against carbohydrate Ags. Thus the concept of directing Ag to FDC and perhaps other cells may provide an adjuvant free delivery system that can be directly applied to the development of safer more efficacious vaccines.

SUMMARY

Successful vaccination strategies typically result in the induction of high-affinity humoral responses that are maintained for long periods of time. A hallmark of long-term Ab responses is that the immunogens are trapped and retained on FDC and that germinal centers form around these Ag-bearing cells. We have cited evidence that Ag and secondary signals associated with FDC play critical roles in eliciting Ab production, expanding specific B cell populations and selecting high-affinity clones of B cells for maintaining Ab production and B cell memory. We also discussed responses that did not appear to involve retained Ag or germinal center formation and have correlated these with low affinity and poor maintenance. With the onset of molecular approaches to vaccine design, we believe that an understanding of events in vivo will provide insight into the effective design of vaccines. For example, we have discussed the concept of targeting Ag to FDC to elicit a high-affinity Ab response that would be maintained. Concepts derived from a basic understanding of microenvironments in vivo may prove important in being able to design safer and more efficacious vaccines.

REFERENCES

1. Britton S and Moller G. Regulation of antibody synthesis against *Escherichia coli* endotoxin. I. Suppressive effect of endogenously produced and passively transferred antibodies. J Immunol 1968; 100:1326-1334.
2. Graf MW and Uhr JW. Regulation of antibody formation by serum antibody. I. Removal of specific antibody by means of immunoadsorption. J Exp Med 1969; 130:1175-1186.
3. Bolton RW, Rozmiarek H and Chorpenning FW. Cyclic antibody formation to polyglycerophosphates in normal and injected rats. J Immunol 1977; 118:1154-1158.
4. Tew JG, Kosco MH and Szakal AK. The alternative antigen pathway. Immunol Today 1989; 10:229-231.

5. Szakal AK, Kosco MH and Tew JG. Microanatomy of lymphoid tissue during the induction and maintenance of humoral immune responses: structure function relationships. Ann Rev Immunol 1989; 7:91-109.
6. Mandel TE, Phipps RP, Abbot A, et al. The follicular dendritic cell: long term antigen retention during immunity. Immunol Rev 1980; 53:29-59.
7. Tew JG and Mandel TE. The maintenance and regulation of serum antibody levels: evidence indicating a role for antigen retained in lymphoid follicles. J Immunol 1978; 120:1063-1069.
8. Szakal AK and Hanna MG. The ultrastructure of antigen localization and virus-like particles in mouse spleen germinal centers. Exp Mol Path 1968; 8:75-89.
9. Klaus GGB and Humphrey JH. The generation of memory cells. I. The role of C3 in the generation of B memory cells. Immunology 1977; 33:31-40.
10. Klaus GGB, Humphrey JH, Kunkl A, et al. The follicular dendritic cell: its role in antigen presentation in the generation of immunological memory. Immunol Rev 1980; 53:3-28.
11. Tew JG, Mandel TE and Miller GA. Immune retention: immunological requirements for maintaining an easily degradable antigen in vivo. Aust J Exp Biol Med Sci 1979; 57:401-414.
12. Jaroslow BN and Nossal GJV. The effect of whole body X-irradiation on antigen localization in lymphoid follicles. Aust J Exp Biol Med Sci 1966; 44:609.
13. Nettesheim P and Hanna MG,Jr.. Radiosensitivity of the antigen-trapping mechanism and its relation to the suppression of immune response. Adv Exp Med Biol 1969; 5:167.
14. Humphrey JH, Grennan D and Sundaram V. The origin of follicular dendritic cells in the mouse and the mechanism of trapping of immune complexes on them. Eur J Immunol 1984; 14:859-864.
15. Szakal AK, Holmes KL and Tew JG. Transport of immune complexes from the subcapsular sinus to lymph node follicles on the surface of nonphagocytic cells, including cells with dendritic morphology. J Immunol 1983; 131:1714-1727.
16. Donaldson SL, Kosco MH, Szakal AK, et al. Localization of antibody-forming cells in draining lymphoid organs during long-term maintenance of the antibody response. J Leukocyte Biol 1986; 40:147-157.
17. Tew JG, Phipps RP and Mandel TE. The maintenance and regulation of the humoral immune response: persisting antigen and the role of follicular antigen-binding dendritic cells as accessory cells. Immunol Rev 1980; 53:175-201.
18. Gray D and Skarvall H. B-cell memory is short lived in the absence of antigen. Nature 1988; 336:70-73.
19. Tew JG, Mandel TE and Burgess AW. Retention of intact HSA for prolonged periods in the popliteal lymph nodes of specifically immunized mice. Cell Immunol 1979; 45:207-212.
20. Tew JG and Mandel TE. Prolonged antigen half-life in the lymphoid follicles of specifically immunized mice. Immunology 1979; 37:69-76.
21. Szakal AK, Kosco MH and Tew JG. A novel in vivo follicular dendritic cell-dependent iccosome-mediated mechanism for delivery of antigen to antigen-processing cells. J Immunol 1988; 140:341-353.
22. Szakal AK, Gieringer RL, Kosco MH, et al. Isolated follicular dendritic cells: cytochemical antigen localization, Nomarski, SEM, and TEM morphology. J Immunol 1985; 134:1349-1359.
23. Dintzis RZ, Middleton MH and Dintzis HM. Studies on the immunogenicity and tolerogenicity of T-independent antigens. J Immunol 1983; 131:2196-2203.

24. Kosco MH, Szakal AK and Tew JG. In vivo obtained antigen presented by germinal center B cells to T cells in vitro. J Immunol 1988; 140:354-360.
25. Tew JG, Self CH, Harold WW, et al. The spontaneous induction of anamnestic antibody responses in lymph node cell cultures many months after primary immunization. J Immunol 1973; 111:416-423.
26. Tew JG, Greene EJ and Makoski MH. In vitro evidence indicating a role for the Fc region of IgG in the mechanism for the long-term maintenance and regulation of antibody levels in vivo. Cell Immunol 1976; 26:141-152.
27. Bystryn JC, Schenkein I and Uhr JW. A model for the regulation of antibody synthesis by serum antibody. In: Amos B. ed. Progress in immunology. N.Y.: Academic Press, 1971:628.
28. Bystryn JC, Graf MW and Uhr JW. Regulation of antibody formation by serum antibody. II. removal of specific antibody by means of exchange transfusion. J Exp Med 1970; 132:1279-1287.
29. Burton GF, Maeda K, Szakal AK, et al. Immunogenicity of follicular dendritic cell (FDC) associated antigen. In: Imai Y, Tew JG and Hoefsmit ECM. eds. Dendritic Cells in Lymphoid Tissue. Elsevier Science, 1990:149-156.
30. Burton GF, Kosco MH, Szakal AK, et al. Iccosomes and the secondary antibody response. Immunology 1991; 73:271-276.
31. Klaus GGB and Kunkl A. The role of germinal centers in the generation of immunological memory. In: Microenvironments in haemopoietic and lymphoid differentiation: CIBA Foundation Symposium 84. London: Pitman Medical, 1981:265-280.
32. Coico RF, Bhogal BS and Thorbecke GJ. Relationship of germinal centers in lymphoid tissue to immunologic memory VI. Transfer of B cell memory with lymph node cells fractionated according to their receptors for peanut agglutinin. J Immunol 1983; 131:2254-2257.
33. Tew JG, Burton GF, Szakal AK, et al. A subpopulation of germinal center B cells differentiate directly into antibody forming cells upon secondary immunization. Adv Exp Med Biol 1988; 237:215-225.
34. Sordat B, Sordat M, Hess MW, et al. Specific antibody within germinal center cells of mice after primary immunization with horseradish peroxidase: a light and electron microscopic study. J Exp Med 1970; 131:77-91.
35. MacLennan ICM. The centre of hypermutation. Nature 1991; 354:352-353.
36. Jacob J and Kelsoe G. In situ studies of the primary immune response to (4-hydroxy-3-nitrophenyl)acetyl. II. a common clonal origin for PALS-associated foci and germinal centers. J Exp Med 1992; 176:679-687.
37. Berek C, Berger A and Apel M. Maturation of the immune response in germinal centers. Cell 1991; 67:1121-1129.
38. Berek C. The development of B-cells and the B-cell repertoire in the microenvironment of the germinal centre. Immunological Rev 1992; 126:5-19.
39. Liu YJ, Joshua D, Williams GT, et al. Mechanism of antigen-driven selection in germinal centres. Nature 1989; 342:929-931.
40. Kosco MH, Burton GF, Kapasi ZF, et al. Antibody-forming cell induction during an early phase of germinal centre development and its delay with ageing. Immunology 1989; 68:312-318.
41. DiLosa RM, Maeda K, Masuda A, et al. Germinal center B cells and antibody production in the bone marrow. J Immunol 1991; 1460:4071-4077.
42. Tew JG, DiLosa RM, Burton GF, et al. Germinal centers and antibody production in bone marrow. Immunol Rev 1992; 126:1-14.

43. Szakal AK, Taylor JK, Smith JP, et al. Kinetics of germinal center development in lymph nodes of young and aging immune mice. Anat Rec 1990; 227:475-485.
44. Gray D, Kosco MH and Stockinger B. Novel pathways of antigen presentation for the maintenance of memory. Int Immunol 1991; 3:141-148.
45. Kosco MH. Follicular dendritic cells induce B cells to express B7/BB1 and upregulate class II resulting in APC activity. Proc 11th Germinal Center Conference 1993; 112.(Abstract)
46. Burton GF, Kupp LI, Szakal AK, et al. Follicular dendritic cells (FDC) and B cell chemotaxis. Proc 11th Germinal Center Conference 1993; 116.(Abstract)
47. Kupp LI, Kosco MH, Schenkein HA, et al. Chemotaxis of germinal center B cells in response to C5a. Eur J Immunol 1991; 21:2697-2701.
48. Benner R, Meima F, Van der Meulen GM, et al. Antibody formation in mouse bone marrow I. Evidence for the development of plaque-forming cells in situ. *Immunology 1974; 26:247-255.*
49. Benner R, Hijmans W and Haaijman JJ. The bone marrow: the major source of serum immunoglobulins, but still a neglected site of antibody formation. Clin Exp Immunol 1981; 46:1-8.
50. Schnizlein CT, Szakal AK and Tew JG. Follicular dendritic cells in the regulation and maintenance of immune responses. Immunobiol 1984; 168:391-402.
51. Burton GF, Conrad DH, Szakal AK, et al. Follicular dendritic cells (FDC) and B cell co-stimulation. J Immunol 1993; 150:31-38.
52. Jacob J, Kassir R and Kelsoe G. In situ studies of the primary immune response to (4-hydroxy-3-nitrophenyl)acetyl. I. the architecture and dynamics of responding cell populations. J Exp Med 1991; 173:1165-1175.
53. MacLennan ICM, Liu YJ and Johnson GD. Maturation and dispersal of B-cell clones during T cell-dependent antibody responses. Immunological Rev 1992; 126:143-161.
54. Jacob J, Kelsoe G, Rajewsky K, et al. Intraclonal generation of antibody mutants in germinal centres. Nature 1991; 354:389-392.
55. Berek C and Ziegner M. The maturation of the immune response. Immunol Today 1993; 14:400-404.
56. Kayhty H, Karanko V, Peltola H, et al. Serum antibodies after vaccination with Haemophilus influenza type b capsular polysaccharide and resonses to reimmunizaiton: no evidence of immunologic tolerance or memory. Pediat 1984; 74:857-865.
57. Weissman IL, Gutman GA, Friedberg SH, et al. Lymphoid tissue architecture III. Germinal center, T cells and thymus-dependent vs thymus-independent antigens. Adv Exp Med Biol 1976; 66:229-237.
58. Nahm MH, Kroese GM and Hoffmann JW. The evolution of immune memory and germinal centers. Immunol Today 1992; 13:438-440.
59. Wilson ME and Hamilton RG. Immunoglobulin G subclass response of localizaed juvenile periodontitis patients to *Actinobacillus actinomycetemcomitans* Y4 lipopolysaccharide. InfectImmun 1992; 60:1806-1812.
60. Lu H, Califano JV, Schenkein HA, et al. Immunoglobulin class and subclass distribution of antibodies reactive with the immunodominant antigen of *Actinobacillus actinomycetemcomitans* serotype b. InfectImmun 1993; 61:2400-2407.

61. Haffajee AD, Socransky SS, Ebeersole JL, et al. Clinical, microbiological and immunological features associated with the treatment of active periodontosis lesions. JClinPerio 1983; 11:600-618.
62. Califano JV, Schenkein HA and Tew JG. Immunodominant antigen of *Actinobacillus actinomycetemcomitans* strain Y4 in high responder patinets. InfectImmun 1989; 57:1582-1589.
63. Lopatin DE, LaBelle D and Lee SW. Measurement of relative avidity of antibodies reactive with *Porphyromonas (Bacteroides) gingivalis* in the sera of subjects having adult periodontitis. JPerioRes 1991; 26:167-175.
64. Kawamura H and Berzofsky JA. Enhancement of antigenic potency in vitro and immunogenicity in vivo by coupling the antigen to anti-immunoglobulin. J Immunol 1986; 136:58-65.
65. Lees A, Morris SC, Thyphronitis G, et al. Rapid stimulation of large specific antibody responses with conjugates of antigen and anti-IgD antibody. J Immunol 1991; 145:3594-3600.
66. Carayanniotis G and Barber BH. Adjuvant-free IgG responses induced with antigen coupled to antibodies against class II MHC. Nature 1987; 327:59-61.
67. Steinman RM. Cytokines amplify the function of accessory cells. Immunol Lett 1988; 17:197-202.
68. Carayanniotis G, Skea DL, Luscher MA, et al. Adjuvant-independent immunization by immunotargeting antigens to MHC and non-MHC determinants in vivo. Mol Immunol 1991; 28:261-267.
69. Mjaaland S and Fossum S. Modulation of immune responses with monoclonal antibodies. I. effects on regional lymph node morphology and on antihapten responses to haptenized monoclonal antibodies. Eur J Immunol 1990; 20:1457-1461.
70. Snider DP, Kaubusch A and Segal DM. Enhanced antigen immunogenicity induced by bispecific antibodies. J Exp Med 1990; 171:1957-1963.

CHAPTER 4

Characteristics of Virus-specific CD8+ T Cell Memory

Peter C. Doherty
Sally R. Sarawar
Ralph Tripp
Sam Hou

INTRODUCTION

The idea that specific immune memory persists following an encounter with antigen is so accepted that it is one of the few generally familiar tenets of immunology. Everyone has been immunized against a variety of pathogens, and expects to be protected as a consequence. The awareness of second-set allograft rejection and the long-term presence of antibody following a virus infection is central to immunological thinking. Despite this, the mechanisms underlying memory have received comparatively little attention until fairly recently.[1-3] The great drive over the past 20 years has been to understand immune recognition, repertoire generation, tolerance and (to a lesser extent) effector function. Memory was, perhaps, seen simply as an extension of the same themes. This is probably correct in essence, but it is becoming very clear that there are questions particular to the nature of memory that demand rigorous experimental analysis.

Many of the tools that we need to dissect the nature of immune memory are already available, or are being developed. We are rapidly gaining a much clearer understanding of the molecular control and signaling events that determine the differentiation status of lymphocytes.[4,5] Categories of lymphocytes can be defined with monoclonal antibodies (mAbs) specific for cell-surface molecules that are variously expressed depending on the differentiation status of the cell.[6-8] Furthermore, utilization of mice that are doubly transgenic for a T cell receptor (TCR) pair[9] recognizing a particular peptide+MHC glycoprotein complex (p+MHC-I or II) will allow differentiation status to be compared for "naive" and primed T cells with the same specificity.

Strategies in Vaccine Design, edited by Gordon L. Ada, D.Sc.

This brief account concentrates on CD8+ T cell memory. Much of the relevant data is based on limiting dilution analysis (LDA)[10] for cytotoxic T lymphocyte precursors (CTLp). Current concepts of the general characteristics of B cell and CD4+ T cell memory have been summarized in recent reviews.[2,3] Contemporary studies of memory for virus-specific B cells and CD4+ T cells are in progress, but it is too soon for a general discussion of this information.

DEFINITION: PROTECTION AND T CELL MEMORY ARE NOT NECESSARILY SYNONYMOUS

The classical way to show immune memory to a pathogen has been to prime and then challenge. This it is obviously the topic of interest when vaccine efficacy is being considered. However protection against secondary exposure measures only some of the characteristics of memory. There are other variables, such as the anatomical site of the infectious process, which influence the protection phenotype but are not a direct consequence of the prevalence of memory T cells. This may be particularly true for respiratory infections, where a high frequency of virus-immune CD8+ CTLp may lead to virus clearance being enhanced by only 1-2 days (see The Recall Response, below).

A good example of the complexity of challenge experiments comes from the lymphocytic choriomeningitis virus (LCMV) model.[11,12] This virus is substantially non-lytic and is carried in nature by mice that are infected *in utero*, live and reproduce normally and in turn pass the infection onto their offspring.[13] An acute immunopathological disease mediated by CD8+ effector T cells develops when LCMV is injected intracerebrally (i.c.) into previously unexposed adults.[14] Death is presumably a consequence of direct CD8+ T cell-mediated damage to LCMV-infected cells[15] in the choroid plexus and meninges. The development of fatal neurological disease can be prevented by the early adoptive transfer of LCMV-specific effector CTLs, which presumably terminate the infectious process before it has gone too far.[16] The same effect is apparent in virus-challenge studies. The "x" line in Figure 1 represents the hypothetical number of virus-infected cells which, if damaged by immune T cells over a fairly short interval, will lead to a physiological crisis and death, the normal consequence of the primary response (dotted histogram, Fig. 1) to i.c. LCMV. When a small dose of virus is given i.c. to mice primed with a vaccinia construct expressing the LCMV CD8+ T cell epitope, the more rapid secondary response (hatched histogram, Fig. 1) terminates the infectious process before the "x" stage is reached (lower diagonal, Fig. 1). However a large i.c. challenge result leads to "x" before effector function develops (upper diagonal, Fig. 1). The consequence when the T cells enter the central nervous system is then more rapid death than in the primary response. Also, the position of the "secondary" histogram (Fig. 1) will move to the right with declining CTLp frequency. The phenotype of memory is either protection or enhanced immunopathology, depending on the way that the experiment is done (Fig. 1).

Thus we simply cannot base speculation on the differentiation status and maintenance of memory lymphocyte populations on virus challenge studies. The results are often too confusing for readers who do not have close familiarity with these complex experimental systems. Furthermore, if

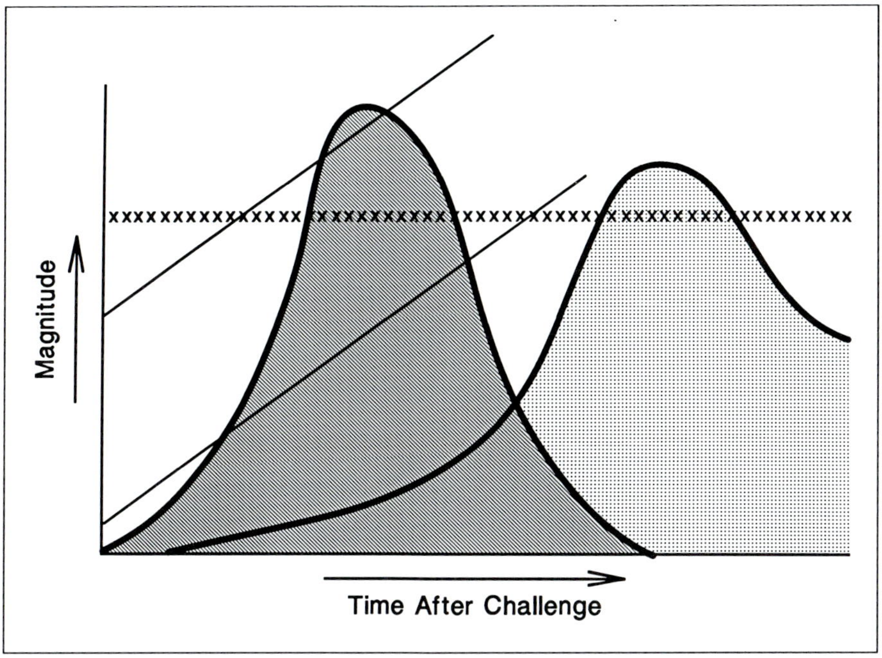

Fig. 1. Murine LCMV is essentially non-lytic and is carried as a clinically-inapparent infection in immunosuppressed mice. Fatal neurological disease results when large numbers of LCMV-infected choroid plexus and meningeal cells are damaged more or less synchronously by CD8⁺ CTL effectors, represented by the histogram (dots) for "primary CD8⁺ CTL response" intersecting the "xxx" line. Mice that are primed only to a p+MHC-I epitope recognized by LCMV-immune CD8⁺ CTLp will generate a potent secondary response on i.c. challenge. This will protect if the challenge dose is low, illustrated by the intersect of the "secondary CD8⁺ CTL response" histogram (hatching) with the lower diagonal, as the infectious process is terminated early and "xxx" is not reached. However, a high dose of virus (upper diagonal) may lead to "xxx" before the secondary CTL effectors become available. Again, the result is death from T cell-mediated immunopathology. Decreasing numbers of LCMV-specific CTLp would be expected to move the "secondary" histogram to the right, which would shift the consequences of the low dose challenge (lower diagonal) from protection to immunopathology. Giving very high titers of LCMV to unprimed mice may paradoxically lead to non-fatal consequences, a phenomenon that is currently drawing attention to the possibility of "immune exhaustion."[91,96]

we use protection as the central characteristic of memory, we exclude a variety of experimental approaches where this type of analysis is not possible. *The definition of T cell memory has to be that there is clear, quantifiable evidence of enhanced response following a previous encounter with antigen.* This may or may not be an accurate predictor of increased resistance. The protection experiment is more relevant if, for example, the virus-specific CTLp frequencies are measured for comparable mice.

CELL-SURFACE PHENOTYPE

The mAb-defined markers that have been assessed for the categorization of naive, effector and memory virus-immune CD8⁺ T cells in the mouse are listed in Table 1. The earliest studies were done with CD44,[8,17,18] which was shown at about the same time to be expressed at high levels on memory (but not naive) alloreactive T cells.[19,20] Taken together, these studies show that the alloreactive T cell population in young adults is not comprised solely of lymphocytes that have been cross-primed to self MHC+non-self peptide. However, as mice age, an increasing proportion of the total T lymphocyte pool becomes CD44-high.[21] This is to be expected as the individual accumulates antigenic experience through life. One problem with using CD44 is that naive T cells in some mouse strains (e.g., BALB/c) constitutively express quite high levels of this glycoprotein,[22] though the intensity of staining is further increased with activation. At this stage, the most useful markers discriminating naive and activated/memory $CD8^+$ T cells in the mouse look to be L-selectin, CD11b, and CD44 (Table 1). Recently activated and memory T cells may, perhaps, be distinguished using CD69 or LFA-1. The CD45 isotypes,[23,24] which have been widely used for the analysis of $CD4^+$ T cell memory (particularly in humans), have yet to be shown to be useful for categorizing murine $CD8^+$ T cells.

Many of the generalizations that look to be particularly helpful for understanding the recirculation characteristics of naive versus memory T cells have been made from experiments that use only patterns of cell-surface glycoprotein expression to discriminate these two broad categories of lymphocytes.[25-27] However, the lack of functional correlation is potentially a problem and such analyses should not yet be considered to have established principles that are engraved in stone. The findings with mice should also be regarded with some circumspection when thinking about the population biology of lymphocytes with different cell-surface characteristics. Laboratory mice are generally maintained in relatively clean environments. Humans, or domestic animals, will inevitably be exposed to a much broader range of pathogens. Also people live much longer than mice, and the consequences of both thymus involution and memory T cell accumulation for future patterns of responsiveness should thus be much greater.

Table 1. Cell-surface markers that have been assessed for virus-immune $CD8^+$ T cells

		Level of expresson on $CD8^+$ T Cells			
Marker	Alternative nomenclature	Naive	Effector	Memory	Reference
CD44	Pgp-1	Low	High	High	6, 17, 18
L-selectin	LECAM-1, Mel-14	High	Low	Low	7, 8
CD11b	Mac-1	Low	High	High	7
LFA-1		Low	High	Low	8
CD45RB		Low/High	Low/High	Low/High	8
CD69		Low	High	Low	a
CD49d	LPAM	Low	High	High	a

[a] Unpublished data from our laboratory

The main utility of the cell-surface marker studies is likely to be for enrichment of particular functional subsets, and for correlation with the differentiation status of the cells. The approach will obviously be of particular value with mice that are transgenic for single TCR α and β chains of known antigen specificity.[9]

DURATION OF CD8⁺ T CELL MEMORY

The idea that T cell memory is long-lived is drawn from a fairly limited information base derived from mouse experiments and observational studies in humans. Much of this is indirect, inferential or even anecdotal. The amount of quantitative information (established by LDA) is minimal. It may be possible to model the cellular basis of immune memory mathematically if we take the trouble to develop more hard data for at least one experimental system. Murine influenza would probably be a good place to start.

INFLUENZA IN THE MOUSE

The influenza A viruses[28] infect a variety of species in nature, not including *Mus musculus*. Some influenza A viruses are quite pathogenic for laboratory mice,[29] and most studies have been done with viruses that kill if given intranasally (i.n.) in a sufficiently high dose. Many of the experiments have utilized A/PR8/34 (PR8, H1N1) and A/HKx31 (HK, H3N2), the latter being a high-growing recombinant[30] that has most of the internal proteins of PR8 but different surface hemagglutinin (H) and neuraminidase (N) glycoproteins. However, normal mice housed in adjacent, unprotected (with filter tops) cages do not become infected when housed near those with a fulminant influenza pneumonitis, and controls placed in the same cage often fail to sero-convert.

Mice that are infected once with an influenza A virus have greatly expanded numbers of influenza-specific CD8⁺ CTLp for life,[10,28,31] though there is a decrease with advanced age.[32-34] The frequency of CTLp specific for a major p+MHC-I determinant changes from <1:100,000 spleen or lymph node WBC to 1:2,000-1:10,000. Estimates of CTLp prevalence in the aged can be increased if irradiated stimulators from young mice are used in the LDA, indicating that the function of antigen-presenting cells declines with longevity.[32] Also there are senescent changes that influence the capacity of the lymphocytes to proliferate but not to differentiate to be CTL effectors.[35]

The long-term nature of murine CD8⁺ T cell memory for the influenza A viruses creates some problems for the currently fashionable idea[2,12,36] that the maintenance of memory is absolutely dependant on antigen persistence. Neither viral RNA nor mRNA could be found by PCR of lung or regional lymph node for more than two weeks after primary infection.[37] Persistent antigen would thus need to take the form of either protein or peptide. One proposal is that protein persists on the surface of follicular dendritic cells (FDC),[38-40] whence it may be "picked off" by B cells expressing the appropriate surface Ig molecule. A possible consequence could be re-stimulation of CD4⁺ T cells following antigen processing and presentation of p+MHC-II on the B lymphocyte. There is evidence that, under some circumstances, soluble protein can be processed through the endogenous pathway leading to the expression of p+MHC-I complexes.[41] Both mechanisms would require that the FDC maintain protein on their surface for 1-2 years after a single episode of influenza infection.

Virus-immune CD8⁺ T cell memory in people

Humans also show evidence of $CD8^+$ T cell memory for the influenza A viruses,[42] the difference from mice being that people are regularly challenged (at least every 2-3 years) by i.n. infection with other influenza A viruses carrying cross-reactive p+MHC-I determinants. Resistance to severe influenza infection is directly correlated with the presence of $CD8^+$ memory T cells in peripheral blood. Loss of effective $CD8^+$ CTLp in the aged,[43,44] and absence of prior priming in the very young, may be the reason for the greater susceptibility of these two populations.

Adults, especially those with small children in day-care, will also be experiencing re-challenge with a variety of respiratory viruses (including paramyxoviruses) at not too distant intervals.[45] All of a panel of adults tested for evidence of $CD4^+$ or $CD8^+$ T cell memory to human parainfluenza virus type 1 (HPIV-1), the cause of croup in small children[45], were circulating $CD4^+$ and/or $CD8^+$ CTLp.[46] Epidemiological evidence indicates that (as with human influenza) prior exposure to HPIV-1 leads to less severe symptoms on natural challenge. However, re-infection with the same virus clearly occurs for this and other paramyxoviruses such as respiratory syncitial virus.

Continuing (or sporadic) re-challenge will also occur with the herpesvirus which characteristically establish latent or persistent infections.[47] *Herpes simplex* virus "hides" in sensory neurons in the trigeminal ganglion. The neurons remain constitutively class I and class II MHC^- and are not recognized by effector $CD4^+$ or $CD8^+$ T cells.[48] Damage to the lip (e.g., sunburn) is thought to cause virus to travel down the axon and instigate a "cold-sore", which will then provide a new antigenic stimulus leading (presumably) to both the development of effector CTL and the boosting of immune memory. Something similar is thought to occur in shingles, when declining immunity in the aged causes the emergence of *Herpes zoster* virus[49] that has presumably been latent in neurons since the individual had chicken-pox as a child. Epstein-Barr virus (EBV) establishes a latent infection in B lymphocytes, characterized by non-expression of the protein providing the peptide targeted by $CD8^+$ effector T cells.[50,51] Individuals that are heavily immunosuppressed may develop EBV-induced B cell lymphomas.

Whether virus-immune $CD8^+$ T cell memory will persist for life in humans without some form of re-stimulation is not clear. Immunization with live-attenuated measles virus again leads to long-term protection.[52] The consequence of subsequent natural challenge might be thought to be neutralization by antibody and antigen presentation only via the class II MHC pathway. This could explain why measles-specific $CD4^+$ CTLp seem to be more prominent than $CD8^+$ CTLp in primed individuals. However, can we really exclude the possibility that there may have been some undetected focus of re-infection in cells at a mucosal surface?

Perhaps the best evidence for long-term maintenance of human virus-specific $CD8^+$ T cell memory in the absence of re-challenge comes from urban northern USA residents who were given vaccinia virus[53] as children.

Such individuals have been shown to be circulating virus-specific CD8+ CTLp for more than 50 years (Demkowicz, W.E. Jr., et al, unpublished data). These were not laboratory workers, and so are unlikely to have been exposed again to vaccinia virus or to a potentially cross-reactive poxvirus.

THE RECALL RESPONSE: CHARACTERISTICS AND LIMITATIONS

Memory T cells, unlike circulating antibody, are not immediately available to deal with a secondary infection. Under in vivo conditions, it takes three to five days for memory CTLp to differentiate to the stage where they mediate effector function.[54,55] Earliest studies of recall in the virus-immune CD8+ T cell response were done with the murine influenza model, using mice that were primed and challenged with variants (e.g., H1N1→H3N2) that shared conserved nucleoprotein (NP) CTL epitopes but did not elicit cross-reactive neutralizing antibody. The inflammatory response in the respiratory tract of such mice is greater in magnitude, more rapid in onset and effector CTL can be found in the lung earlier. Evidence of virus clearance is detected by day 5 (rather than day 7 or day 8 in the primary response) and the mice survive challenge with 10-times the dose that causes lethal pneumonia in immunologically naive animals. The kinetics of cytokine gene expression in both the regional lymph node and lung are also enhanced following secondary challenge.[56]

The use of recombinant vaccinia viruses carrying genes coding for proteins that provide peptides recognized by CD8+ CTL has often been disappointing from the aspect of protection against respiratory infection,[57,58] though there have been encouraging results with a peptide vaccine[59] in the Sendai virus (murine PIV1) pneumonia model. Greater success has been achieved in, for instance, preventing fatal LCMV immunopathology[60,61] when an appropriate dose of challenge virus is used (Fig. 1). This may be telling us that the recall of CD8+ T cell memory is more effective in the operational sense for virus infections of solid tissues than for those at mucosal surfaces. However mice primed i.n. with an influenza A virus were only able to resist high-dose i.c. injection of a vaccinia virus-influenza NP construct at the stage that effector CTL were present, though in vivo re-stimulation of memory CTLp with influenza virus as little as eight hours before i.c. challenge was also protective.[62] This is another example of the fine-tuning of immunity that can determine the clinical outcome of the race between virus growth and host response, illustrated in a different context in Figure 1.

The normal situation in the primary response to Sendai virus or to an influenza A virus is that the CD8+ CTLp differentiate in the nurturing environment of the draining mediastinal lymph node (MLN) before exiting to the lung.[8,63] Massive stimulation via the clonotypic TCR as a consequence of encountering large numbers of virus-infected respiratory epithelial cells then induces the rapid development of CTL activity, with consequent virus clearance. A similar sequence of events (with more rapid kinetics) also occurs in the secondary response.[55] It is possible that the effectiveness of a proportion of the recirculating memory CTLp, which lack the lymph node homing receptor (L-selectin), may be minimized because they localize immediately to the site of inflammatory pathology rather than to the MLN. This might be advantageous if the lymphocytes are held in a circumscribed anatomical niche, such as the cerebrospinal fluid or liver tissue. However, T cells that have exited too soon into the lung lumen could potentially be moved on by protective physiological mechanisms (ciliary movement, mucus flow) before they become effectors. When thinking of immunization strategies to prevent (rather than clear) infection at mucosal barriers, it seems important to emphasize mechanisms that will promote the local availability of neutralizing antibody.[64,65]

MAINTENANCE OF CD8⁺ T CELL MEMORY

We know that naive and memory CD8⁺ T cells are phenotypically different (Table 1). Memory T cells are L-selectin-low: lack of expression of L-selectin on cell surface following in vitro stimulation reflects that the molecule is being cleaved at the cell surface as a consequence of a protein kinase C-dependant process.[66] Memory T cells are also easier to induce to effector function, requiring much less exogenous cytokine[6,67] in the culture medium. The key characteristics of virus-immune T cell memory seem to be the number of precursors is increased, generally at least 10-fold, the CTLps are in some sense "activated", the CTLps are not terminally differentiated. Also, sufficient contact with the appropriate p+MHC-I complex will drive such lymphocytes to become effector CTL. Many other important issues, such as the rate of lymphocyte turn-over[68] (if any), are currently open. How are these memory T cell populations maintained? Several possibilities are currently being considered.

PERSISTENT ANTIGEN

The strict antigenic-fundamentalists of immunology[2,12,36] believe that, as the stimulation of naive virus-specific CD8⁺ CTLp is driven by the interaction between the clonotypic TCR and the appropriate p+MHC-I complex, a comparable mechanism must also be involved in the maintenance of memory. The possibility of re-infection, or reactivation of latent virus obviously fulfills this criterion. However long-term T cell memory has been demonstrated in situations where virus challenge is unlikely and, at least for the murine influenza model, persistence of viral genome cannot be demonstrated (see "Duration", above). The underlying assumption would then have to be that sufficient peptide is being leached (at intervals?) into the class I MHC processing pathway to allow some degree of re-stimulation via the clonotypic TCR though not, perhaps, to the extent that the lymphocytes differentiate to be effector CTL. What is the evidence for this idea? Two contradictory interpretations are currently available, both derived from experiments with the LCMV model.

The analysis of Oehen et al[12] demonstrates quite clearly that the generation of LCMV-specific CD8⁺ CTLp is antigen-dose dependant. A "parking" experiment where memory spleen populations were injected into normal recipients showed that, unless these mice were further infected with LCMV, all evidence for the persistence of virus-specific CTLp quickly disappeared. Both sets of data are considered to support the idea that persistence of antigen is required to maintain T cell memory.

The contrary position has been taken by Ahmed and colleagues,[69] who have done careful "parking" experiments giving Thy1.1⁺ FACS-separated

LCMV-immune $CD8^+$ CTLp to irradiated, bone marrow-reconstituted $Thy1.2^+$ recipients. The donor cell populations were further checked by PCR to ensure that there was no carry-over of potentially reactivatable virus. Sequential LDA analysis has shown that the LCMV-specific CTLp are maintaining in the long-term, and even increasing in frequency, in the absence of further exposure to antigen.

We are in the process of repeating these studies for Sendai-virus-specific CTLp. The experiments are not yet complete. Transfer of $Thy1.1^+$ H-$2K^b$+Sendai virus NP-specific memory CTLp to lethally-irradiated (but non-thymectomized), bone marrow reconstituted $Thy1.2^+$ recipients leads to the long-term persistence of memory CTLp, at a very low frequency that has maintained for five months so far. The $Thy1.1^+$ CTLp can, however, be routinely demonstrated by bulk culture. Mice given a vaccinia virus-Sendai NP construct relatively soon after cell transfer showed greatly increased numbers of CTLp by day 8 after secondary challenge, which presumably reflects proliferation and an increase in clonal burst size. This interpretation is illustrated in Figure 2. Other parking experiments using thymectomized, irradiated normal and β2-microglobulin disrupted (β2-m, -/-) recipient mice[70] are also showing that the virus-specific CTLps persist in the absence of antigen, though the latest time point examined to date is 50 days.

The true test of the antigen-persistence model is to take $Thy1.2^+$ mice that are either normal or who have recovered from a primary virus infection,

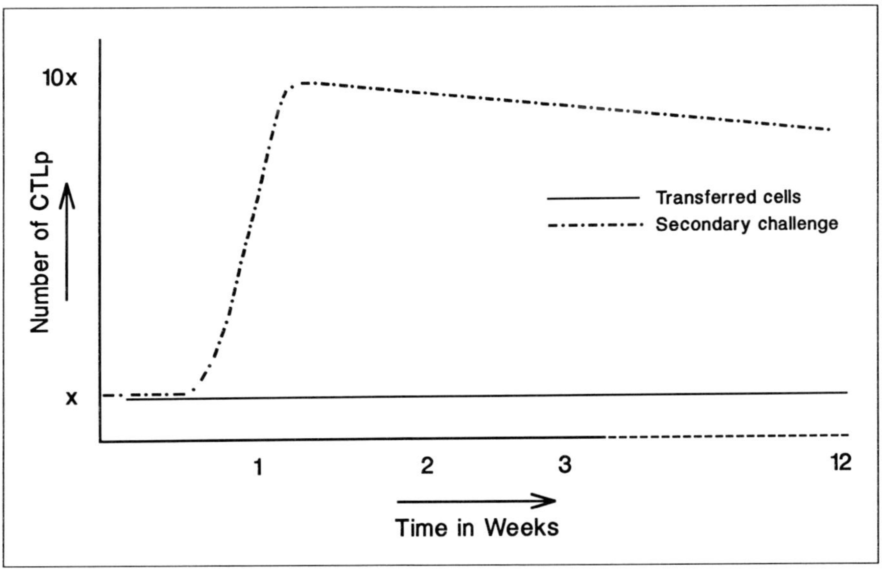

Fig. 2. This illustrates the experiment considered by some investigators to favor the idea that antigen persistence is required for the maintenance of T cell memory. Memory T cells are adoptively transferred into recipients that are, or are not, given another dose of antigen. Our analysis with the Sendai virus model indicates that secondary challenge causes acute proliferation and a greatly increased frequency of $CD8^+$ CTLp. This experiment has generally been misinterpreted, as it is inherently unable to distinguish between the consequences of increasing the clonal burst size and the possible contribution of antigen persistence. Memory $CD8^+$ CTLp are also maintained for several months, though at much lower frequency, in the recipients that are not given antigen.

deplete with an mAb to Thy1.2 (to provide "lebensraum") and then transfer Thy1.1$^+$ virus-immune CTLp. This should allow the postulated "pool" of persistent antigen to remain intact. We have just started this experiment.

Cross-reactive stimulation

Another clonotypic TCR-dependant strategy for maintaining T cell memory relies on the fact that memory CTLp are already partially "activated" and inducible with less "signal."[71] The idea is that low affinity TCR-mediated recognition of self or other non-self p+MHC-I will be sufficient to keep the memory T cells "ticking-over" without differentiating to be effectors. Our experiment where we have "parked" Sendai virus-specific CD8$^+$ CTLp in an antigen-free β2-m (-/-) environment should tell us whether cross-reactive recognition of p+MHC-I on professional antigen-presenting cells is required, though it will not exclude the possibilities that other T cells are able to fulfil this role or that p+MHC-IIs can function in this way for CD8$^+$ CTLp. The former tends to emphasize the role of self p+MHC-I and could lead into "network-type" arguments. Also, T cell-T cell recognition may result in "veto" effects rather than a re-enforcing stimulus.[72] The p+MHC-II possibility seems unlikely; the CD8-MHC-I interaction is considered to enhance the avidity of cell-cell contact,[73] which should be particularly important for low affinity TCR recognition.

Activated environments

The idea is that sporadic clonotypic TCR-independent exposure in cytokine-rich environments will help to maintain the "activated" phenotype of memory CD8$^+$ CTLp. Secondary lymphoid tissue is subject to regular antigenic challenge, resulting in massive, nonspecific recruitment of circulating T and B lymphocytes.[8,74,75] Memory T cells will not normally enter the lymph node by the L-selectin-dependant high endothelial venule route,[76] but they do traffic through lymph nodes via the afferent lymph[25] and are found also in the spleen.

The numbers of cells transcribing mRNA for a variety of cytokine genes (including IL-2 and IL-4) in the MLN of mice infected primarily (H3N2) or secondarily (H1N1) with influenza A viruses are considerably in excess of the expected frequencies for antigen-specific CD4$^+$ or CD8$^+$ CTLp.[56] The kinetics are enhanced following H1N1→H3N2 challenge, indicating that virus-specific memory T cells are being re-stimulated in this site. Thus, exposure to cytokines produced by both nonspecific (NK cells, macrophages) and specific (T cells, B cells) components of the host response may provide sufficient "signal(s)" to induce transcriptional activity in other lymphocytes that are in proximity but are not being directly engaged via their clonotypic TCR. One prediction of this model would be that CD4$^+$ T cells, which tend to produce more lymphokine,[77] help to maintain CD8$^+$ T cell memory by maximizing generalized "activation" in antigenically-stimulated lymphoid tissue.

Foci of inflammatory process and pathology also provide "activated environments".[74,78,79] Most of the CD8$^+$ T cells that can be lavaged from the lungs of mice with Sendai virus or influenza virus pneumonia are not specific for the inducing pathogen, and have a CD44-high, L-selectin-low phenotype.[8] Furthermore the CD8$^+$ set is consistently LFA-1-high, CD69-high (the characteristic of effector rather than memory T cells, Table 1) at the time that there is maximal cellular extravasation. There is clearly a great deal of "bystander" activation occurring in this and in other sites of virus-induced inflammatory pathology. A key question is whether such T cells can return to the recirculating pool (see "Mechanisms for Loss of $CD8^+$ T Cell Memory", below).

Constitutive differentiation

A minimalist version of the antigen-independent, "activated environment" model is that memory $CD8^+$ CTLp have differentiated to a state that allows long-term survival (and turn-over?) in the absence of signaling events other than those encountered under physiological conditions. However, lymphocytes are clearly not living in an "inert" milieu when there is little antigenic challenge. Recirculating T cells traffic, for instance, through normal bone marrow, which is a site of constant cytokine production for hemopoiesis.[80] Mature T cells are also found in the thymus where, again, dynamic processes are occurring.

Constitutive differentiation is, of course, a characteristic of tumors. However lymphomas tend to show "immature" phenotypes, and substantial genetic abnormalities.[81] Oncogenic change can happen with mature human T cells in Sezary syndrome, or following infection with HTLV-1, but both conditions are rare.[82,83] Bovine $CD4^+$ and $CD8^+$ T cells infected with the apicomplexan (like malaria) parasite, *Theileria parva,* assume a transformed phenotype and are the cause of the leukosis central to the wasting disease, East Coast Fever.[84] These parasitized T cells grow-out in tissue culture medium without any need for antigen or added lymphokine. Treatment of such cultures with a drug that kills the parasite, but is not directly cytotoxic for the lymphocyte, also leads to the death of the T cell as a consequence of eliminating the agent inducing the constitutive activation.[85] In general, the fact that it is necessary to provide antigen and/or lymphokine to maintain memory $CD8^+$ T cells under conditions of in vitro culture indicates that the lymphocytes are still subject to normal growth control mechanisms.

MECHANISMS FOR LOSS OF $CD8^+$ T CELL MEMORY

The profiles of cell-surface marker expression indicate, as discussed above (see "Activated Environments"), that memory T cells accumulate preferentially in sites of inflammatory process. We showed some years back that influenza-specific $CD8^+$ CTLps were at higher frequency in a vaccinia-virus-induced meningitis than in lymphoid tissue.[86] This analysis is currently being repeated for the viral pneumonia models. The obvious question is whether "bystander" memory CTLps that enter a focus of pathology are lost to the immune system or later return to the circulation and resume their surveillance function. Loss would seem a distinct possibility in the viral pneumonias, as the inflammatory exudate is (in the course of time) presumably "coughed-up".

A better understanding of the extent of CTLp proliferation following secondary challenge[87,88] also needs to be developed. At least some of the CTLp will be driven to effector CTL function which may, perhaps, represent a stage of terminal differentiation leading to apoptosis.[89] Are the numbers of memory CTLp increased concurrently, or is the potential pool of responders being drained? We do know that substantial clonal expansion, which translates into prolonged memory, occurs when limiting numbers of memory CTLps are adoptively-transferred into recipients that are then challenged with antigen. However, it is not clear that an analogous process operates when the frequency is high and the CTLp may not need to be expanded to achieve the numbers of effectors that are required to terminate the infectious process. Limited epidemiological evidence for human influenza indicates that secondary challenge is likely to increase CTLp frequency.

Experiments with the LCMV model have shown that naive mice given very high doses of some virus variants,[90,91] particularly those known to infect a small proportion of the $CD4^+$ subset,[92] develop a transient CTL response which is then "exhausted." The mice survive without showing evidence of severe immunopathology (Fig. 1). The idea is that there are simply too many virus-infected cells around for the available CTL which, due to persistent engagement via the clonotypic TCR, are driven to apoptotic cell death. However, cell transfer experiments with primed CTLp indicate that "immune exhaustion"[91] is not a factor for LCMV-specific memory $CD8^+$ CTLp.[93,94] Also, people persistently infected with HIV-1 circulate effector $CD8^+$ CTL for months or years.[95] How much the "immune exhaustion" idea can be generalized from the non-cytopathic LCMV model remains to be seen.[96] Lytic viruses generally kill their hosts if key elements of the immune response are suppressed though, at least for some viruses, there are alternatives to $CD8^+$ T cell-mediated clearance mechanisms.[97]

PERSPECTIVE

The definition of immunological memory must be that there is rigorous, quantifiable evidence of enhanced response following a prior encounter with the inducing antigen. Analysing protection against virus challenge is a very complicated way of addressing the basic problem, which may or may not provide a conceptually accessible measure of memory (Fig. 1). Rational in vivo dissection of the cellular and molecular basis of virus-immune $CD8^+$ T cell memory requires that we concentrate on CTLp frequencies, and on defining the functional status of the lymphocytes. Both approaches have been greatly facilitated by the availability of a range of mAbs to cell-surface markers. Questions such as the need (or otherwise) for antigen persistence should yield to rigorous, quantitative experimental analysis. Some key advances in understanding are likely to result from the rational use of transgenic mice with a monoclonal TCR phenotype, providing the un-primed T cells are truly representative of normal naive populations. However, it will still be important to factor in the range of affinity/avidity constraints, and the concurrent operation of other lymphocyte subsets that characterize normal immune responses. More attention needs to be given to the human situation, as people live so much longer than mice, though there is the difficulty that the antigenic history is generally obscure.

ACKNOWLEDGMENTS

Experiments mentioned from this laboratory were funded by USPHS grants AI29579, AI31596, CA21765, GM37759 and by the American Lebanese Syrian Associated Charities. We thank Dr. Francis A. Ennis for helpful discussion.

References

1. Yin XM, Vitetta ES. The lineage relationship between virgin and memory B cells. Int Immunol 1992; 4:691-698.
2. Gray D. Immunological memory. Annu Rev Immunol 1993; 11:49-77.
3. Bradley LM, Croft M, Swain SL. T-cell memory: New perspectives. Immunol Today 1993; 14:197-199.
4. Perlmutter RM, Levin SD, Appleby MW, et al. Regulation of lymphocyte function by protein phosphorylation. Annu Rev Immunol 1993; 11:451-499.
5. Fraser JD, Straus D, Weiss A. Signal transduction events leading to T-cell lymphokine gene expression. Immunol Today 1993; 14:357-362.
6. Tabi Z, Lynch F, Ceredig R, et al. Virus-specific memory T cells are Pgp-1+ and can be selectively activated with phorbol ester and calcium ionophore. Cell Immunol 1988; 113:268-277.
7. McFarland HI, Nahill SR, Maciaszek JW, et al. CD11b (Mac-1): A marker for CD8+ cytotoxic T cell activation and memory in virus infection. J Immunol 1992; 149:1326-1333.
8. Hou S, Doherty PC. Partitioning of responder CD8+ T cells in lymph node and lung of mice with Sendai virus pneumonia by LECAM-1 and CD45RB phenotype. J Immunol 1993; 150:5494-5500.
9. Pircher H, Burki K, Lang R, et al. Tolerance induction in double specific T-cell receptor transgenic mice varies with antigen. Nature 1989; 342:559-561.
10. Owen JA, Allouche M, Doherty PC. Limiting dilution analysis of the specificity of influenza-immune cytotoxic T cells. Cell Immunol 1982; 67:49-59.
11. Oehen S, Hengartner H, Zinkernagel RM. Vaccination for disease. Science 1991; 251:195-198.
12. Oehen S, Waldner H, Kündig TM et al. Antivirally protective cytotoxic T cell memory to lymphocytic choriomeningitis virus is governed by persisting antigen. J Exp Med 1992; 176:1273-1281.
13. Buchmeier MJ, Welsh RM, Dutko FJ et al. The virology and immunobiology of lymphocytic choriomeningitis virus infection. Adv Immunol 1980; 30:275-331.
14. Doherty PC, Zinkernagel RM. T-cell-mediated immunopathology in viral infections. Transplant Rev 1974; 19:89-120.
15. Baenziger J, Hengartner H, Zinkernagel RM, et al. Induction or prevention of immunopathological disease by cloned cytotoxic T cell lines specific for lymphocytic choriomeningitis virus. Eur J Immunol 1986; 16:387-393.
16. Allan JE, Doherty PC. Immune T cells can protect or induce fatal neurological disease in murine lymphocytic choriomeningitis. Cell Immunol 1985; 90:401-407.
17. Lynch F, Chaudhri G, Allan JE, et al. Expression of Pgp-1 (or Ly24) by subpopulations of mouse thymocytes and activated peripheral T lymphocytes. Eur J Immunol 1987; 17:137-140.
18. Ceredig R, Allan JE, Tabi Z, et al. Phenotypic analysis of the inflammatory exudate in murine lymphocytic choriomeningitis. J Exp Med 1987; 165:1539-1551.
19. Budd RC, Cerottini JC, Horvath C, et al. Distinction of virgin and memory T lymphocytes. Stable acquisition of the Pgp-1 glycoprotein concomitant with antigenic stimulation. J Immunol 1987; 138:3120-3129.
20. Budd RC, Cerottini JC, MacDonald HR. Phenotypic identification of memory cytolytic T lymphocytes in a subset of Lyt-2+ cells. J Immunol 1987; 138:1009-1013.
21. Green-Johnson JM, Wade AW, Szewczuk MR. Regional accumulation of Pgp-1+ memory cells in senescent mucosal immune system. Reg Immunol 1992; 4:175-185.

22. Lynch F, Ceredig R. Mouse strain variation in Ly-24 (Pgp-1) expression by peripheral T cells and thymocytes. Implications for T cell differentiation. Eur J Immunol 1989; 19:223-229.
23. Michie CA, McLean A, Alcock C, et al. Lifespan of human lymphocyte subsets defined by CD45 isoforms. Nature 1992; 360:264-265.
24. Beverley PC. Functional analysis of human T cell subsets defined by CD45 isoform expression. Semin Immunol 1992; 4:35-41.
25. Mackay CR, Marston WL, Dudler L. Naive and memory T cells show distinct pathways of lymphocyte recirculation. J Exp Med 1990; 171:801-817.
26. Mackay CR, Marston W, Dudler L. Altered patterns of T cell migration through lymph nodes and skin following antigen challenge. Eur J Immunol 1992; 22:2205-2210.
27. Sprent J. Lifespans of naive, memory and effector lymphocytes. Curr Opin Immunol 1993; 5:433-438.
28. Ada GL, Jones PD. The immune response to influenza infection. Curr Top Microbiol Immunol 1986; 128:1-54.
29. Kawaoka Y. Equine H7N7 influenza A viruses are highly pathogenic in mice without adaptation: potential use as an animal model. J Virol 1991; 65:3891-3894.
30. Kilbourne ED. Future influenza vaccines and the use of genetic recombinants. Bull World Health Organ 1969; 41:643-645.
31. Askonas BA, Mullbacher A, Ashman RB. Cytotoxic T-memory cells in virus infection and the specificity of helper T cells. Immunology 1982; 45:79-84.
32. Effros RB, Walford RL. The effect of age on the antigen-presenting mechanism in limiting dilution precursor cell frequency analysis. Cell Immunol 1984; 88:531-539.
33. Effros RB, Walford RL. Diminished T-cell response to influenza virus in aged mice. Immunology 1983; 49:387-392.
34. Bender BS, Johnson MP, Small PA. Influenza in senescent mice: impaired cytotoxic T lymphocyte activity is correlated with prolonged infection. Immunology 1991; 72:514-519.
35. Perillo NL, Naeim F, Walford RL, et al. The in vitro senescence of human T lymphocytes: failure to divide is not associated with a loss of cytolytic activity or memory T cell phenotype. Mech Ageing Dev 1993; 67:173-185.
36. Gray D, Matzinger P. T cell memory is short-lived in the absence of antigen. J Exp Med 1991; 174:969-974.
37. Eichelberger MC, Wang M, Allan W, et al. Influenza virus RNA in the lung and lymphoid tissue of immunologically intact and CD4-depleted mice. J Gen Virol 1991; 72:1695-1698.
38. Tew JG, Kosco MH, Burton GF, et al. Follicular dendritic cells as accessory cells. Immunol Rev 1990; 117:185-211.
39. Mandel TE, Phipps RP, Abbot A, et al. The follicular dendritic cell: long term antigen retention during immunity. Immunol Rev 1980; 53:29-59.
40. Van Rooijen N. Follicular dendritic cell-B cell interactions in virus disease. Common localization but different cell damage caused by antibody immobilized virus? Arch Virol 1992; 122:215-218.
41. Rayachaudhuri S, Morrow WJW. Can soluble antigens induce $CD8^+$ cytotoxic T cell responses? A paradox revisited. Immunol Today 1993; 14:344-348.
42. McMichael AJ, Gotch FM, Dongworth DW, et al. Declining T-cell immunity to influenza, 1977-82. Lancet 1983; 2:762-764.
43. Powers DC. Influenza A virus-specific cytotoxic T lymphocyte activity declines with advancing age. J Am Geriatr Soc 1993; 41:1-5.

44. Mbawuike IN, Lange AR, Couch RB. Diminished influenza A virus-specific MHC class I-restricted cytotoxic T lymphocyte activity among elderly persons. Viral Immunol 1993; 6:55-64.
45. Welliver RC, Ogra PL. Immunology of respiratory viral infections. Annu Rev Med 1988; 39:147-162.
46. Slobod KS, Allan J. Both $CD4^+$ and $CD8^+$ parainfluenza type 1 virus-specific cytotoxic T cell precursors recirculate in adults. Clin Exp Immunol 1993;93: 363-369.
47. Banks TA, Rouse BT. Herpesviruses-Immune escape artists. Clin Infect Dis 1992; 14:933-941.
48. Joly E, Mucke L, Oldstone MB. Viral persistence in neurons explained by lack of major histocompatibility class I expression. Science 1991; 253:1283-1285.
49. Sharp M, Terada K, Wilson A, et al: Kinetics and viral protein specificity of the cytotoxic T lymphocyte response in healthy adults immunized with live attenuated varicella vaccine. J Infect Dis 1992; 165:852-858.
50. Murray RJ, Kurilla MG, Brooks JM, et al. Identification of target antigens for the human cytotoxic T cell response to Epstein-Barr virus (EBV): implications for the immune control of EBV-positive malignancies. J Exp Med 1992; 176:157-168.
51. Moss DJ, Misko IS, Sculley TB, et al. Immune regulation of Epstein-Barr virus (EBV): EBV nuclear antigen as a target for EBV-specific T cell lysis. Springer Semin Immunopathol 1991; 13:147-156.
52. Dhib-Jalbut S, Jacobson S. Cytotoxic T cells in paramyxovirus infections of humans. Curr Top Microbiol Immunol 1993; in press.
53. Demkowicz WE, Jr., Ennis FA. Vaccinia virus-specific $CD8^+$ cytotoxic T lymphocytes in humans. J Virol 1993; 67:1538-1544.
54. Bennink J, Effros RB, Doherty PC: Influenza pneumonia: early appearance of cross-reactive T cells in lungs of mice primed with heterologous type A viruses. Immunology 1978; 35:503-509.
55. Allan W, Carding SR, Eichelberger M, et al. hsp65 $mRNA^+$ macrophages and gd T cells in influenza virus-infected mice depleted of the $CD4^+$ and $CD8^+$ lymphocyte subsets. Microb Pathog 1993; 14:75-84.
56. Carding SR, Allan W, McMickle A, et al: Activation of cytokine genes in T cells during primary and secondary murine influenza pneumonia. J Exp Med 1993; 177:475-482.
57. Andrew ME, Coupar BE, Boyle DB, et al. The roles of influenza virus haemagglutinin and nucleoprotein in protection: analysis using vaccinia virus recombinants. Scand J Immunol 1987; 25:21-28.
58. Connors M, Kulkarni AB, Collins PL, et al. Resistance to respiratory syncytial virus (RSV) challenge induced by infection with a vaccinia virus recombinant expressing the RSV M2 protein (Vac-M2) is mediated by $CD8^+$ T cells, while that induced by Vac-F or Vac-G recombinants is mediated by antibodies. J Virol 1992; 66:1277-1281.
59. Kast WM, Roux L, Curren J, et al. Protection against lethal Sendai virus infection by in vivo priming of virus-specific cytotoxic T lymphocytes with a free synthetic peptide. Proc Natl Acad Sci U S A 1991; 88:2283-2287.
60. Battegay M, Oehen S, Schulz M, et al. Vaccination with a synthetic peptide modulates lymphocytic choriomeningitis virus-mediated immunopathology. J Virol 1992; 66:1199-1201.
61. Klavinskis LS, Whitton JL, Oldstone MB: Molecularly engineered vaccine which expresses an immunodominant T- cell epitope induces cytotoxic T lymphocytes that confer protection from lethal virus infection. J Virol 1989; 63:4311-4316.

62. Doherty PC, Allan W, Boyle DB, et al. Recombinant vaccinia viruses and the development of immunization strategies using influenza virus. J Infect Dis 1989; 159:1119-1122.
63. Hou S, Doherty PC, Zijlstra M, et al. Delayed clearance of Sendai virus in mice lacking class I MHC-restricted CD8+ T cells. J Immunol 1992; 149:1319-1325.
64. Mazanec MB, Kaetzel CS, Lamm ME, et al. Intracellular neutralization of virus by immunoglobulin A antibodies. Proc Natl Acad Sci USA 1992; 89:6901-6905.
65. Mbawuike IN, Wyde PR, Anderson RR. Enhancement of the protective efficacy of inactivated influenza A virus vaccine in aged mice by IL-2 liposomes. Vaccine 1990; 8:347-352.
66. Jung TM, Dailey MO: Rapid modulation of homing receptors (gp90MEL-14) induced by activators of protein kinase C. Receptor shedding due to accelerated proteolytic cleavage at the cell surface. J Immunol 1990; 144:3130-3136.
67. Kos FJ, Mullbacher A. IL-2-independent activity of IL-7 in the generation of secondary antigen-specific cytotoxic T cell responses in vitro. J Immunol 1993; 150:387-393.
68. Freitas AA, Rocha BB. Lymphocyte lifespans: homeostasis, selection and competition. Immunol Today 1993; 14:25-29.
69. Ahmed R. Immunological memory against viruses. Semin Immunol 1992; 4:105-109.
70. Zijlstra M, Bix M, Simister NE, et al. Beta 2-microglobulin deficient mice lack CD4-8+ cytolytic T cells. Nature 1990; 344:742-746.
71. Beverley PC. Is T-cell memory maintained by crossreactive stimulation? Immunol Today 1990; 11:203-205.
72. Fink PJ, Shimonkevitz RP, Bevan MJ. Veto cells. Annu Rev Immunol 1988; 6:115-137.
73. Tanabe M, Karaki S, Takiguchi M, et al. Antigen recognition by the T cell receptor is enhanced by CD8 alpha-chain binding to the alpha 3 domain of MHC class I molecules, not by signaling via the cytoplasmic domain of CD8 alpha. Int Immunol 1992; 4:147-152.
74. Doherty PC, Allan JE, Lynch F, et al. Dissection of an inflammatory process induced by CD8+ T cells. Immunol Today 1990; 11:55-59.
75. Allan W, Tabi Z, Cleary A, et al: Cellular events in the lymph node and lung of mice with influenza. Consequences of depleting CD4+ T cells. J Immunol 1990; 144:3980-3986.
76. Butcher EC: Cellular and molecular mechanisms that direct leukocyte traffic. Am J Pathol 1990; 136:3-11.
77. Kelso A. Cytokines: structure, function and synthesis. Curr Opin Immunol 1989; 2:215-225.
78. Nahill SR, Welsh RM. High frequency of cross-reactive cytotoxic T lymphocytes elicited during the virus-induced polyclonal cytotoxic T lymphocyte response. J Exp Med 1993; 177:317-327.
79. Sarawar SR, Carding, SR, Allan W et al. Cytokine profiles of bronchoalveolar lavage cells from mice with influenza pneumonia: consequences of CD4+ and CD8+ T cell depletion. Regional Immunology 1993; 5:142-150.
80. Tew JG, DiLosa M, Burton GF, et al. Germinal centers and antibody production in bone marrow. Immunol Rev 1992; 126:99-112.
81. Rabbitts TH. Translocations, master genes, and differences between the origins of acute and chronic leukemias. Cell 1991; 67:641-644.

82. Kono DH, Baccala R, Balderas RS, et al. Application of a multiprobe RNase protection assay and junctional sequences to define V beta gene diversity in Sezary syndrome. Am J Pathol 1992; 140:823-830.
83. Srivastava BI, Banki K, Perl A. Human T-cell leukemia virus type I or a related retrovirus in patients with mycosis fungoides/Sezary syndrome and Kaposi's sarcoma. Cancer Res 1992; 52:4391-4395.
84. Morrison WI, Goddeeris BM. Cytotoxic T cells in immunity to Theileria parva in cattle. Curr Top Microbiol Immunol 1990; 155:79-93.
85. Ole-MoiYoi OK. Theileria parva: an intracellular protozoan parasite that induces reversible lymphocyte transformation. Exp Parasitol 1989; 69:204-210.
86. Hurwitz JL, Korngold R, Doherty PC. Specific and nonspecific T-cell recruitment in viral meningitis: possible implications for autoimmunity. Cell Immunol 1983; 76:397-401.
87. Allan JE, Doherty PC. Consequences of cyclophosphamide treatment in murine lymphocytic choriomeningitis: evidence for cytotoxic T cell replication in vivo. Scand J Immunol 1985; 22:367-374.
88. Rouse BT, Hartley D, Doherty PC. Consequences of exposure to ionizing radiation for effector T cell function in vivo. Viral Immunol 1989; 2:69-78.
89. Kabelitz D, Pohl T, Pechold K. Activation-induced cell death (apoptosis) of mature peripheral T lymphocytes. Immunol Today 1993; 14:338-339.
90. Doherty PC, Zinkernagel RM, Ramshaw IA. Specificity and development of cytotoxic thymus-derived lymphocytes in lymphocytic choriomeningitis. J Immunol 1974; 112:1548-1552.
91. Moskophidis D, Lechner F, Pircher H, et al. Virus persistence in acutely infected immunocompetent mice by exhaustion of antiviral cytotoxic effector T cells. Nature 1993;362:758-761.
92. Ahmed R, King CC, Oldstone MB. Virus-lymphocyte interaction: T cells of the helper subset are infected with lymphocytic choriomeningitis virus during persistent infection in vivo. J Virol 1987; 61:1571-1576.
93. Jamieson BD, Butler LD, Ahmed R. Effective clearance of a persistent viral infection requires cooperation between virus-specific Lyt2⁺ T cells and nonspecific bone marrow-derived cells. J Virol 1987;61:3930-3937.
94. Oldstone MB, Blount P, Southern PJ, et al. Cytoimmunotherapy for persistent virus infection reveals a unique clearance pattern from the central nervous system. Nature 1986; 321:239-243.
95. Rowland-Jones S, McMichael A. Cytotoxic T lymphocytes in HIV infection. Semin Virol 1993; 4:83-94.
96. Doherty PC. Immune exhaustion: driving virus-immune CD8⁺ T cells to death. Trends Microbiol 1993; 1:207-209.
97. Doherty PC. Virus infections in mice with targeted gene disruptions. Curr Opin Immunol 1993; 5:479-483.

CHAPTER 5

Role of CD8⁺ Cytotoxic T Cells in Viral Infections

Hikmat Hayder
Robert Blanden

In viral infections, the virus is usually cleared from host tissues as a result of the concerted efforts of several cells of the immune system. The original observation that T lymphocytes play a major role in limiting viral infections[1] was followed by the discovery of major histocompatibility (MHC) restriction of T lymphocytes.[2] Cytotoxic T lymphocytes (Tc or CTL) from lymphocytic choriomeningitis virus (LCMV)-infected mice were shown to kill target cells in a virus-specific and MHC-restricted manner, and the MHC molecules involved in Tc responses were identified as MHC class I molecules.[3] Since these seminal discoveries, there has been considerable investigation of the role of Tc cells in host defence mechanisms against viral infections.

Influenza virus has proved to be particularly useful in the detailed analysis of Tc response in vivo and in vitro.[4] Initially, it was assumed that Tc cells recognized viral proteins inserted into the host cell membrane. However, Tc cells against serologically distinguishable influenza virus subtypes, were highly cross-reactive. The antigens recognized by influenza cross-reactive Tc cell clones were identified as non-membrane-associated proteins.[5] Further, it was also shown that Tc cells recognized transfectants that express fragments of influenza virus nucleoprotein, and that different mouse strains responded to different regions of nucleoprotein.[6] These experiments clarified the nature of the antigen recognized by Tc cells. Target antigens were identified as complexes of viral peptide and MHC class I molecule.[7]

Antigen binding by Tc cells is accomplished by a heterodimeric structure, the T cell receptor, composed of disulfide-linked α and β chains. Both chains are clonally variable and assemble via gene rearrangement during T cell differentiation. Tc cells express the surface molecule CD8 which is usually required as a co-receptor, binding to a conserved region of the

Strategies in Vaccine Design, edited by Gordon L. Ada, D.Sc.

MHC class I heavy chain. A Class I MHC molecule consists of two non-covalently bound chains, the heavy chain with two polymorphic domains and β2 microglobulin, a conserved light chain. In the endoplasmic reticulum (ER), both chains assemble with a peptide into a stable complex which is then transported to the cell surface.

Peptides are generated from proteins in the cytosol, possibly by a protease complex with MHC-encoded subunits, known as a proteasome. The peptides are then thought to be transported into the lumen of the ER by ATP-dependent MHC-encoded peptide transporters (TAP) located in the ER membrane.[8,9] Physical association of peptides with MHC class I molecules was visualized by X-ray crystallography. In these images the peptide could be seen bound in the groove made up of a β-pleated sheet floor and two walls formed by α helices of the two membrane distal polymorphic domains of the heavy chain.[10] Naturally processed viral peptides were isolated from influenza virus and vesicular stomatitis virus-infected murine tumor cells by reversed-phase high performance liquid chromatography (HPLC). Sequencing of these peptides has revealed a usual length of eight or nine amino acids and a characteristic allele-specific motif involving at least two amino acids which represents the minimal requirement for binding of peptides by a particular MHC class I molecule.[11]

Most exogenous antigens enter the endosomal pathway and are presented by MHC class II but not class I molecules. However, there have been reports of stimulating Tc cell responses in vivo using viral proteins, and non-infectious bacteria and protozoa.[12] The conditions under which such antigens can also be presented by class I MHC are not yet fully defined. Structural and chemical properties of the antigen affect the way in which it interacts with antigen-presenting cells (APC) and influence its presentation by MHC molecules.[13]

In addition to the antiviral activity of MHC class I-restricted CD8$^+$ Tc cells; it is likely that they are involved in regulating the class of immune response.[14] However, once generated effector Tc cells can control viral infections by lysis of infected cells, provided this occurs before assembly of progeny virions and by secretion of cytokines which mediate various antiviral mechanisms.[15-18] The extent to which direct cytolytic activity and cytokines released by CD8$^+$ Tc cells contribute to resolving viral infections may vary among viruses. The fact that MHC class I molecules are expressed on almost all cells, gives Tc cells the powerful potential to contribute to clearance of various viral infections. On the other hand, under certain circumstances, Tc cells can also be harmful to the host. The pathology associated with LCMV infection in mice, where the virus is noncytopathic, is caused by the Tc response rather than the virus.[19]

Tc CELL GENERATION AND ROLE OF ANTIGEN-PRESENTING CELLS

A number of questions arise concerning requirements for the initial induction of virus-specific Tc cells in vivo and their migration around the body. For example, where does the first encounter between the precursor Tc cells and the antigen take place? What type of APC is required for the induction of Tc cells? How do effector Tc cells migrate to the site of infection? What are the mechanisms involved in downregulation of the Tc response after virus clearance? What are the characteristics of memory Tc cells and the requirements for induction and maintenance of memory? What are the roles of $CD4^+$ helper T cells in $CD8^+$ Tc cell responses? The answers to these questions are incomplete and may vary with different virus-host combinations.

Recent findings point to regional lymph nodes as the site of primary immune response in mice infected with influenza virus intranasally.[20] In this example, the cellularity of the mediastinal lymph nodes is massively increased within the first two days of virus infection. Because the virus does not replicate productively in the lymph nodes, it is believed that antigen-loaded APC entering the afferent lymph from respiratory tissues are involved in the primary exposure of Tc cells to antigen. Dendritic cells (DC) are specialized cells with abundant cell surface MHC molecules as well as the B7 molecule required for naive Tc cell induction.[21] The characteristic clustering of naive T cells around DC probably provides the environment in which the Tc cell response is initiated. It is also speculated that effector Tc cells may be involved in removal of the antigen-presenting DC in the lymphoid tissue as a downregulation mechanism for the Tc cell response,[21] as could be inferred from class I MHC-restricted negative feedback effects on Tc responses caused by effector Tc cell injection into ectromelia-infected mice.[22]

Whether other types of APC are able to initiate virus-specific response in vivo is unclear. In vitro experiments with alloantigens suggest that the APC function for induction of naive Tc cells is dependent on DC with little or no contribution from macrophages.[23] DC infected in vitro or in vivo with influenza virus and cultured with T cells from lymph nodes of normal specific pathogen-free mice resulted in the generation of influenza-specific effector Tc cells.[24] When peritoneal exudate macrophages infected with influenza virus were used as APC, no primary Tc cell response was induced. However, both influenza-infected macrophages and DC were capable of inducing a secondary Tc cell response in spleen T cells from influenza virus-primed mice. The role of different cytokines in Tc cell induction in vivo has not been fully elucidated yet. However, primary influenza virus-specific Tc cells were induced by stimulation of mouse spleen cells with a synthetic peptide derived from nucleoprotein in the presence of interleukin-7.[25]

Evidence from experimental systems using other viral and non-viral antigens also indicates that DCs are the principal APC for primary Tc cell induction.[26] DCs are believed to be non-phagocytic since the endocytic tracer colloidal carbon, when injected intravenously into mice, is cleared exclusively by cells identified in situ as phagocytic macrophages and not by DC.[27] Therefore, the ability of DC to acquire peptides for MHC class I presentation in cases where the antigen is non-infectious seems to be limited.[28] On the other hand there is evidence that DCs entering the afferent lymph from the tissues contain large amounts of antigen.[21] When the soluble hen egg lysozyme was coupled to beads, DCs did not ingest the beads but nonetheless processed the protein for presentation.[29] In addition, peptide fragments were detected in the supernatant after incubation of the intact protein with DCs but not macrophages or B cell blasts. A potent Tc cell response against ovalbumin was achieved by using DCs incubated with intact protein packaged in pH-sensitive liposomes.[30]

TARGET CELL LYSIS BY Tc CELLS

Available evidence points to at least two major mechanisms for target cell killing by MHC class I-restricted T cells.[31,32] The first involves the exocytosis of perforin-containing granules by activated Tc cells. In the second mechanism, Tc cells trigger programmed cell death (apoptosis) in target cells possibly by surface molecule signaling.

PERFORIN-MEDIATED CELL LYSIS

Cytoplasmic granules, which are usually observed in Tc cells at the site of contact with target cells, have been isolated and shown to contain calcium-dependent cytolytic activity.[33] These lytic granules contain a pore-forming protein, perforin, which causes complement-like lesions on target cells. Purified perforin lyses various target cells in a calcium-dependent fashion. Perforin binds to phosphorylcholine moieties on target cell membranes and polymerizes after insertion into the lipid bilayer. Polymerized perforin appears as tubular inserts in target cell membranes. Because there does not seem to be binding specificity for perforin, it is possible that membrane lesions can occur in effector cells as well as targets with implications for the life span of activated effector Tc cells. In addition to causing membrane lesions, perforin may also be involved in DNA fragmentation of target cells.[33] Serine proteases contained in Tc cell granules have been implicated in DNA fragmentation. Granzyme A binds to nuclear proteins suggesting a mechanism for exposing the DNA to endogenous nucleases.[34]

A link between acquisition of cytocidal activity and perforin expression was demonstrated. Perforin anti-sense oligonucleotides partially inhibited the cytotoxic effect of activated Tc cells.[35] Direct evidence for the role of perforin in Tc cell antiviral effector function came from perforin-knock out mice[36] which do not express the perforin protein and fail to clear LCMV infection. These mice showed no defects in lymphocyte migration, lymphokine secretion by Tc cells, and MHC class II-disparate allograft rejection. These observations argue strongly for an essential role of perforin-mediated target cell killing via cell-to-cell contact in control of LCMV infection. Tc cells secrete lymphokines including IFN-γ which exerts pleiotropic effects, such as activation of macrophages and natural killer cells and upregulation of MHC expression. However, the normal levels of lymphokines produced in perforin knock-out mice are clearly not sufficient for achieving clearance of LCMV infection. It will be of great interest to infect perforin knock-out mice with a variety of other viral and non-viral pathogens.

Target cell lysis by Tc cells in vivo has also been inferred recently from experiments with LCMV.[37] An internal virus protein, nucleoprotein, appeared in the sera of LCMV-infected mice immediately after $CD8^+$ Tc cell transfer and was not present in the sera of mice depleted of $CD8^+$ T cells. Normally, viral nucleoprotein released in vivo by Tc cells is bound and masked by anti-nucleoprotein antibodies in the serum. However, depletion of $CD4^+$ T cells in these mice prevented generation of antibodies and allowed detection of nucleoprotein. Since LCMV is not cytopathic and does not cause cell lysis, the nucleoprotein appeared to be released in vivo as a result of lysis of infected cells by Tc cells.

Granule-independent target cell lysis

Because target cell lysis caused by Tc cells has been observed under conditions where calcium-dependent perforin/granule exocytosis does not occur, at least one other mechanism of cytotoxicity clearly exists. Cell surface molecules are likely to be involved in triggering apoptosis in target cells. Apoptosis is characterized by cell shrinkage, nuclear collapse and cleavage of chromatin into nucleosomal fragments.[38] Fas is a cell transmembrane member of the tumor necrosis factor receptor family. Experiments with mice carrying a mutation in the Fas protein led to the conclusion that Fas was involved in transduction of a cytotoxic signal.[39] Fas-linked mechanisms probably account for most calcium-independent cytotoxicity while calcium-dependent target cell lysis does not appear to require Fas. Perforin-mediated cell lysis and DNA fragmentation appear to be independent since inhibition of DNA fragmentation does not inhibit membrane lysis. DNA fragmentation, a hallmark of apoptosis, occurs within minutes of Tc cell encounter with target cells,[32] suggesting that de novo protein synthesis may not be required in killing all target cell types.

Why are there two mechanisms for target cell destruction? Although direct evidence for increased susceptibility of apoptotic cells to membrane lysis is lacking, it has been suggested that extensive DNA fragmentation, by preventing complete DNA repair, allows rapid and effective cell lysis.[38] Viral DNA may also be fragmented in Tc cell-mediated apoptosis as has been shown for polyomavirus.[38] This may ensure that infectious viral DNA is not released after lysis of target cells and may reduce the risk of cell transformation by certain viruses.

TYPES OF VACCINES

Prevention of infectious diseases through vaccination represents the ultimate goal in global efforts to control such diseases. A number of approaches, some more successful than others, have been attempted.[40] Although there are general principles that determine vaccine efficacy, such as the strength and duration of protection, ease of delivery and safety of the vaccine, there are requirements unique to each vaccine. These depend largely on characteristics of the virus and the type of immune response which can protect against the virus. Types of vaccines are discussed in relation to Tc cell responses.

Live attenuated virus vaccines

Historically, live attenuated virus vaccines have been the most successful in controlling human and animal virus infections. These include vaccinia (which achieved the unique feat of eliminating smallpox), polio, mumps, measles, rubella, and yellow fever. This type of vaccine has the advantage of resembling a natural infection resulting in the induction of appropriate classes of immune response. Virus proteins synthesized endogenously by infected host cells stimulate Tc cell responses. Attenuated viruses still allow sufficient virus replication to provide a large pool of proteins, including non-structural proteins, as a source of peptides suited for binding various MHC types. One potential hazard of live virus vaccine is reversion of the attenuated vaccine strain to the wild type, virulent virus. Also, the vaccine itself may cause disease which may lead to serious complications especially in immunocompromized individuals.

The process of virus attenuation is not fully understood and many attempts to generate attenuated strains, which are immunologically effective, have failed. Also the risks associated with introducing some live viruses may be judged to outweigh the advantages. The limited shelf life of some live viruses is another disadvantage; the special storage and transportation requirements of live virus vaccines may not be available in some parts of the world.

Whole, inactivated virus vaccines

Another example of successful vaccination has been achieved through the use of heat-inactivated or formaldehyde-inactivated viruses. The main advantage of this type of vaccine is that the risk of reversion to virulent virus does not exist. Because Tc cell responses are generated against peptides derived from cytosolic proteins (often non-structural viral proteins), killed viral vaccines may not induce strong Tc cell responses. Incorporation of inactivated viruses into agents that ensure delivery of the antigens to the cytosol can enable induction of Tc cell responses to these vaccines, but only to structural viral proteins. Another disadvantage of killed virus vaccines is a requirement for optimization of dose of virus and multidose regimens, since the inoculum will not replicate in the host.

Subunit vaccines

Technical advances in the last decade have provided the tools for identifying viral proteins which can stimulate a protective immune response. Synthetic peptides spanning such identified regions have been used for immunization. These subunit vaccines have some advantages such as stability and safety for use even in immunocompromized hosts. However, the limited diversity of antigen may fail to protect all individuals in outbred populations. The phenomenon of non-responder inbred mouse strains, though more acutely evident than in heterozygous or outbred populations, is related to the ability of a given peptide to bind to a particular MHC molecule and to immunoregulation associated with self tolerance.[41] This will ultimately affect the efficacy of peptide-based vaccines in human populations. In addition, studies with animal models showed the need for immunological adjuvants in combination with peptides to induce a strong immune response. Another problem with peptide vaccines may be even more fundamental. In vivo injection of a peptide from LCMV led to an initial proliferation of peptide-specific Tc cells followed by a decline to undetectable levels.[42] This was in contrast to the efficient induction of effector and memory Tc cells after infection with live LCMV. Furthermore, the reduced number of Tc cells in peptide-immunized mice was shown to be due to the death of these peptide-specific cells. Similarly, in vivo administration of MHC class I-specific peptides from influenza virus induces specific Tc cell hyporesponsiveness.[43]

Recently, immunization with a soluble fragment made of 272 amino acids of the large tumor antigen of simian virus 40 (SV40) without adjuvants was shown to prime mouse Tc cells.[44] This peptide appears to be capable of entering the cytosol and being processed in the endogenous pathway which requires peptide transport from the cytosol to the lumen of the ER. RMA-S cells, which are transport-defective were not able to present this antigen. Analysis of this protein revealed hydrophobic moieties and the ability to bind palmitic acid tightly. These characteristics presumably promote fusion of the protein with plasma membranes of APC allowing entry to the cytosol.[44] Priming of Tc cells was also obtained in experiments using APC pulsed with chicken egg ovalbumin (OVA) linked with beads but not with soluble OVA.[45] Such experiments indicate alternative mechanisms for entry to the class I processing pathway.

The requirement for $CD4^+$ MHC class II-restricted T helper (Th) cells for Tc cell response has been studied in model systems where animals were depleted of the Th cell subset or by using animals where disruption of the CD4 gene prevents Th cell development. In general, the results of these experiments indicate the ability of these animals to develop an effective Tc cell response in absence of Th cells.[46,47] Recently however, evidence emerged suggesting that such Tc cell response is limited in duration leading to the eventual loss of Tc cells generated in absence of Th cells.[48] These Tc cells can be rescued from deletion by restimulation in the presence of Th cells. It will be interesting to see if these findings apply generally to antiviral Tc cell responses and effects on memory Tc cell induction and persistence.

Although the humoral response against viruses has been considered separately from the Tc cell response, Tc cells may be required for optimal humoral responses. Recently, it was shown that an absence of influenza virus-specific Tc cells in β2-microglobulin-deficient mice resulted in a 10-fold lower antibody response than in presence of these cells.[49] These results may reflect the important role of lymphokines produced by Tc cells or the ability of Tc cells to provide viral antigens, by lysing target cells, for generating antibodies. Therefore inclusion of Tc epitopes should be considered even when the vaccine is intended to induce a humoral response.

Live Recombinant Vectors

Due to the success of vaccinia virus in stimulating a powerful protective immune response, responsible for the eradication of smallpox, many recombinant vaccinia vectors encoding one or more proteins of other viruses have been produced and investigated. These experiments have provided an enormous amount of information on the role of different viral proteins in immunity. This was particularly useful for generating Tc cell responses, and identifying sources of Tc cell determinants in a wide range of viruses.

The fundamental observation that viral internal antigens can be recognized by Tc cells was made using a vaccinia vector.[50] The level of expression of genes varies depending on the promoter used. Viral proteins expressed from the early-late 7.5K vaccinia promoter were successfully recognized by Tc cells whereas proteins controlled by a late promoter were not.[51] Although substantial amounts of protein were expressed using the late promoter, vaccinia-encoded serine proteinase inhibitors (serpins) may prevent antigen processing and generation of immunogenic peptides. Proteins expressed from the late promoter may not be immunodominant as they have to compete with more peptides. Such proteins are available after the shut down of host cell protein synthesis which results in limiting the supply of MHC molecules. Because of potential hazards associated with vaccinia virus, modifications of the virus are needed to ensure the safety of vaccines. One novel approach is to include various cytokine genes in the recombinant genome resulting in attenuation of the virus.[52] However, this approach has not been successful in enhancing Tc cell activity.[53]

The avian-specific poxviruses, fowlpox and canarypox, are currently being evaluated as recombinant vaccine vectors.[54] These viruses do not replicate productively in non-avian species and function as a vehicle for introducing the foreign genes efficiently into the host cells. The results obtained from these vaccines are encouraging.

Adenovirus, which causes a mild respiratory infection in humans, is an attractive vaccine vector candidate. The unattenuated vaccine is administered orally and may provide protection at mucosal surfaces.[54] The inability of human adenoviruses to infect monkey cells prevents primate trials, however some adenovirus mutants have been adapted to growth in monkey cells. Adenovirus replicates in the nucleus of infected cells and therefore transcripts of virus genes may be modified in a way that interferes with generation of protective determinants. However, constructs expressing simian immunodeficiency virus (SIV) gene products were properly processed.[55] Bacterial vectors are also potential candidates for virus vaccines.[56] Studies on the relationships between these vectors and the type of immunity they induce in the host will be necessary for determining their suitability for future vaccines.

Naked DNA vaccines

The recently reported success in expressing foreign DNA injected into host tissue is currently held as a promising approach to vaccination. Influenza virus nucleoprotein, cloned into expression plasmid DNA, was injected intramuscularly into mice.[57] These mice developed a Tc cell response which appeared to protect them from a lethal challenge with a serologically unrelated influenza virus. Even though the plasmid DNA does not replicate and does not appear to require integration into the host genome, transcription and translation of the plasmid DNA occurs. The cytosolic location of the synthesized proteins allows efficient presentation by class I MHC molecules. Viral proteins expressed in this way also have the advantage of providing a wide selection of peptide determinants to associate with different MHC class I molecules. A detailed analysis of the mechanism involved in the induction of the immune responses after naked DNA injection is required before rational evaluation of its future vaccine potential can be undertaken.

THE USE OF ADJUVANTS IN VACCINES

An inherent difficulty with non-infectious virus vaccines is their poor immunogenicity, often requiring the use of adjuvants, which are compounds able to enhance the immune response. In humans, aluminum hydroxides and phosphates, often referred to as alum, have been used. However, alum is not active with all antigens and mostly stimulates antibody responses. New adjuvants are needed that are safe for clinical use and that can help achieve the appropriate type of response to each vaccine. The biological properties of the adjuvant are responsible for influencing the antigen uptake by particular APC and contribute to the induction of particular classes of immunity. This topic has been analyzed by comparing alum and Freund's complete adjuvant (FCA), in mice. FCA, which consists of a water-in-oil emulsion containing killed mycobacteria, stimulated mostly T helper cells involved in delayed-type hypersensitivity (Th1), while alum stimulated T cells of the type associated with antibody response (Th2).[58]

In general, adjuvants can be divided into three groups depending on their source: vegetal, chemical or bacterial. Saponin, in the presence of cholesterol, forms distinct structures called immunostimulating complexes (ISCOMs). ISCOMs have been used to stimulate immune responses to many antigens including Tc cell responses to noninfectious antigens.[59] The ability of ISCOMs to introduce antigens into the cytosol for class I MHC presentation can be explained by the intercalation of saponin into cholesterol membranes.[58]

Another approach to introduce antigens into the cytoplasm involves the use of lipid tails. A synthetic peptide of influenza virus nucleoprotein covalently linked to a lipid (tripalmitoyl-S-glyceryl cysteinyl-seryl-serine (P3CSS) efficiently primed influenza virus-specific Tc cells in vivo.[60] The ability of the lipopeptide to induce high affinity Tc cells is in contrast to the response obtained from immunization with peptide alone. Although lipopeptides appear to be successful in stimulating Tc cells, the general problem of peptide selectivity in outbred populations must be taken into account. Using multipeptides linked to lipid may overcome this problem and provide universal vaccine candidates.

DETERMINANT SELECTION FOR Tc CELLS

In virus-infected cells, immunogenic peptides can be derived from any viral protein synthesized inside the cell regardless of its function. Some viral proteins are produced in large enough quantities and early during the infection to provide peptides dominantly represented as Tc determinants. In adenovirus-infected cells, two early proteins E1 and E2 have been shown to contain immunodominant Tc cell determinants in association with H-2K^k and H-2D^b MHC class I molecules in mice.[61]

Nucleoproteins of many viruses appear to contain immunodominant determinants for Tc cells. In contrast to the diversity of a given viral envelope protein in viruses such as influenza and HIV, most internal proteins are conserved. Combined knowledge of conserved virus protein sequences and MHC class I allele-specific motifs, as predicted from naturally processed peptides, may allow rational design of vaccines containing multiple determinants for outbred populations. Many peptides have been identified from HIV gag, env and pol protein sequences as Tc cell determinants.[62]

VIRUS STRATEGIES TO EVADE TC CELL RESPONSE

Antigen recognition by Tc cells involves binding of the T cell receptor to a complex of a class I MHC molecule and an antigenic peptide. A number of viruses have evolved mechanisms which allow them to avoid induction of, or escape detection by, Tc cells by interfering with the interaction of these components. These mechanisms fall under four strategies:
(i) downregulation of cell surface expression of MHC class I molecules,
(ii) downregulation of viral proteins containing T cell determinants,
(iii) inhibition of peptide generation,
(iv) emergence of virus antigenic variants non-reactive to existing Tc responses.

Interference with MHC molecules can be achieved by decreasing transcription or translation of MHC class I mRNA. Another mechanism involves viral proteins which interfere with class I MHC assembly or transport to the cell surface. Adenovirus E3 19-kDa protein binds in allele-specific fashion to newly synthesized class I MHC molecules and retains them in the ER. The E3-gene product(s) also appears to downregulate E1A, the viral protein from which Tc cell determinants are generated.[63] Human cytomegalovirus (HCMV) genome encodes a protein that can bind to β2 microglobulin and may prevent assembly of MHC class I.[64]

Emergence of Tc cell-evading antigenic variants during a viral infection has been reported.[65] Mutations in viral genes coding for Tc cell determinants may modify the peptide determinant directly or interfere with antigen processing and, thus allowing virus-infected cells to evade Tc cells. Tc cell-driven variant selection, unlike antibody-driven selection, is relevant only in the context of the individual's MHC. However, such a mechanism could play a role in establishing virus persistence in the infected host.

MEMORY TC RESPONSE

At the heart of vaccine efficacy is the ability to generate memory cells which can mediate strong secondary responses. Two important features which determine the strength of immunological memory Tc are the frequency and the persistence of antigen-reactive memory cells. Following infection with influenza virus, mice develop a life-long ability to recall enhanced, anti-influenza Tc cell responses. The frequency of influenza virus-reactive Tc precursor cells increases 30-fold within one week after priming.[20] The influenza virus genome was not detectable in these mice after the primary infection was cleared; thus, continuing viral protein synthesis was not necessary to maintain memory Tc cells. The possibility that proteins or peptides may be sequestered in host tissu o maintain a cytosolic depot for processing in the class I MHC pathway was directly addressed in adoptive transfer experiments.[66] T cells from influenza virus-primed or -unprimed mice were transferred to irradiated hosts which had been previously infected with influenza or to uninfected mice. After 4-25 weeks these recipients were challenged with a heterologous influenza virus. The kinetics of Tc cell responses of splenocytes from mice that received memory Tc cells was typical of a secondary response regardless of whether that recipient had been infected previously or not, thus demonstrating that Tc memory to influenza virus was maintained in the absence of antigen. In an experimental system which measured the capacity of secondary Tc responses to protect against lethal challenge with LCMV, it was found that priming with LCMV induced Tc memory which protected mice against a lethal challenge 14 weeks after priming.[67] Mice primed with recombinant vaccinia virus expressing LCMV proteins, however, were not protected against a lethal challenge but 80% of the primed mice survived a lower challenge dose of LCMV. These results suggest that properties of the priming virus may influence the strength and duration of Tc memory.

The heterogeneity of pathogenesis of viral diseases and the MHC differences between individuals in outbred human populations is a challenge to vaccine development directed at achieving consistent T cell responses.

However, increased insight into patterns of cellular interactions in the immune system and technological advances in the fields of immunology and virology should have a positive effect on our future approach to vaccines. In most viral infections Tc cell responses are beneficial to the host. Specific requirements for inducing effective and durable Tc cell responses against viruses, such as the nature of vaccine, dose, and route of vaccination need to be defined more clearly.

REFERENCES

1. Blanden RV. T cell response to viral and bacterial infection. Transplant Rev 1974; 19:56-88.
2. Zinkernagel RM and Doherty PC. H-2 compatibility requirement for T-cell mediated lysis of target cells infected with lymphocytic choriomeningitis virus. J Exp Med 1975; 141:1427-36.
3. Blanden RV, Doherty PC, Dunlop MBC et al. Genes required for cytotoxicity against virus infected target cells in K and D regions of H-2 complex. Nature 1975; 254:269-70.
4. Ada GL, Leung KN, and Ertl H. An analysis of effector T cell generation and function in mice exposed to influenza A or Sendai viruses. Immunol Rev 1981; 58:5-24.
5. Townsend ARM, McMichael AJ, Carter NP et al. Cytotoxic T cell recognition of the influenza nucleoprotein and hemagglutinin expressed in transfected mouse L cells. Cell 1984; 39:13-25.
6. Townsend ARM, Gotch FM and Davey J. Cytotoxic T cells recognize fragments of influenza nucleoprotein. Cell 1985; 42:457-67.
7. Townsend ARM., Rothbard J, Gotch FM et al. The epitopes of influenza nucleoprotein recognized by cytotoxic T lymphocytes can be defined with short synthetic peptides. Cell 1986; 44:959-68.
8. Heemels M-T. and Ploegh H. Untapped peptides. Curr Biol 1993; 3: 380-3.
9. Howard JC and Seeling A. Peptides and the proteasome. Nature 1993; 365:211-67.
10. Bjorkman PJ, Saper MA, Samraoui B et al. Structure of the human class I histocompatibility antigen, HLA-A2. Nature 1987; 329:506-12.
11. Rotzchke O and Falk K. Naturally occurring peptide antigens derived from the MHC class I-restricted processing pathway. Immunol. Today 1991; 12:447-55.
12. Raychaudhuri S and Morrow WJW. Can soluble antigens induce CD8+ cytotoxic T-cell responses? A paradox revisited. Immunol. Today 1993; 14:344-7.
13. Scott P and Kaufmann HE. The role of T cell subsets and cytokines in the regulation of infection. Immunol Today 1991; 12:346-48.
14. Bretscher PA. The regulatory functions of CD4+ and CD8+ T-cell subsets in immune class regulation. Res Immunol 1991; 142:45-50.
15. Glasgow LA. Cellular immunity in host resistance to viral infections. Arch Intern Med 1970; 126:125-34.
16. Blanden RV. Mechanism of recovery from a generalized viral infection: mouse pox. II Passive transfer of recovery mechanism with immune lymphoid cells. J Exp Med 1971; 133:1074-89.
17. Blanden RV. Mechanism of recovery from a generalized viral infection: mouse pox. III. Regression of infectious foci. J Exp Med 1971; 133:1090-104.
18. Ramsay A, Ruby J and Ramshaw I. A case for cytokines as effectors in the resolution of virus infection. Immunol Today 1993; 14:155-7.

19. Doherty PC and Zinkernagel RM. T-cell mediated immunopathology in viral infection. Transplant Rev 1974; 19:89-120.
20. Doherty PC, Allan W and Eichelberger M. Roles of αβ and γδ T cell subsets in viral immunity. Ann Rev Immunol 1992; 10:123-50.
21. Knight SC, and Staff AJ. Antigen-presenting cell types. Cur Opin Immunol 1993; 5:374-82.
22. Pang T and Blanden RV. Regulation of the T-cell response to ectromelia virus infection. I. Feedback suppression by effector T cells. J Exp Med 1976; 143:469-81.
23. Inaba K, Young JW and Steinman RM. Direct activation of $CD8^+$ cytotoxic T lymphocytes by dendritic cells. J Exp Med 1987; 166:182-94.
24. Macatonia SE, Taylor PM, Knight, SC, and Askonas, BA. Primary stimulation by dendritic cells induces antiviral proliferative and cytotoxic T cell response in vitro. J Exp Med 1989; 169:1255-64.
25. Kos F and Müllbacher A. Induction of primary anti-viral cytotoxic T cells by in vitro stimulation with a short synthetic peptide and interleukin-7. Eur J Immunol 1992; 22:3183-5.
26. Crowley M, Inaba K and Steinman RM. Dendritic cells are the principal cells in mouse spleen bearing immunogenic fragments of foreign proteins. J Exp Med 1990; 172:383-6.
27. Witmer-Pack MD, Crowley MT, Inaba K and Steinman RM. Macrophages, but not dendritic cells, accumulate colloidal carbon following administration in situ. J Cell Sciences 1993; 105:965-73.
28. Nonacs R, Humborg C, Tam JP, and Steinman RM. Mechanisms of mouse spleen dendritic cell function in the generation of influenza-specific cytotoxic T lymphocytes. J Exp Med 1992; 176:519-29.
29. De Bruijn MLH, Nieland JD, Harding CV and Melief CJM. Processing and presentation of intact hen egg lysozyme by dendritic cells. Eur J Immunol1992; 22:2347-52.
30. Nair S, Zhou F, Reddy R, Huang L and Rouse BT. Soluble proteins delivered to dendritic cells via pH-sensitive liposomes induce primary cytotoxic T lymphocyte response in vitro. J Exp Med 1992; 175:609-12.
31. Berke G. T-cell-mediated cytotoxicity. Curr Opin Immunol 1991; 3:320-25.
32. Taylor MK and Cohen JJ. Cell-mediated cytotoxicity. Curr Opin Immunol 1992; 4:338-43.
33. Tschopp J and Nabholz M. Perforin-mediated target cell lysis by cytolytic T lymphocytes. Annu Rev Immunol 1990; 8:279-302.
34. Apasov S, Redegeld F and Sitkovsky M. Cell-mediated cytotoxicity: contact and secreted factors. Curr Opin Immunol 1993; 5:404-10.
35. Acha-Orbea H, Scarpellino L, Hertig S et al. Inhibition of lymphocyte mediated cytotoxicity by perforin antisense oligenucleotides. EMBOJ 1990; 9:3815-9.
36. Kägi D, Ledermann B, Bürki K et al. Function of CD8 positive T lymphocytes and NK cells in perforin deficient mice (Abstract). EMBO Workshop on cell-mediated cytotoxicity, Weizmann Institute of Science, 29 August-1 September; 1993.
37. Kyburz D, Speiser DE, Battegay et al. Lysis of infected cells in vivo by antiviral cytolytic T cells demonstrated by release of cell internal viral proteins. Eur J Immunol 1993; 23:1540-5.
38. Cohen JJ, and Duke RC. Apoptosis and programmed cell death in immunity. Annu Rev Immunol 1992; 10:267-93.
39. Rouvier E, Luciani M-F and Goldstein P. Fas involvement in Ca^{2+}-independent T cell-mediated cytotoxicity. J Exp Med 1993; 177:195-200.

40. Ada, GL. Vaccines. In: Paul WE, ed. Fundamental Immunology. 2nd ed. New York: Raven, 1989: 985-1032.
41. Müllbacher A, Blanden RV and Brenan M. Neonatal tolerance of major histocompatibility complex antigens alters Ir gene control of the cytotoxic T cell response to vaccinia virus. J Exp Med 1983; 157:1324-38.
42. Kyburz D, Aichele P, Spieser DE et al. T cell immunity after a viral infection versus T cell tolerance induced by soluble viral peptides. Eur J Immunol 1993; 23:1956-62.
43. Müllbacher A, and Tha Hla R. In vivo administration of major histocompatibility complex class I-specific peptides from influenza virus induced specific cytotoxic T cell hyporesponsiveness. Eur J Immunol 1993; (in press).
44. Schirmbeck R, Zerrahn J, Kuhröber A et al. Immunisation of mice with the N-terminal (1-272) fragment of simian virus 40 large T antigen (without adjuvants) specifically primes cytotoxic T lymphocytes. Eur J Immunol 1993; 23:1528-34.
45. Kovacsovics-Bankowski M, Clark K, Benacerraf B and Rock KL. Efficient major histocompatibility complex class I presentation of exogenous antigen upon phagocytosis by macrophages. Proc Natl Acad Sci 1993; 90:4942-6.
46. Liu Y and Müllbacher A. The generation and activation of memory class I MHC-restricted cytotoxic T cell responses to influenza A virus in vivo do not require CD4+T cells. Immunol Cell Biol 1989; 67:413-20.
47. Rahemtulla A, Fung-Leung WP, Schilham MW et al. Normal development and function of CD8+ cells but markedly decreased helper cell activity in mice lacking CD4. Nature 1991: 353:180-4.
48. Kirberg J, Bruno L, and von Boehmer H. CD^{4+8-} help prevents rapid deletion of CD8+ cells after transient response to antigen. Eur J Immunol 1993; 23:1963-7.
49. Epstein SL, Misplon JA, Lawson CM et al. β2-microglobulin-deficient mice can be protected against influenza A infection by vaccination with vaccinia-influenza recombinants expressing hemagglutinin and neuraminidase. J Immunol 1993; 150:5484-93.
50. Yewdell JW, Bennink JR, Smith GL. and Moss B. Influenza virus nucleoprotein is a major target antigen for cross-reactive anti-influenza A cytotoxic T lymphocytes. Proc Nat Acad Sci 1988; 82: 1785-89.
51. Coupar BEH Andrew ME, Both GW and Boyle DB. Temporal regulation of influenza hemagglutinin expression in vaccinia. Eur J Immunol 1986; 16:1479-87.
52. Ramshaw IA, Andrew ME, Phillips SM et al. Recovey of immunodefficient mice from a vaccinia virus/ IL2 recombinant infection. Nature 1987; 329:545-6.
53. Müllbacher A, Ramshaw IA and Coupar BEH. Vaccinia-interleukin 2 recombinant virus or exogenous interleukin 2 does not alter the magnitude or immune response gene defects of the cytotoxic T cell response to vaccinia virus in vivo. Scan J Immunol 1989; 29:1-6.
54. Connell N, Stever CK, and Jacobs WR. Old microbes with new faces: molecular biology and the design of new vaccines. Curr Opin Immunol 1992; 4:442-8.
55. Cheng S-M, Lee S-G, Ronchetti-Blume, M et al. Robust expression of the SIV envelope protein by a recombinant human adenovirus host-range mutant. In: Vaccines New York: Cold Spring Harbour Laboratory,1991:145-50.
56. Schödel F. Prospects for oral vaccination using recombinant bacteria expressing viral epitopes. Adv Virus Res 1992; 41:409-26.
57. Ulmer JB, Donnelly JJ, Parker SE et al. Heterologous protection against influenza by injection of DNA encoding a viral protein. Science 1993; 259:1745-9.

58. Audibert FM and Lise LD. Adjuvants: current status, clinical perspectives and future prospects. TiPs. 1993; 14:174-8.
59. Takahashi J, Takeshita T, Morein B et al. Induction of CD8+ cytotoxic T cells by immunization with purified HIV-1 envelope protein in ISCOMs. Nature 1990; 344:873-5.
60. Deres K, Schild H, Wiesmüller, KH et al. In vivo priming of virus-specific cytotoxic T lymphocytes with synthetic lipopeptide vaccine. Nature 1989; 342: 561-4.
61. Müllbacher A, Bellett AJD, and Tha Hla RT. The murine cellular immune response to adenovirus type 5. Immunol Cell Biol 1989; 67:31-9.
62. Nixon DF, Broliden K, Ogg G, Broliden P-A. Cellular and humoral antigenic epitopes in HIV and SIV. Immunol 1992; 76:515-34.
63. Müllbacher A. Viral escape from immune recognition:multiple strategies of adenovirus. Immunol Cell Biol 1992; 70:59-63.
64. Grundy JE, Mckeating JA and Griffiths PD. Cytomegalovirus strain AD169 binds β2 microglobulin in vitro after release from cells. J Gen Virol 1982; 68:777-84.
65. Pircher H, Moskophidis D, Rohrer U et al. Viral escape by selection of cytotoxic T-cell-resistant virus variants in vivo. Nature 1990; 346:629-33.
66. Müllbacher A. The long term maintenance of cytotoxic T cell memory does not require persistence of antigen. J Exp Med 1993 (in press).
67. Oehen S, Waldner J, Kündig TM. Antivirally protective cytotoxic T cell memory to lymphocytic choriomeningitis virus is governed by persisting antigen. J Exp Med 1993; 176:1273-81.

CHAPTER 6

The Contribution of CD8⁺ Cytolytic T Cells to the Control of Bacterial and Parasitic Infections

Jörg Arnoldi
Stefan H. E. Kaufmann

INTRODUCTION

Intracellular pathogens such as *Mycobacterium tuberculosis*/*M. bovis*, *M. leprae*, *Salmonella typhi*/*S. paratyphi*, *Listeria monocytogenes*, *Leishmania sp.*, *Plasmodium sp.*, *Toxoplasma sp.* and *Trypanosoma cruzi* are responsible for some of the most prevalent infectious diseases globally. Tuberculosis, for example, afflicts 10 million people and causes 3 million cases of death annually. A common reason for the pathogenicity of these microbes is their permanent intracellular living in host cells which reduces their extracellular stages almost completely. Although a wide variety of host cells is invaded by these pathogens, mononuclear phagocytes (MP) are preferentially infected. Resistance to phagocytosis and killing by macrophages enables these parasites to multiply in a kind of "trojan horse", in which they are effectively protected from humoral defense mechanisms. As a corollary, these pathogens tend to cause chronic infections which may last for years. Because intracellular pathogens avoid direct contact with antibodies, their elimination requires recognition of infected host cells. Focus on infected host cells rather than on the pathogen per se frequently accounts for T cell mediated pathology. Parasite antigens which are presented by infected host cells in the context of gene products of the major histocompatibility complex (MHC) are detected by distinct T lymphocyte subsets. Depending on the type of

Strategies in Vaccine Design, edited by Gordon L. Ada, D.Sc.

pathogen, the relative contribution of these T cell subsets to protection or pathogenesis may vary. In this review, emphasis is laid upon the role of $CD8^+$ α/β T cells and their cytolytic potential in defense against intracellular bacteria and protozoa. By doing so we do not exclude participation of other T cell populations—particularly $CD4^+$ T cells—and of other functions primarily MP activation via interferon-γ (IFN -γ) secretion—in immunity against intracellular pathogens.

T CELL SUBSETS IN IMMUNITY AGAINST INTRACELLULAR PATHOGENS

Postthymic T cells segregate into three distinct subsets according to their use of T cell-receptors (TCR) and accessory molecules which interact with MHC gene products on target cells. The major population of T cells expresses an α/β TCR and either the CD4 or the CD8 molecule in a mutually exclusive way. Adoptive transfer experiments have shown that both $CD4^+$ and $CD8^+$ T cells contribute to protection against numerous intracellular pathogens.[1] A second, minor T cell population expresses a different TCR composed of a γ– and a δ-chain. These γ/δ T cells rarely express the CD4 or the CD8 molecule and hence are generally double-negative.

$CD4^+$ T cells recognize antigenic peptides in the context of MHC class II molecules which are constitutively expressed on the surface of a restricted cell population including MP and B cells. These $CD4^+$ T cells further segregate into functionally distinct T helper 1 (Th1) cells and T helper 2 (Th2) cells. The former ones produce IL-2 and IFN-γ and frequently express cytolytic activities while the latter ones secrete IL-4, IL-5, IL-6, and IL-10 and are rarely cytolytic. Different effector functions of these two T cell subsets also determine their relative contribution to antimicrobial defense.[2,3]

$CD8^+$ T cells are characterized by their cytolytic activity and the secretion of IFN-γ. They recognize antigenic peptides in the context of MHC class I molecules which are constitutively expressed by almost all nucleated cells with the notable exception of terminally differentiated neurons. This feature enables $CD8^+$ T cells to survey almost all cells which may be abused by intracellular bacteria or protozoa. As to be discussed in this review, numerous experimental animal systems have demonstrated an important contribution of $CD8^+$ T cells to the induction and regulation of antimicrobial protection. Although in humans, indications for $CD8^+$ T cells in resistance against intracellular bacteria and protozoa are less convincing, their importance is most likely.[4-6]

γ/δ T cells represent a minor fraction among T cells in lymphoid organs and blood of man and mouse. However, they make up a significant proportion among the intraepithelial lymphocytes (IEL) in mucosal tissue sites such as lung and gut. Interestingly, a high proportion of these intraepithelial γ/δ T cells express the CD8 molecule on their surface. Since many pathogens enter their hosts through mucosal tissues, γ/δ T cells may provide an early line of defense.[1] After appropriate activation, they secrete IFN-γ and develop strong cytolytic activities which are generally MHC-nonrestricted. Although it has been demonstrated that γ/δ T cells are induced by components of many intracellular bacteria and protozoa, recent studies indicate an accessory rather than an effector role of γ/δ T cells in antimicrobial immunity.[7,8]

ANTIGEN PRESENTATION TO CD8 T CELLS

Protein antigens of intracellular pathogens including cell wall antigens and secreted proteins are strong inducers of T cell responses. To induce T cells these proteins have to be processed and presented by their host cells in an MHC restricted manner (Fig. 1). Cells which have no nucleus are MHC class I and class II negative and cannot become positive. These are erythrocytes which are the target cells for malaria at certain parasite stages. Thus, these cells are not seen by $CD4^+$ nor by $CD8^+$ T cells. However, they are phagocytosed by liver macrophages and then parasite antigens may be presented.

Antigen association with MHC class I structures (HLA-A, B, C in man, H-2K, D, L in mice) is normally focused to endogenous proteins which are newly synthesized by the cell. Proteins are degraded into peptides, transported into the endoplasmic reticulum, bound to MHC class I molecules and translocated to the cell membrane. Using this classical MHC class I pathway, virus-infected cells are recognized by $CD8^+$ cytolytic T cells and destroyed. In contrast, antigens which are taken up via endocytosis are termed exogenous antigens and are primarily presented through the endosomal MHC class II restricted way. Nevertheless, several situations have been discovered where exogenous antigens are presented by MHC class I molecules. Using specific cytolysins, particularly listeriolysin, *L. monocytogenes* evades from the endosome into the cytoplasm.[9] Consequently, proteins which are secreted by *L. monocytogenes* in the cytosol are introduced into the endogenous pathway of antigen processing and presentation by MHC class I gene products.[10,11] Similarly, recent studies suggest that

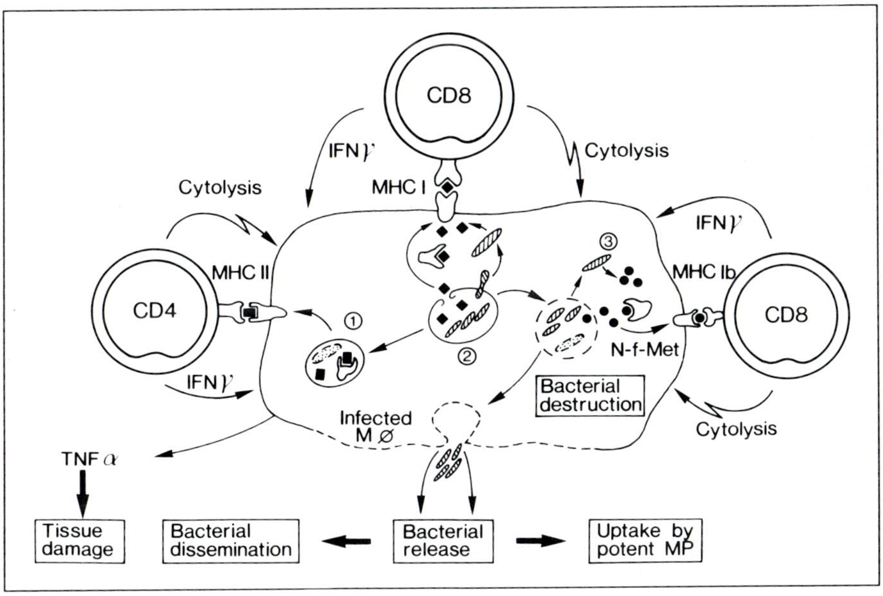

Fig. 1. Possible consequences of T cell–macrophage interactions in infections with intracellular pathogens. Inside the host cell, different ways of antigen processing and antigen presentation proceed: 1. MHC class II restricted endosomal pathway. 2. MHC class I restricted cytosolic pathway. 3. alternative MHC class Ib restricted pathway for N-f-Met peptides.

virulent *M. tuberculosis* strains produce cytolysins which are capable of lysing cellular membranes and thus promote evasion into the cytoplasm.[12] Another mechanism was recently demonstrated in *T. gondii* infection. After fusion of the parasite membrane and the vacuolar membrane of the host cell, a major surface antigen, p30, of *T. gondii* is able to enter the cytoplasm. This antigen was shown to be introduced into the cytosolic MHC class I restricted pathway.[13] Introduction into the cytosolic way may be one important but not exclusive mechanism of MHC class I antigen presentation of microbial proteins. Even in case of intracellular bacteria such as *M. bovis* and *S. typhimurium* which remain in the endosome and mainly contact the MHC class II pathway, antigenic peptides are also presented by MHC class I molecules.[14] This enables $CD8^+$ T cells to recognize cells, invaded by these pathogens. In this case peptide translocation from the endosome into the cytoplasm, perhaps by specific transporter systems, may be involved.[15] Some antigens of *L. major*, normally residing in the phagolysosome, seem to be introduced into the MHC class I pathway by similar mechanisms which results in the activation of specific $CD8^+$ T cells.

Besides this classical MHC class I pathway, a second intracellular processing mechanism from the endosome to the endoplasmic reticulum has been described recently.[16] It is likely that this type of antigen-presentation is not restricted by conventional MHC class I molecules but rather involves a conserved MHC class Ib gene product. These nonclassical, nonpolymorphic MHC products present N-formylated-peptides.[17] Since the N-f-Met sequence provides a signal for protein secretion in bacteria, MHC class Ib molecules may be specialized for presentation of secreted bacterial polypeptides.

FUNCTIONS OF CD8 T CELLS

Many intracellular pathogens such as *L. monocytogenes*, *M.leprae* and *P. falciparum* are not restricted to macrophages but preferentially invade nonprofessional phagocytes, e.g., hepatocytes which are primarily MHC class II negative (Table 1). These cells lack potent antimicrobial effector mechanisms and represent a niche which promotes parasite survival. MHC class I restricted $CD8^+$ T cells may provide an important mechanism for combating intracellular pathogens by identifying infected MHC class II negative host cells and mobilizing appropriate effector functions.

Cytolysis. Receptor-mediated killing of infected MHC class II positive or negative cells seem to be a major task of $CD8^+$ T cells in infectious diseases.[18] Target cell killing involves different mechanisms by which pores are inserted into cell membranes causing circular lesions in the surface of target cells. To achieve this task, cytolytic T cells contain numerous electron-dense secretory granules in their cytoplasm which are secreted by exocytosis and release perforins into the intracellular space after receptor-mediated cell-cell binding.[19] In addition, $CD8^+$ T cells are capable of inducing cell necrosis by secretion of TNF-β. Finally, $CD8^+$ T cells can cause apoptosis in infected cells. After contact with $CD8^+$ T cells, target cells undergo shrinkage, the nucleus collapses, the cromatin is cleaved into nucleosomal fragments and the DNA is fragmented. Subsequently, these apoptotic cells are disposed of by MP without releasing their pathogenic load.[20] Recent evidence suggests that MHC class I antigens are involved in T cell induced signal transduction in target cells, leading to apoptosis.[21]

Table 1. Major facultative and obligate intracellular bacteria and protozoa

Pathogen	Disease	Preferred target cell	Survival strategies of the pathogen	Comments
Mycobacterium tuberculosis	Tuberculosis	Macrophages	Inhibition of phagosome-lysosome fusion, interference with ROI, evasion into cytoplasm (?)	Preferentially affects the lung
Mycobacterium bovis	Tuberculosis (rare)	Macrophages	Inhibition of phagosome-lysosome fusion, interference with ROI	Preferentially affects the lung BCG as attenuated vaccine strain
Mycobacterium leprae	Leprosy	Macrophages, Schwann cells and many other cells	Interference with ROI, evasion into cytoplasm(?), infection of nonprofessional phagocytes	Preferentially affects skin and nerves
Listeria monocytogenes	Listeriosis	Macrophages, hepatocytes	Evasion into cytoplasm, infection of nonprofessional phagocytes	Rare in humans; widely used as experimental mouse model
Salmonella typhi/S.paratyphi	Typhoid	Macrophages	Inhibition of phagosome-lysosome fusion, interference with ROI	Preferred entry through the gut
Plasmodium sp.	Malaria	Hepatocytes, erythrocytes	Infection of MHC^- erythrocytes and of nonprofessional phagocytes	Preferentially affects spleen, liver and erythrocytes,
Leishmania sp.	Leishmaniosis	Macrophages	Interference with ROI, resistance to lysosomal enzymes	Preferentially affects skin
Toxoplasma gondii	Toxoplasmosis	Macrophages	Encapsulation by necrotic tissue wall, inhibition of parasitophorous vacuole-lysosome fusion	Rapidly multiplying tachyzoites affect liver and brain, slowly multiplying bradyzoites persist in tissue cysts in brain and muscles

IFN-γ. The main effector cells in defense against intracellular parasites are MPs which upon appropriate activation produce reactive radicals including oxygen and nitrogen intermediates which are toxic for most microbial pathogens. For this purpose, MPs have to be activated by cytokines, in particular IFN-γ. In vitro activation of murine MP by IFN-γ induces growth inhibition of *M. tuberculosis* and killing of most other intracellular pathogens.[22] IFN-γ is produced by $CD4^+$ T cells, $CD8^+$ T cells, γ/δ T cells and natural killer cells. Recent studies have shown upregulation of MHC class I expression in the infected host by IFN-γ from $CD8^+$ T cells.[23] Certain MHC class II negative cells, like Schwann cells become MHC class II positive after IFN-γ treatment and are then accessible to $CD4^+$ T cell-mediated effector mechanisms.[24]

IN VIVO STUDIES

Animal models. The relative contribution of $CD8^+$ T cells to acquired resistance against intracellular pathogens has been analyzed in two ways: first by adoptive transfer of antigen-specific $CD8^+$ T cells from infected donor mice and second by in vivo elimination of $CD8^+$ T cells by treatment with monoclonal antibodies (mAb). More recently, "knock out" mice in which defined genes had been deleted have been employed for this type of analysis.

Role of CD8 T Cells In Vivo

In murine listeriosis, these approaches have revealed a dominant role for $CD8^+$ T cells with some contribution by $CD4^+$ T cells and γ/δ T cells.[25-27] Adoptive transfer of anti-listerial resistance by $CD8^+$ T cells can be enhanced by simultaneous administration of recombinant IL-2 which seems to be an important factor in the development and activation of $CD8^+$ T cells.[28,29]

In contrast, *M. bovis BCG* and *S. typhimurium* only induce low $CD8^+$ T cell responses while depletion of $CD4^+$ T cells causes dramatic increases in bacterial numbers. In contrast, depletion of $CD8^+$ T cells has only small effects on the course of infection.[2] Reasons for the preferential induction of strong $CD4^+$ T cell responses may be (i) these pathogens remain within the endosomal compartment of their host cells and (ii) that MPs are able to kill their invaders effectively.

Resistance of mice against tuberculosis equally depends on $CD4^+$ T cells and $CD8^+$ T cells.[30,31] Tubercle bacilli only reside in MHC class II positive macrophages and are highly resistant to intracellular killing. Therefore, both activation and cytolysis are required which can be best afforded by $CD4^+$ and $CD8^+$ T cells.[32] The strong dependence on $CD8^+$ T cells in antituberculous protection, therefore, needs to be analyzed in more detail.

In order to characterize the role of T cell subsets in protective immunity to *Leishmania sp.*, susceptible Balb/c mice were depleted of either $CD4^+$ or $CD8^+$ T cells. Not only $CD4^+$ but also $CD8^+$ T cell-depleted mice were highly susceptible to infection, indicating that $CD8^+$ T cells at least partly contribute to efficient control of parasitemia. Th1 and Th2 $CD4^+$ T cells which secrete different cytokines and represent the main effector cells in primary infection, may either suppress or activate $CD8^+$ T cell-mediated anti-leishmanial immunity.[33,34] $CD8^+$ T cell depletion enhanced disease in resistant and susceptible mice as assessed by lesion size and, more importantly, abrogated the induction of resistance to reinfection.[35,36] Taken together, these findings demonstrate the importance of $CD8^+$ T cells in immunity against leishmania parasites.[37-39] In murine toxoplasmosis, treatment with anti $CD8^+$ mAb enhanced cyst formation in resistant and susceptible mouse strains, indicating $CD8^+$ T cell regulation of pathologic tissue reactions against *Toxoplasma sp.*[40] Although there is a substantial role for both the $CD4^+$ and $CD8^+$ T cell subset in resistance against this pathogen, $CD8^+$ T cells appear to be the major mediators of protective immunity against toxoplasmosis.[41] Adoptive transfer experiments, using cytolytic $CD8^+$ T cell clones from mice immunized with *Plasmodium sp.* sporozoites, demonstrate the importance of $CD8^+$ T cells in immunity against this stage of malaria.[42] In the liver stage the recognition and elimination of infected hepatocytes depends on MHC class I restricted $CD8^+$ cytolytic T cells.[43] In contrast, protective immunity against blood stage malaria primarily depends on $CD4^+$ Th1 and Th2 cells. Thus, the dominance of $CD8^+$ T cells or $CD4^+$ T cells varies depending on the stage of disease.

More recently mutant mice have been generated by homologous genetic recombination in which the beta2-microglobulin (β2m) gene, as part of the MHC class I complex had been deleted.[44,45] These mice lack functional $CD8^+$ α/β T cells and therefore are a valuable model for studying the role of $CD8^+$ T cells in vivo. These mice were found to be extremely susceptible to *L. monocytogenes* and *M. tuberculosis* infection.[46,47] The β2m-deficient mice also suffer slightly from infection with *M. bovis BCG* (unpublished). In experimental murine tuberculosis, susceptibility is histologically manifested by the development of multiple caseous liquefied lesions.[47] In listeriosis formation of lesions in the liver is delayed (Arnoldi et al., unpublished). These findings suggest a role for $CD8^+$ T cells in granuloma formation both in tuberculosis and listeriosis and substantiate the central role of MHC class I dependent mechanisms in murine listeriosis and tuberculosis and the minor contribution of these mechanisms in murine *M. bovis BCG* infection. Similarly, β2m-deficient mice suffer markedly from infection with *T. cruzi.* These mice produced high levels of $CD4^+$ T cell-derived cytokines including IL-2 and IFN-γ.[45] This indicates an important role of $CD8^+$ T cells in cytokine regulation and induction of infiltrative inflammatory cells. However, in blood-stage malarial infection with β2m deficient mutants recent studies suggest an accessary rather than an essential role of $CD8^+$ T cells.[48]

Human studies. Participation of $CD8^+$ T cells in immunity to intracellular pathogens in humans is suggested by immunohistological studies. In lesions of tuberculoid leprosy patients, $CD8^+$ T cells, expressing a putative differentiation marker of cytolytic T cells, have been identified.[49] Evidence also exists for the activation of antigen-specific $CD8^+$ T cells in tuberculosis and malaria.[50,51] Taken together, these observations provide first evidence for the participation of $CD8^+$ T cells in human immune responses to intracellular microbes.

Role of IFN-γ In Vivo

Both $CD4^+$ T cells and $CD8^+$ T cells are potent IFN-γ producers. The major role of IFN-γ in acquired resistance of mice against intracellular pathogens has been demonstrated by several in vivo studies. Administration of recombinant IFN-γ (rIFN-γ) protects mice against *L. monocytogenes, M. tuberculosis* and *Plasmodium sp.* infection.[52-54] Application of rIFN-γ into lepromatous skin lesions causes local upgrading of cell-mediated immunity, represented by granuloma formation at the site of injection, paralleled by a reduction in the number of viable bacteria.[55] Conversely treatment with anti-IFN-γ mAb significantly influences the course of various microbial infections. In murine listeriosis and tuberculosis, IFN-γ neutralization exacerbates disease.[56,57] During malaria infection, parasitemia was elevated after IFN-γ neutralization with mAb.[58] In leishmaniasis, neutralization of IFN-γ at the time of reinfection reduced Leishmania-specific delayed-type hypersensitivity (DTH) responses, suggesting that IFN-γ is involved in recall of immunological memory to *Leishmania sp.* in vivo.[59] The protective activity of adoptively transferred $CD8^+$ T cells against murine toxoplasmosis was completely ablated by anti-IFN-γ treatment.[60] These findings strongly suggest that $CD8^+$ T cells contribute to protection by IFN-γ secretion. Recent experiments by Harty et al. however contradict an essential requirement for IFN-γ in protection against listeriosis.[61] These studies demonstrated effective protection against listeriosis by $CD8^+$ T cells despite IFN-γ neutralization, indicating an IFN-γ-independent mechanism. Nevertheless, the important role of IFN-γ in antimicrobial immunity is not doubtful and has been verified by the recent demonstration that "knock out" mice deficient in the genes for IFN-γ or the IFN-γ receptor are highly susceptible to infection with *L. monocytogenes, M. bovis* and *M. tuberculosis.*[62-64]

CD8 T CELL CLONES IN VITRO

$CD8^+$ T cell clones which express cytolytic activities in vitro and transfer protection in vivo have been isolated from listeria-infected mice.[65] One T cell clone has been shown to be specific for listeriolysin which is involved in translocation of the parasite into the cytoplasm.[65] Other T cell clones, recognizing N-f-Met protein sequences which are presented by MHC class Ib molecules, have recently been identified.[66] Mycobacteria-reactive $CD8^+$ T cell clones with cytolytic activity have also been established from mice after immunization with killed *M. tuberculosis* or viable *M. bovis.*[67] After restimulation in vitro, these clones were capable of lysing mycobacteria-primed macrophages in an antigen-specific way. After appropriate stimulation, IFN-γ was produced by several of these T cell lines.[14,68]

Although antigens of *S. typhimurium* only induce weak cytolytic T cell responses, recombinant *S. typhimurium*, expressing a dominant *Plasmodium sp.* circumsporozoite (CS) antigen, induce strong protective immunity against challenge with *Plasmodium sp.* sporozoites in the absence of antibodies. In vitro studies suggest that protective immunity depends on induction of antigen-specific MHC class I restricted $CD8^+$ T cells.[69] Several $CD8^+$ T cell clones were derived from spleen cells of sporozoite-immune mice, all displaying apparently identical epitope specificity. These clones induced high levels of cytolysis in vitro upon exposure to peptide-primed MHC-compatible target cells.[6]

In experimental toxoplasmosis, $CD8^+$ T cell clones with reactivity against a purified membrane protein of *T. gondii* have been generated.[70] Interestingly, a subset of responder T cells was directly parasiticidal to extracellular *T. gondii* and exhibited cytotoxicity, independent from antibody opsonization, lymphokine secretion and MHC involvement.[5] Yet, MHC-restricted cytolysis appears to be a characteristic feature of CD8+ T cells in toxoplasmosis.

In vitro studies indicate that *Leishmania sp.* parasites are not affected by destruction of their host cells by cytolytic T cell clones. Nevertheless, cocultures of infected macrophages with CD8+ T cells expressed enhanced leishmanicidal activity. These results indicate that parasite killing was attributable to macrophage activation, resulting from cytokine secretion by these T cells.[71]

IMMUNOPATHOLOGICAL MECHANISMS IN SITU

CD8+ T cells, undoubtful important cells in the protection against intracellular parasites, frequently are also responsible for pathologic sequelae of infection. Tissue damage often occurs as a result of CD8+ T cell involvement. IFN-γ secretion by CD8+ T cells causes activation in MP not only of antiparasitic functions but also of TNF-α secretion which may then harm surrounding tissue sites. Cytolytic activities of CD8+ T cells will also cause tissue destruction. For example, Schwann cells provide a major habitat for *M. leprae*, and destruction of these cells represents a dominant pathomechanism in leprosy.[72] Similarly, destruction of hepatocytes by CD8+ T cells appears to promote liver damage in murine listeriosis as indicated by increased liver enzyme levels.[73]

Target cell lysis of infected cells facilitates dissemination of facultatively intracellular parasites which may be beneficial or disastrous for the host. Coordination of lysis with activation of professional phagocytes allows transmission of parasites from a protective recess to aggressive assailants. First, pathogens become accessible to humoral immune mechanisms and, second can be phagocytosed by highly competent MP. On the other hand, dissemination after target cell lysis promotes microbial spreading which facilitates infection of secondary tissue sites and other individuals.

Granulomatous lesions represent the histologic focus of defense against intracellular pathogens. Composed of mononuclear phagocytes, CD4+ T cells, surrounded by an outer mantle of CD8+ T cells, the granuloma fulfills an important role in antimicrobial protection by containing the pathogens within discrete foci and preventing them from spreading. During tuberculosis, however, chronic granulomas develop in the lung which represent a protective niche for persistent tubercle bacilli. In this situation, lysis could become an important prerequisite for sterile microbial elimination.

Release of bacteria into the environment of a hypoxic necrotic granulomatous center may promote microbial growth inhibition and elimination. In productive granulomas, monocytes with high antimicrobial potential are present which inhibit bacterial spreading to secondary tissue sites. CD8+ T cells, recently suggested to be an important factor in the formation and persistence of productive granulomas are capable of lysing uncapacitated tissue macrophages and facilitating bacterial release and uptake by more efficient newly immigrant monocytes, activated by IFN-γ.[29]

CD8 T CELLS IN ANTIMICROBIAL IMMUNITY

The involvement of CD8+ T cells in infections with intracellular pathogens ranges from dominant CD8+ T cell response, balanced CD4+–CD8+ T cell activation to marginal $CD8^+$ T cell participation. In mice, particularly strong activation of $CD8^+$ T cells has been noted in infections with *L. monocytogenes*, *P. falciparum* and *T. cruzi*. These pathogens preferentially invade MHC class II negative cells and hence are best combated in an MHC class II-independent way. Immunity of mice against *M. tuberculosis* seems to depend on a balanced ratio between $CD4^+$ and $CD8^+$ T cells.[67] Since tubercle bacilli are primarily located within MP which express MHC class II molecules constitutively, mycobacterial antigens can be presented to $CD4^+$ Th1 lymphocytes. Nevertheless, participation of $CD8^+$ T cells is required for the defense against this pathogen. *M. tuberculosis* is able to deactivate macrophages, and consequently remains unaffected by IFN-γ activated macrophages. Furthermore, various tissue macrophages, such as Kupffer cells in the liver, are highly refractory to cytokine activation. In this situation, cytolytic $CD8^+$ T cells are capable of effectively inducing cellular immunity.

CD8 T CELLS AND VACCINATION

MHC-determined mechanisms of antigen processing and presentation enable the host to mount appropriate defense mechanisms against microbes residing in cellular recesses. Obviously, antigens which induce appropriate T cell responses represent possible vaccine candidates. Hence, the identification of relevant peptides is of major interest for research related to control of infectious diseases.

Soluble "exogenous" protein antigens which are administered in pure form are preferentially internalized by MHC class II positive antigen-presenting cells. Because these antigens are presented in an MHC class II restricted manner they generally induce strong $CD4^+$ T cell and only marginal $CD8^+$ T cell responses. Interestingly, peptides can be loaded directly into the pocket of MHC class I molecules on the cell surface in vivo. Because this direct loading allows bypassing of MHC restricted processing, $CD8^+$ T cell responses can be induced efficiently by peptide vaccination. However, distinct MHC haplotypes are "specific" for distinct peptides. Hence, peptide immunization is extremely restricted in its scope. Because N-f-Met-containing peptides are presented by the nonpolymorphic MHC class Ib molecules, this restriction may be overcome provided that N-f-Met-containing peptides are efficiently recognized by $CD8^+$ T cells of humans. Otherwise, whole proteins need to be introduced into the MHC class I pathway by appropriate means. These include certain adjuvants such as ISCOM which is capable of translocating integrated proteins through the plasma membrane and viable carrier systems able to deliver recombinant proteins into the cytoplasmic compartment.[74] Either system allows introduction of soluble proteins into the MHC class I pathway.

Recent research concerned with viable carriers has focused on two bacterial systems as vaccines against intracellular pathogens: recombinant *M. bovis BCG* and aroA- *S. typhimurium*. Both strains have been shown to be potent inducers of humoral and cellular immunity comprising both $CD4^+$ and $CD8^+$ T cell responses.[75,76] Yet, from what has been said before, both vaccine candidates, in their current stage, are poor stimulators of $CD8^+$ T cells. To promote MHC class I restricted antigen presentation, translocation through the phagosomal membrane of recombinant proteins expressed by *M. bovis BCG* or aroA- *S. typhimurium* has to be improved. This may be achieved by integrating genes which facilitate eggression from the phagosomal into the cytoplasmic compartment such as listeriolysin from *L. monocytogenes.*[77]

CONCLUDING REMARKS

In this review, emphasis was laid upon the function and role of $CD8^+$ T cells in protective immunity against intracellular pathogens. Without doubt, $CD8^+$ T cells, together with $CD4^+$ T cells and γ/δ T cells, form an integral part of the network that is required for optimal T cell responses. Although $CD8^+$ T cells are capable of working independently, numerous experimental data suggest the requirement for a crossstalk between different T cell subsets in order to achieve optimal protection. Since many intracellular pathogens invade MHC class II negative host cells, MHC class I restricted $CD8^+$ T cells may play a unique part in the defense against these invaders which cannot be fulfilled by $CD4^+$ T cells and partially compensated by γ/δ T cells. Their capacity to activate macrophages by IFN-γ secretion paired with their ability to directly lyse infected host cells may make $CD8^+$ T lymphocytes particularly effective mediators of antimicrobial defense. Because numerous intracellular pathogens rapidly develop resistance against antibiotics novel vaccination strategies based on the activation of the complete "T cell network" including $CD8^+$ T cells are urgently required.

ACKNOWLEDGMENTS

S.H.E.K. gratefully acknowledges financial support from SFB 322 and Landesforschungsschwerpunkt. Many thank to Mrs. R. Mahmoudi for her excellent help.

REFERENCES

1. Kaufmann SHE. Immunity to intracellular bacteria. Ann Rev Immunol 1993; 11: 129-163
2. Pedrazzini T, Hug K, Louis JA. Importance of $L3T4^+$ and $Lyt\text{-}2^+$ cells in the immunologic control of infection with *Mycobacterium bovis* strain Bacillus Calmette-Guérin in mice. J Immunol 1987; 139: 2032-2037
3. Magee DM, Wing EJ. Cloned $L3T4^+$ T lymphocytes protect mice against *Listeria monocytogenes* by secreting IFN-γ. J Immunol 1988; 141: 3203-3207
4. Kaufmann SHE. $CD8^+$ T lymphocytes in intracellular microbial infections. Immunol Today 1988; 9: 168-174
5. Khan IA, Smith KA, Kasper LH. Induction of antigen-specific parasiticidal cytotoxic T cell splenocytes by a major membrane protein (P30) of *Toxoxplasma gondii.* J Immunol 1988; 141: 3600-3605
6. Rodrigues MM, Cordey AS, Arreaza G, Corradin G, Romero P, Maryanski JL, Nussenzweig RS, Zavala F. $CD8^+$ T cell clones derived against the *Plasmodium yoelii* circumsporozoite protein protect against malaria. Int Immunol 1991; 3: 579-585
7. Munk ME, Gatrill A, Kaufmann SHE. Antigen-specific target cell lysis and interleukin-2 secretion by *Mycobacterium tuberculosis*-activated γ/δ T cells. J Immunol 1990; 145: 2434-2439
8. Mombaerts P, Arnoldi J, Russ F, Tonegawa S, Kaufmann SHE. Different roles of α/β and γ/δ T cells in immunity against an intracellular bacterial pathogen. Nature 1993; 365: 53-56

9. Portnoy DA, Chakraborty T, Goebel W, Cossart P. Molecular determinants of *Listeria monocytogenes* pathogenisis. Infect Immun 1992; 60: 1263-1267
10. Moore MW, Carbone FR, Bevan MJ. Introduction of soluble protein into the class I pathway of antigen processing and presenting. Cell 1988; 54: 777
11. Brown ML, Fields PE, Kurlander RJ. Metabolic requirements for macrophage presentation of *Listeria monocytogenes* to immune CD8 cells. J Immunol 1992; 148: 555-561
12. King CH, Mundayoor S, Crawford JT, Shinnick TM. Expression of contact-dependent cytolytic activity by *Mycobacterium tuberculosis* and isolation of the genomic locus that encodes the activity. Infect Immun 1993; 61: 2708-2712
13. Yano A, Ohno S, Norose K, Baba T, Yamashita K, Aosai F, Segawa K. Antigen presentation by Toxoplasma-infected cells: Antigen entry through cell membrane fusion. Int Arch Allergy Immunol 1992; 98: 13-17
14. De Libero G, Flesch IEA, Kaufmann SHE. Mycobacteria-reactive Lyt-2$^+$ T cell lines. Eur J Immunol 1988; 18: 59-66
15. Pfeifer JD, Wick MJ, Roberts RL, Findlay K, Normark SJ, Harding CV. Phagocytic processing of bacterial antigens for class I MHC presentation to T cells. Nature 1993; 361: 359-362
16. Pamer EG, Wang C-R, Flaherty L, Fischer Lindahl K, Bevan MJ. H-2M3 presents a *Listeria monocytogenes* peptide to cytotoxic T lymphocytes. Cell 1992; 70: 215-223
17. Fischer-Lindahl K, Hermel E, Loveland BE, Wang C-R. Maternally transmitted antigen of mice: A model transplantation antigen. Ann Rev Immunol 1991; 9: 351-372
18. Hakim FT, Gazzinelli RT, Denkers E, Hieny S, Shearer GM, Sher A. CD8$^+$ T cells from mice vaccinated against *Toxoplasma gondii* are cytotoxic for parasite-infected or antigen-pulsed host cells. J Immunol 1991; 147: 2310-2316
19. Young DB, Nathan CF, Palladino MA, Cohn ZA. Functional channel formation associated with cytotoxic T cell granules. Proc Natl Acad Sci USA 1986; 83: 150-154
20. Gao XM, Quinn CL, Bell JI, Mc Michael AJ. Expression and function of HLA-B27 in lipid-linked form: implications for cytotoxic T lymphocyte-induced apoptosis signal transduction. Eur J Immunol 1993; 23: 653-658
21. Cohen JJ, Duke RC, Fadok VA, Sellins KS. Apoptosis and programmed cell death in immunity. Ann Rev Immunol 1992; 10: 267-293
22. Flesch IEA, Kaufmann SHE. Mycobacterial growth inhibition by Interferon gamma-activated bone marrow macrophages and differential susceptibility among strains of *Mycobacterium tuberculosis.* J Immunol 1987; 138: 4408-4413
23. Joly E, Mucke L, Oldstone MBA. Viral persistance in neurons explained by lack of major histocompatibility class I expression. Science 1991; 253: 1283-1285
24. Steinhoff U, Wand-Würtenberger A, Bremerich A, Kaufmann SHE. *Mycobacterium leprae* renders Schwann cells and mononuclear phagocytes susceptible or resistant against killer cells. Infect Immun 1991; 59: 684
25. Baldridge JR, Barry RA, Hinrichs DJ. Expression of systemic protection and delayed-type hypersensitivity to *Listeria monocytogenes* is mediated by different T-cell subsets. Infect Immun 1990; 58: 654-658
26. Czuprynski CJ, Brown JF. Effects of purified anti-Lyt-2 mAb treatment on murine listeriosis: comparative roles of Lyt-2$^+$ and L3T4$^+$ cells in resistance to

primary and secondary infection, delayed-type hypersensitivity and adoptive transfer of resistance. Immunol 1990; 71: 107-112

27. Mielke MEA, Ehlers S, Hahn H. T-cell subsets in delayed-type hypersensitivity, protection, and granuloma formation in primary and secondary Listeria infection in mice: superior role of Lyt-2+ cells in aquired immunity. Infect Immun 1988; 56: 1920-1925
28. Haak-Frendscho M, Czuprynski CJ. Use of recombinant interleukin-2 to enhance adoptive transfer of resistance to *Listeria monocytogenes* infection. Infect Immun 1992; 60: 1406-1414
29. Maraskovsky E, Chen WF, Shortman K. IL-2 and IFN-γ are two necessary lymphokines in the development of cytolytic T cells. J Immunol 1989; 143: 1210-1214
30. Leveton C, Barnass S, Champion B, Lucas S, De Souza B, Nicol M, Banarjee D, Rook G. T-cell-mediated protection of mice against virulent *Mycobacterium tuberculosis.* Infect Immun 1989; 57: 390-395
31. Flory CM, Hubbard RD, Collins FM. Effects of in vivo T lymphocyte subset depletion on mycobacterial infections in mice. J Leukoc Biol 1992; 51: 225-229
32. Ottenhoff TH, Mutis T. Specific killing of cytotoxic T cells and antigen-presenting cells by CD4+ cytotoxic T cell clones. A novel potentially immunoregulatory T-T cell interaction in man. J Exp Med 1990; 171: 2011-2024
33. Hill JO, Awwad M, North RJ. Elimination of CD4+ suppressor T cells from susceptible BALB/c mice releases CD8+ T lymphocytes to mediate protective immunity against Leishmania. J Exp Med 1989; 169: 1819-1827
34. Hill JO. Reduced numbers of CD4+ suppressor cells with subsequent expansion of CD8+ protective T cells as an explanation for the paradoxical state of enhanced resistance to Leishmania in T-cell deficient BALB/c mice. Immunol 1991; 72: 282-286
35. Müller I, Pedrazzini T, Kropf P, Louis J, Milon G. Establishment of resistance to *Leishmania major* infection in susceptible BALB/c mice requires parasite-specific CD8+ T cells. Int Immunol 1991; 3: 587-597
36. Murray HW, Squires KE, Miralles CD, Stoeckle MY, Granger AM, Granelli-Piperno A, Bogdan C. Acquired resistance and granuloma formation in experimental visceral leishmaniasis. Differential T cell and lymphokine roles in initial versus established immunity. J Immunol 1992; 148: 1858-1863
37. Milon G, Titus RG, Cerottini J-C, Marchal G, Louis JA. Higher frequency of *Leishmania major*-specific L3T4+ T cells in susceptible BALB/c as compared with resistant CBA mice. J Immunol 1986; 136: 1467-1471
38. Titus RG, Milon G, Marchal G, Vassalli P, Cerottini J-C, Louis JA. Involvement of specific Lyt-2+ T cells in the immunological control of experimentally induced murine cutaneous leishmaniosis. Eur J Immunol 1987; 17: 1429-1433
39. Farrell JP, Müller I, Louis JA. A role for Lyt-2+ T cells in resistance to cutaneous leishmaniosis in immunized mice. J Immunol 1989; 142: 2052-2056
40. Brown CR, McLeod R. Class I MHC genes and CD8+ T cells determine cyst number in *Toxoplasma gondii* infection. J Immunol 1990; 145: 3438-3441
41. Suzuki Y, Remington JS. Dual regulation of resistance against *Toxoplasma gondii* infection by Lyt-2+ and Lyt-1+, L3T4+ T cells in mice. J Immunol 1988; 140: 3943-3946
42. Romero P, Maryanski JL, Cordey AS, Corradin G, Nussenzweig RS, Zavala

F. Isolation and characterization of protective cytolytic T cells in a rodent malaria model system. Immunol Lett 1990; 25: 27-31
43. Hoffman SL, Weiss W, Mellouk S, Sedegah M. Irradiated sporozoite vaccine induces cytotoxic T lymphocytes that recognize malaria antigens on the surface of infected hepatocytes. Immunol Lett 1990; 25: 33-38
44. Zijlstra M, Bix M, Simister NE, Loring JM, Raulet DH, Jaenisch R. ß2-microglobulin deficient mice lack $CD4^-$ $CD8^+$ cytolytic T cells. Nature 1990; 344: 742
45. Tarleton RL, Koller BH, Latour A, Postan M. Susceptibility of ß2-microglobulin-deficient mice to *Trypanosoma cruzi* infection. Nature 1992; 356: 338-340
46. Roberts AD, Ordway DJ, Orme IM. *Listeria monocytogenes* infection in ß2-microglobulin-deficient mice. Infect Immun 1993; 61: 1113
47. Flynn JL, Goldstein MM, Triebold KJ, Koller B, Bloom BR. Major histocompatibility complex class I-restricted T cells are required for resistance to *Mycobacterium tuberculosis* infection. Proc Natl Acad Sci USA 1992; 89: 12013-12017
48. Heyde van der HC, Manning DD, Roopenian DC, Weidanz WP. Resolution of blood-stage malarial infections in $CD8^+$ cell-deficient ß2m $^{0/0}$ mice. J Immunol 1993; 151: 3187-3191
49. Modlin RL, Melancon-Kaplan J, Young SMM, Pirmez C, Kino H, Convit J, Rea TH, Bloom BR. Learning from lesions: Patterns of tissue inflammation in leprosy. Proc Natl Acad Sci USA 1988; 85: 1213-1217
50. Rossi GA, Balbi B, Manca F. Evidence for selective presence of PPD-specific T-lymphocytes at site of inflammation in the early phase of infection. Am Rev Respir Dis 1987; 136: 575-579
51. Sinigaglia F, Matile H, Pink JRL. *Plasmodium falciparum*-specific human T cell clones: evidence for helper and cytotoxic activities. Eur J Immunol 1987; 17: 187-192
52. Kiderlen AF, Kaufmann SHE, Lohmann-Matthes M-L. Protection of mice against the intracellular bacterium *Listeria monocytogenes* by recombinant immune interferon. Eur J Immunol 1984; 14: 964-967
53. Denis M. Involvement of cytokines in determining resistance and aquired immunity in murine tuberculosis. J Leuk Biol 1991; 50: 495-501
54. Weidanz WP, Melancon-Kaplan J, Cavacini LA. Cell-mediated immunity to the asexual blood stages of malarial parasites: animal models. Immunol Lett 1990; 25: 87-96
55. Kaplan G, Cohn ZA. Leprosy and cell-mediated immunity. Curr Opin Immunol 1991; 3: 91-96
56. Buchmeier NA, Schreiber ND. Requirement of endogenous interferon-γ production for resolution of *Listeria monocytogenes* infection. Proc Natl Acad Sci USA 1985; 82: 7404-7408
57. Denis M. Growth of *Listeria monocytogenes* in murine macrophages and its modulation by cytokines: activation of bactericidal activity by interleukin-4 and interleukin-6. Can J Microbiol 1991; 37: 253-257
58. Schofield L, Villaquiran J, Ferreira A, Schellekens H, Nussenzweig R, Nussenzweig V. Gamma interferon, $CD8^+$ T cells and antibodies required for immunity to malaria sporozoites. Nature 1987; 330: 664-667
59. Müller I, Kropf P, Etges RJ, Louis JA. Gamma Interferon response in sec-

ondary *Leishmania major* infection: role of CD8[+] T cells. Infect Immun 1993; 61: 3730-3738
60. Suzuki Y, Remington JS. The effect of anti-IFN-γ antibody on the protective effect of Lyt-2[+] immune T cells against toxoplasmosis in mice. J Immunol 1990; 144: 1954-1956
61. Harty JT, Screiber RD, Bevan MJ. CD8 T cells can protect against an intracellular bacterium in an interferon-γ-independent fashion. Proc Natl Acad Sci USA 1992; 89: 11612-11616
62. Dalton DK, Pitts-Meek S, Keshav S, Figari IS, Bradley A, Stewart TA. Multiple defects of immune cell function in mice with disrupted interferon-γ genes. Science 1993; 259: 1739-1742
63. Huang S, Hendriks W, Althage A, Hemmi S, Bluethmann H, Kamijo R, Vilcek J, Zinkernagel RM, Aguet M. Immune response in mice that lack the IFN-γ receptor. Science 1993; 259: 1742-1745
64. Cooper AM, Dalton DK, Stewart TA, Griffin JP, Russell DG, Orme IM. Disseminated tuberculosis in interferon-gamma gene disrupted mice. J Exp Med 1993; in press
65. Kaufmann SHE, Simon MM, Hahn H. Specific Lyt 123 T cells are involved in protection against *Listeria monocytogenes* and in delayed-type hypersensitivity to listerial antigens. J Exp Med 1979; 150: 1033-1038
66. Kaufmann SHE, Rodewald HR, Hug E, De Libero G. Cloned *Listeria monocytogenes* specific non-MHC restricted Lyt2[+] T cells with cytolytic and protective activity. J Immuniol 1988; 140: 3173-3179
67. Kaufmann SHE, De Libero G. Cytolytic T cells in *M. tuberculosis* infections. In: Bendinelli M, Friedman H, ed. Mycobacterium Tuberculosis. Plenum Publishing Corporation, 1988: 151-170
68. Flesch IEA, Kaufmann SHE. Attempts to characterize the mechanisms involved in mycobacterial growth inhibition by gamma-Interferon-activated bone marrow macrophages. Infect Immun 1988; 56: 1464-1469
69. Aggarwal A, Kumar S, Jaffe R, Hone D, Gross M, Sadoff J. Oral Salmonella: Malaria circumsporozoite recombinants induce specific CD8[+] cytotoxic T cells. J Exp Med 1990; 172: 1083-1090
70. Kasper LH, Khan IA, Ely KH, Buelow R, Boothroyd JC. Antigen-specific (p30) mouse CD8 T cells are cytotoxic against *Toxoplasma gondii*-infected peritoneal macrophages. J Immunol 1992; 148: 1493-1498
71. Smith LE, Rodrigues M, Russell DG. The interaction between CD8[+] cytotoxic T cells and Leishmania-infected macrophages. J Exp Med 1991; 174: 499-505
72. Steinhoff U, Kaufmann SHE. Specific lysis by CD8[+] T cells of Schwann cells expressing *Mycobacterium leprae* antigen. Eur J Immunol 1988; 18: 969-972
73. Sasaki T, Mieno M, Udono H, Yamaguchi K, Usui T, Hara K, Shiku H, Nakayama E. Roles of CD4[+] and CD8[+] T cells, and the effect of administration of recombinant murine interferon-gamma in listerial infection. J Exp Med 1990; 171: 1141-1154
74. Morein B, Sundquist B, Hoglund S, Dalsgaard K, Osterhaus A. Iscom, a novel structure for antigenic presentation of membrane proteins from enveloped viruses. Nature 1984; 308: 457-460

75. Aldovini A, Young RA. Humoral and cell-mediated immune responses to live recombinant BCG-HIV vaccines. Nature 1991; 351: 479-482
76. Hoffman SL, Isenbarger D, Long GW, Sedegah M, Szarfman A, Waters L, Hollingdale MR, van der Meide P, Finbloom DS, Ballou WR. Sporozoite vaccine induces genetically restricted T cell elimination of malaria from hepatocytes. Science 1989; 244: 1078-1081
77. Hess J, Kaufmann SHE. Vaccination strategies against intracellular microbes. FEMS 1993; 7: 95-104

CHAPTER 7

Requirements and Basis for Efficacious Vaccination by a Low Antigen Dose Regimen

Against Intracellular Pathogens Uniquely Susceptible to a Cell-mediated Attack

Peter A. Bretscher

INTRODUCTION

Certain intracellular parasites, including those responsible for the leishmaniases,[1] leprosy[2] and tuberculosis,[3] are only contained by a cell-mediated, as opposed to an antibody-mediated, immune response. One approach to achieving efficacious vaccination against these parasites is to define those parasite-dependent "protective" antigens, against which a cell-mediated response is required to achieve containment of the parasite, and to find ways of priming individuals to ensure that a vigorous cell-mediated immune response is mounted against these "protective" antigens following natural infection. This approach is clearly valid, but may in practice be difficult to achieve, given the biochemical complexity of the parasites involved, the likelihood that there are several or many protective antigens, that protection may require that immunity is expressed against a combination of the protective antigens, and that different protective antigens will exist in different individuals, due to polymorphic host genes, MHC genes in particular.

We have been exploring an approach to vaccination against these intracellular parasites that we believe bypasses the requirement for identifying

Strategies in Vaccine Design, edited by Gordon L. Ada, D.Sc.

protective antigens. We assume, on the basis of reported clinical observation, that cell-mediated immunity is protective, and that a failure to obtain containment upon natural infection is due to an inadequate cell-mediated response, usually associated with the production of antibody.[1-3] Exclusivity between the induction of strong cell-mediated and humoral immunity appears to be the rule in the immune response to diverse antigens such as proteins,[4] xenogeneic red cells,[5] and unicellular and multicellular parasites.[1-3,6] This exclusivity reflects the fact that the class of immune response induced against different epitopes presented on one physical entity tends to be coordinately regulated. This tendency for coordinate regulation is referred to as coherence. It would not be generally possible to ensure a cell-mediated response against protective antigens of a parasite, by finding conditions optimal for the induction of cell-mediated immunity against the parasite as a whole, if coherence did not exist.

We have thus explored whether it is possible to expose individuals to parasite antigens in a manner that causes an imprint upon the immune system that ensures a strong and stable cell-mediated response upon subsequent infection with the parasite. Such immunization should ensure protection and limited disease upon infection. Our central aim is to develop a standard form of exposure to parasite antigens that can be universally efficacious in generating such an imprint in all individuals despite the genetic diversity of animal and human populations, a diversity that is known to affect the nature of immune responses. We shall consider, towards the end of this contribution, a potential solution to the problem posed by this genetic diversity.

One major uncertainty needs to be acknowledged at the outset to avoid confusion. Available evidence strongly supports the view that pathogen-specific Th1-like delayed-type hypersensitivity (DTH)-mediating $CD4^+$ T cells are required for the containment of some intracellular parasitic infections, and that the induction of such cells is downregulated during a Th2-like antibody response by $CD4^+$ T cells.[6,7] The regulation controlling the induction of the other major subclass of cell-mediated immunity, namely $CD8^+$ cytotoxic T lymphocytes (CTL), is less clear. This uncertainty is unfortunate as CTLs are most probably important in providing protection against a number of viral and possibly other intracellular parasitic infections. It seems probable, given the relative kinetics of the CTL and antibody response following viral infection, with the CTL response appearing before antibody is produced and declining as antibody production peaks,[8] the similarity of these kinetics to the relative kinetics of the DTH and antibody responses,[7] and the similarity of the cytokine profile of $CD8^+$ T lymphocytes and $CD4^+$ Th1-like cells,[9] to suppose that the induction of $CD8^+$ T cells and $CD4^+$ Th1-like cells come under similar negative regulation during the course of a Th2-like antibody response. This conjecture is assumed to be valid for the purposes of this discussion. If this conjecture is valid, our strategy is likely to apply to vaccination against HIV-1 independently of whether $CD8^+$ CTL and/or $CD4^+$ Th1-like cells are required to contain the infection.[10]

REGULATION OF THE CLASS OF IMMUNITY INDUCED BY NONREPLICATING ANTIGENS

I briefly outline here some of the considerations we have borne in mind in our attempts at developing strategies of efficacious vaccination.

CELLULAR AND MOLECULAR REGULATION ENSURING EXCLUSIVITY OF CELL-MEDIATED AND ANTIBODY RESPONSES

It was discovered in the early 1960s that the induction of antibody to an antigen "A" rendered animals specifically unresponsive for the induction of DTH to "A", a phenomenon referred to as immune deviation.[11] Conversely, it was shown in the early 1970s that the induction of DTH to an antigen could result in unresponsiveness for the induction of antibody.[4] In particular, the administration of low doses of antigen, below that immunogenic for the induction of antibody, resulted both in the induction of DTH and unresponsiveness for the induction of antibody.[4,12,13] This phenomenon is referred to as cell-mediated low-zone immune deviation.

I proposed a Theory of Immune Class Regulation in the early 1970s that attempted to provide a description of the antigen-mediated interactions between leukocytes that control the class of immunity induced, and to explain such phenomena as immune deviation.[14,15] Tests of this theory have provided a partial explanation for the exclusivity between the induction of distinct classes of immunity. Thus, we found that mice immunized to produce antibody expressed no DTH but harbored antigen-specific $CD4^+$ $CD8^-$ T cells that suppress the induction of DTH.[16,17] These cells are referred to as TsDTH cells. Further work showed that this population of cells coordinately inhibits the DTH and facilitates the antibody response, i.e., they switch the response induced by antigen from a cell-mediated to a humoral mode.[18,19] Such coordinate regulation supports their central role in immune class regulation. We also demonstrated that mice, induced to express a strong DTH response and unresponsive for the induction of antibody, harbor antigen-specific $CD4^-$ $CD8^+$ T cells that inhibit the antibody response.[17,20] These cells are referred to as TsAb cells. Further work showed that this population of cells coordinately inhibits the antibody and facilitates the DTH response, i.e. they switch the response induced by antigen from a humoral to a cell-mediated mode.[21] Such coordinate regulation again supports a central role for such cells in immune class regulation.

The exclusivity of DTH and antibody responses can to a certain extent be accounted for by the generation of TsAb and TsDTH cells coordinately with the induction of DTH and antibody responses respectively. However, the existence of these cells raises further questions. Firstly, what ensures their exclusivity? It was proposed that these cells directly or indirectly inhibit each other's induction, so that when one starts winning, it inhibits its adversary, thereby becoming dominant.[14,15] This still seems to be a reasonable proposal that is yet to be critically tested.[22] A role for IFN-γ in promoting Th1-like responses, and of IL-4 and IL-10 in promoting Th2-like responses, seems probable, and these lymphokines may well contribute to the mutual inhibition of the generation of two sets of T cells, one characteristically associated with cell-mediated and the other with antibody responses.[22-24] However, the postulated mutual inhibition of these two sets gives rise to a second question, namely what conditions of antigen stimulation give the induction of each set an edge over its opponent?

THE DECISION CRITERION CONTROLLING WHETHER ANTIGEN INDUCES A CELL-MEDIATED OR AN ANTIBODY RESPONSE

I shall attempt to answer the question of what is the nature of this criterion through a description of experiments aimed at testing a particular hypothesis.

Mice, irradiated and reconstituted with unprimed spleen cells and challenged with a dose of foreign red blood cells that induces antibody in intact animals, can mount either a DTH or an antibody response. The class induced depends upon the number of unprimed spleen cells used for reconstitution. Reconstitution with a large number, comparable to that present in the spleen of a normal mouse, results in the induction of IgG antibody

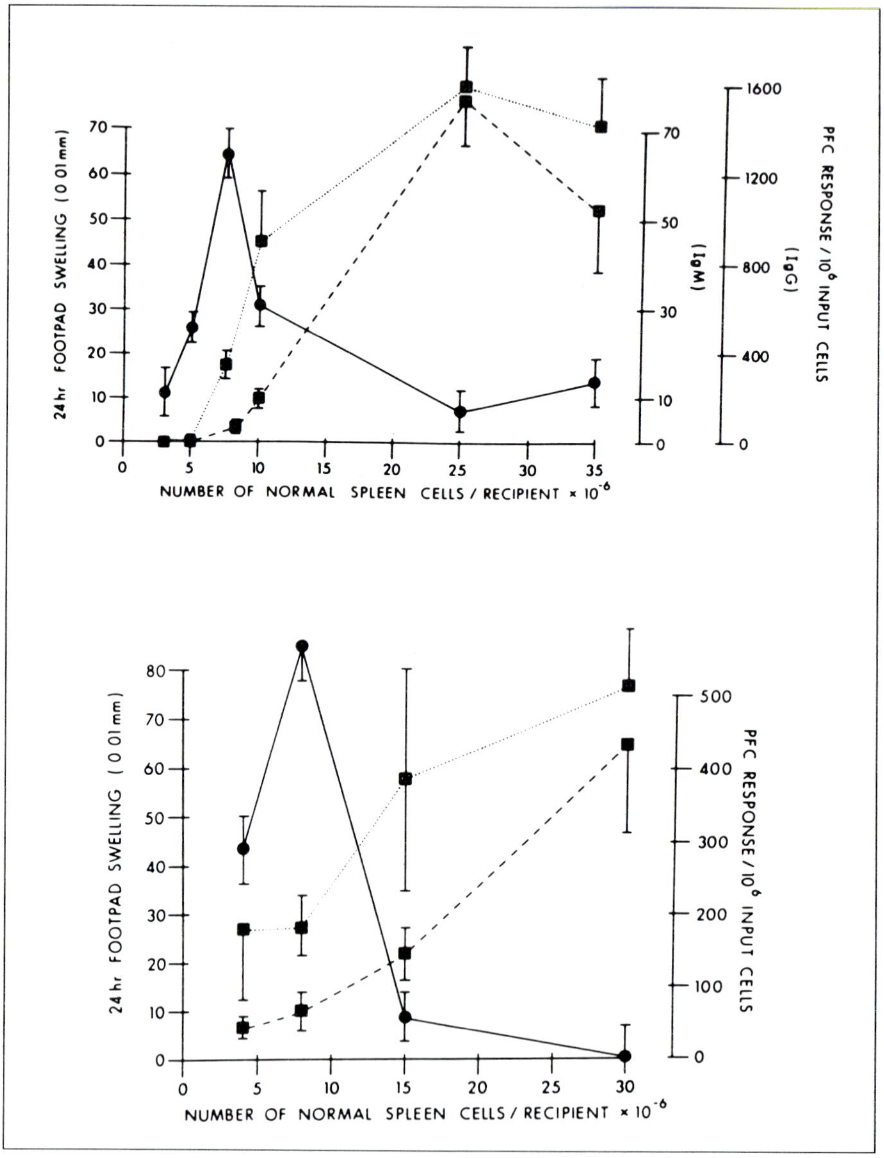

Fig. 1. The DTH (unbroken line), IgM (dotted line) and IgG (broken line) responses mounted by various numbers of normal spleen cells to the antigen donkey RBCs (Figure 1a) and chicken RBCs (Figure 1b) when these cells are used to reconstitute lethally irradiated recipients and are challenged with a standard dose of antigen. The normalized responses are shown. This provides a direct measure of the efficiency with which the lymphocyte precursor cells, that can give rise to various effector cells of different classes of immunity, are induced. (Courtesy of Academic Press, Inc., ref. 19)

and insignificant DTH, whereas reconstitution with a smaller number can result in the induction of DTH with little IgG antibody production, see Figure 1. Clearly, something "more" is needed to induce an IgG than a DTH response. We denote the number of normal spleen cells required to reconstitute the irradiated mice so that the antigen induces only a DTH response as M (for medium), and the number required so that antigen induces only IgG antibody as L (for large). Mice reconstituted with M normal spleen cells, and (L-M) normal spleen cells depleted of T cells, support the antigen-dependent induction of a DTH but not an antibody response,[19] see Table 1. Clearly, it is the greater number of T cells in the population of L normal spleen cells, than the smaller number present in the population of M normal spleen cells, that is responsible for the lack of induction of DTH, and the facilitation of the induction of IgG antibody, that occurs when irradiated mice are reconstituted with L normal spleen cells and are challenged with antigen.

In addition, we examined the effect of giving mice, before irradiation and reconstitution with M normal spleen cells and antigen challenge, increasing numbers of spleen cells obtained from mice immunized to produce antibody. Mice given no cells before irradiation, reconstitution and challenge, mounted a DTH response. The donation of immune spleen cells before irradiation switched the response from a cell-mediated (DTH) to a humoral (IgG) mode in an antigen-specific manner, see Figure 2. The cells responsible were T cells, bearing the Ly1 but not the Ly2 antigen, probably corresponding to $CD4^+$ T cells, see Table 2 and Table 3. The donation of increasing numbers of these antigen-specific $CD4^+$ T cells before irradiation, reconstitution and challenge, resulted in a progressive suppression of the DTH response and coordinately a progressive facilitation of the induction of IgG antibody.[19]

Various conclusions can be drawn from these experiments. Firstly, the same population of normal spleen cells can support the antigen-dependent induction of DTH or antibody responses, depending upon the number of these cells used to reconstitute irradiated mice. This finding demonstrates

Table 1. The higher number of T cells present in a large as opposed to a medium inoculum of unprimed spleen cells is responsible for the humoral response and lack of DTH reactivity

No. of unprimed cells given[a] ($x10^{-6}$)	DTH ± SE	Response[b] (PFC/10^6 input ± SE) IgM	IgG
7.5	78 ± 7	17 ± 7	10 ± 4
7.5 + 27.5 Anti-Thy-1 treated	84 ± 5	20 ± 6	19 ± 4
7.5 + 27.5 C′ treated	22 ± 3	117 ± 16	750 ± 146
7.5 + 27.5 untreated	24 ± 4	107 ± 12	973 ± 44

[a] Yield of cells after C′ treatment 82%, after anti-Thy-1 treatment 52%.

[b] Normalized response to CRBC (i.e., activity from the same number of input precursor cells), assuming C′ treatment kills no cells, and anti-Thy-1 treatment kills all T but no B cells.

(Courtesy of Academic Press, Inc. ref. 19)

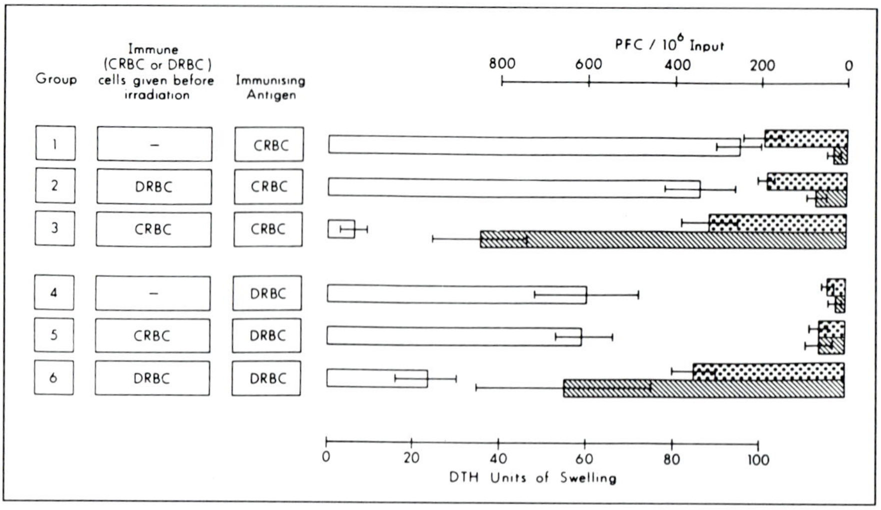

Fig. 2. Illustration of a strategy by which a standard vaccination procedure can be efficacious in a genetically diverse population of individuals. For explanation, see text.

that it is not the ratio of two different kinds of cells present that determines whether a cell-mediated or antibody response is induced, as this ratio will be the same in a population of M or L normal spleen cells. This conclusion is supported by parallel in vitro studies, in which the density of normal spleen cells determines whether antigen induces a DTH or an optimal IgM response.[18] Thus, we cannot "explain" the preferential induction of antibody over a cell-mediated response when L normal spleen cells are stimulated by antigen by supposing that the antigen does so because it interacts more effectively with B cells than macrophages under these circumstances, and that this in turn preferentially results in the induction of Th2-like cells. This "explanation" does not explain why reconstituting irradiated mice with M normal spleen cells and challenging with antigen results in the preferential induction of DTH. Clearly, the observation that reconstitution of irradiated mice with different numbers of unprimed spleen cells results in the induction of different classes of response following antigen challenge demonstrates the importance of quantitative considerations in understanding the nature of the decision criterion. Indeed, the observation that it is the greater number of T cells present in a number L than in the number M of normal spleen cells that allows L to support the antigen-dependent induction of IgG antibody, without the induction of substantial DTH, suggests that the immune system assesses in some manner the number of T cells (or number of a subset of T cells) in the process of determining whether a DTH or an antibody response is induced. Furthermore, the coordinate suppression of the DTH and facilitation of the induction of antibody, by increasing numbers of antigen-specific helper T cells, supports a similar possibility. This possibility I refer to as the **Threshold Hypothesis.**[14,15] This hypothesis states that the induction of all precursor cells requires an antigen-dependent interaction with helper T cells, and that different precursor cells require different numbers of these helper T cell-dependent signals to be induced, i.e., they have different inductive thresholds. The finding of a

Table 2. Cells are responsible for the switch in class induced

No. of normal cells given[a] ($x10^{-6}$)	2×10^7 nylon-passed immune cells	DTH ± SE	PFC/10^6 input ± SE[b]	
			IgM	IgG
8	—	43 ± 3	196 ± 28	446 ± 90
8	Anti-Thy-1 + C′ treated	41 ± 4	354 ± 32	550 ± 145
8	C′ treated	3 ± 3	1003 ± 340	3164 ± 805

[a] Cells, from the spleen of irradiated mice 7 days after reconstitution with 3.5 x 107 spleen cells and CRBC, were passed through a nylon wool column. Recovery of cells from the columns was 12%. Recipient mice were given the equivalent of 2×10^7 immune cells that were treated with either guinea pig compliment (yield 65%) or anti-Thy-1 and complement (yield 20%)

[b] Assayed 7 days after reconstitution.

(Courtesy of Academic Press, Inc. ref. 19)

Table 3. The T cells responsible for the switch in class induced are Ly-1⁺ and LY-2⁻

No. of normal cells given[a] ($x10^{-6}$)	2×10^7 nylon-passed[a] cells	DTH ± SE	PFC/10^6 input ± SE	
			IgM	IgG
7	—	68 ± 3	30 ± 9	13 ± 2
7	Untreated	26 ± 4	116 ± 3	208 ± 40
7	Anti-Ly-1 treated	66 ± 3	45 ± 13	44 ± 18
7	Anti-Ly-2 treated	29 ± 7	83 ± 22	282 ± 81

[a] Cells, from the spleen of irradiated mice 7 days after reconstitution with 35×10^6 normal spleen cells and DRBC, were passed through nylon wool columns. Recovery of cells from columns was 20%. Cells were either untreated or anti-Ly-1.1 or anti-Ly-2.1 and complement treated before being given to mice 24 h before irradiation and reconstitution with 7×10^6 normal spleen cells and DRBC. The number of cells given per mouse before irradiation was derived from 2×10^7 immune cells before passage through the nylon wool column.

(Courtesy of Academic Press, Inc. ref. 19)

requirement for helper T cells in the induction of those T cells that can be induced to give rise to DTH-mediating T cells[25] is consistent with the threshold hypothesis. It is expected on this hypothesis that conditions resulting in the generation of relatively few helper T cell-dependent signals results in the induction of DTH, TsAb cells and Th1-like cells, whereas the generation of more results in the induction of IgG antibody, TsDTH cells and Th2-like cells. The Threshold Hypothesis predicts that the presence of more helper T cells is required to induce IgG than DTH responses under conditions where the antigen concentration is kept constant, and the observations already described and recorded in the tables and figures are consistent with this prediction. Consider what we would expect to happen on this hypothesis if we have conditions adequate to support the induction of antibody and if we then systematically lower the antigen concentration.

Lowering the antigen concentration will reduce the efficiency of helper T cell induction and the delivery of their signals to precursor cells, which is an antigen-dependent process. We would expect, following the Threshold Hypothesis, that the signals generated on systematically lowering the antigen concentration would at some point be insufficient for the induction of antibody but would result in the induction of DTH. This is indeed found to be the case in a number of systems,[4,5] and is crucial to our approach to vaccination.

Locked states

The induction of antibody in rodents prevents the subsequent induction of DTH,[11] a phenomenon already referred to as immune deviation. Various conditions have been delineated by which the parenteral administration of antigen to immunocometent animals renders them unresponsive for the induction of antibody. These are the administration of doses of antigen sub- and supra-immunogenic for the induction of antibody, the administration of antigens with few foreign sites, and the administration of antigen in a manner that would induce antibody but for the co-administration of an immuno-suppressive drug. These four conditions also result in the generation of antigen-specific T cells that inhibit the induction of antibody. In addition, these four conditions of antigen administration also result in the induction of DTH. It was this correlation of conditions that led to the proposal that these unresponsive states reflect regulation whose physiological purpose is to ensure that antibody is not induced during the course of a strong cell-mediated response.[14,15] It seems natural, in view of the finding that mice given low or high doses of antigen can be both rendered unresponsive at the level of antibody production and induced to express DTH to the antigen, that these unresponsive states be referred to as cell-mediated low-zone and high-zone immune deviation respectively.[26] The existence of states in which animals do not mount antibody responses but express cell-mediated immunity, and in which their immune response to the antigen appears to be locked into a cell-mediated mode, is central to our vaccination strategy.

Establishment of stable cell-mediated immunity that renders "susceptible" BALB/c mice resistant to Leishmania major

BALB/c mice have been generally regarded as intrinsically susceptible to *L. major* because they inevitably mount an ineffective antibody response upon substantial infection.[27] We thought it likely that mice, given a sufficiently low number of parasites, would induce stable cell-mediated immunity, if the parasites did not replicate too fast. We therefore examined whether BALB/c mice had a progressive infection when injected subcutaneously into the foot with very low doses of parasites. We found that many mice showed no evidence of lesion as detected by increase in foot size; some showed a small lesion that resolved with time. We therefore thought it possible that a cell-mediated response was mounted and that low-zone immune deviation might have been established. Challenge of these mice between two and a half and eighteen months after exposure to a low dose of parasites with a high, normally pathogenic dose of parasites, shows that the low dose exposed mice have become resistant.[27]

The hypothesis we favored to explain these observations was that exposure of "susceptible" mice to low doses of parasites had resulted in the establishment of low-zone immune deviation to the antigens of *L. major* and hence in resistance to the parasite. We successfully tested several predictions of this hypothesis. Firstly, infection with low numbers of parasites induced only a cell-mediated response; infection with higher doses induced a transient cell-mediated response that decayed as IgG antibody was produced. Secondly, we found a remarkable correlation between the expression of DTH and IgG_1 antibody production and the production of IFN-γ and IL-4, respectively, by spleen cells of infected animals upon stimulation with parasite antigens (Bretscher et al[27] and J.N. Menon and P.A.Bretscher, in preparation).

Thirdly, exposure of mice to a low dose of parasites a few months before challenge with a high dose dramatically affected the nature of the immune response to this high dose; a prolonged DTH response occurred, parasite-specific IgG_1 antibody production was decreased roughly 10-fold, and parasite-specific IgG_{2a} antibody production was increased very substantially. These changes are reflected in the cytokines produced; IFN-γ production is sustained over a period of at least 12 weeks, and the ratio of IFN-γ/IL-4 production is at 10 weeks post challenge about 60 times that in normal animals challenged with a high dose of parasites (ref. 27 and J.N. Menon and P.A. Bretscher, in preparation). This increase in IFN-γ production probably explains the increased production of parasite-specific IgG_{2a} antibody, as the production of this subclass appears to be facilitated by IFN-γ.[28]

Some features of this system appear noteworthy in the context of attempts to understand the nature of the immune response in other infectious diseases. Firstly, it is possible, by carefully titrating in small increments the number of parasites used for infection, to find a dose that results in a "subclinical infection" in about 50% of the animals, and in a prolonged and chronic form of the disease in most of the other mice. Giving a three-fold lower dose of parasites results in most mice experiencing a subclinical infection, whereas giving a three-fold higher dose results in most mice experiencing progressive disease. Mice expressing chronic disease express DTH over a period of months, and produce parasite specific antibody of both IgG_1 and IgG_{2a} subclasses. They appear to be mounting a stable, mixed Th1 and Th2 response, or one intermediate between these two extremes (P.A. Bretscher and G. Wei, in preparation). We appear to have experimentally defined a state that we call borderline leishmaniasis in view of its similarity to the human condition of borderline leprosy, in which both anti-parasite antibody is produced and anti-parasite DTH is expressed. This model may be valuable in examining what immunological manipulations can result in a cure of borderline disease. Such manipulations that are able in general to bend on-going responses from a humoral, Th2-type to a cell-mediated, Th1-type mode may provide treatments for diseases caused by the class of pathogen susceptible only to a cell-mediated attack.

Secondly, mice given very low doses of parasites mount a substantial DTH response that decays after about three months. We believe this decay reflects the death of most of the parasites, such that the parasite antigen is not produced at a level sufficient to maintain the induction of a DTH response. However, these mice are highly resistant. Their spleen cells contain protective cells as assayed by their ability to confer protection to normal mice when given to such mice close to the time of infection with a high and normally pathogenic dose of parasites. These protective cells express negligible DTH to parasite antigens but give rise to a potent DTH response when the mice, given these protective cells, are challenged with a high dose of parasites. Interestingly, spleen cells from mice with chronic, borderline leishmaniasis express DTH but do not contain potent protective cells. In this case, the existence of protective cells is associated with an absence of expression of DTH and is associated with the capacity to generate an anamnestic DTH response. I have argued elsewhere, partly on the basis of these observations, that the long-term induction of PPD-skin sensitivity that usually follows BCG vaccination may represent the induction of borderline immunity and may not result in the efficient generation of protective cells. This line of argument suggests it may be possible to dramatically increase the efficacy of BCG vaccination against tuberculosis and leprosy just by lowering the dose of BCG employed for vaccination.[26]

Is it likely that the establishment of resistance in "susceptible" BALB/c mice against L. major provides a general approach to vaccination against those parasites uniquely susceptible to cell-mediate attack?

a) Is the dependence of the induction of cell-mediated, Th1-type versus the induction of antibody, Th2-type responses likely to be generally dependent upon antigen/parasite dose?

We have argued above that this dose-dependence follows from inherent characteristics of cells of the immune system, namely the difference in the threshold of helper T cell-dependent signals required to induce different classes of precursor cells. From this perspective, the manner in which the dose affects the class induced will always be the same. This argument is supported by observation. It seems likely that both HIV-1 and the mycobacteria responsible for leprosy and tuberculosis are uniquely contained by a cell-mediated attack.[2,3] We have preliminary but strong evidence that there is a similar dose dependence of the class induced against both live BCG given intravenously to BALB/c mice and in the response of these same mice to dead HIV administered intraperitoneally (Bretscher et al, unpublished observations).

b) Can cell-mediated low-zone immune deviation be generally established for any antigen?

The safe answer is that time will tell. Nevertheless, I should like to put forward an interpretation of certain observations that implies that such imprinting has been successfully achieved many times by people working in the field of tumor immunology.

Many studies, particularly the systematic studies by North, have explained some paradoxes of tumor immunology. Observations have shown that the inoculation of a lethal dose of tumor cells into animals usually induces a protective, cell-mediated response. The question of why these animals die was most clearly demonstrated when North and his colleagues showed that expression of this protective immunity decayed as tumor-specific $CD4^+$ T cells were generated that were able to inhibit the induction/expression of the protective cell-mediated response.[29] Thus, a protective, cell-mediated, presumably Th1-like response is first induced against the tumors studied, and this protective response decays as tumor-specific CD4+ T cells are generated that inhibit this cell-mediated response. The kinetic pattern of appearance and interaction between these two classes of T cells is highly analagous to what one sees in mice susceptible to *L. major* and given a pathogenic challenge of parasites; a protective cell-mediated response is induced first, that decays as antibody is induced, and this decay is associated with the appearance of Th2-like cells. We believe that these Th2-like cells inhibit the protective Th1 response. Partly based upon this similarity, I suggest that it is useful to identify the tumor-specific CD4+ T cells, able to inhibit the induction/expression of the tumor-specific cell-mediated response, as Th2-like cells.

The most generally efficacious way of vaccinating mice against tumors is to inject a lethal dose of tumor cells either intradermally or subcutaneously and wait for about nine days, when they have a diameter of about 1 mm, and then to surgically remove the large bulk of the tumor mass. Such mice, if challenged some weeks after excision of the tumor, are resistant. Such excision-priming involves surgically removing the tumor around that time when a maximal, Th1-like cell-mediated response has been mounted. I suggest that removal of the bulk of the tumor at this time abrogates the further development of the immune response and the generation of Th2-like cells that suppress the protective response. Thus these excised mice become, with time, resistant. Their state seems to be analagous to the state we have achieved by exposing "susceptible" BALB/c mice to low doses of parasites. This low dose of parasites also only induces a protective cell-mediated response. If this analogy is truly valid, it follows that effective imprinting has been achieved many times in mice against different kinds of tumors.

c) Is there a strategy of vaccination such that a standard vaccination procedure can be universally efficacious despite the genetic diversity of the human population?

Most mouse strains are said to be resistant to *L. major*. However, old observations show that some "resistant" strains, if infected with a very large number of parasites, are susceptible, and that this susceptibility is associated with an antibody response exclusive of significant DTH.[30] These old observations support our recently formulated proposal that resistance and susceptibility are not absolute but conditional traits. They also support the suggestion that in both "resistant" and "susceptible" mice the dose of parasites determines whether a protective or non-protective immune response is induced, with lower doses favoring protection. What differentiates different strains is not the pattern of dependence of class of immunity induced upon parasite dose, but the absolute scale of this dependence. This idea is expressed in Figure 3.

Consider what we would expect to happen if the three strains of mice, whose immune response characteristics are indicated in Figure 3, were immunized with dose "A" of parasite antigen. An antibody response would be induced in all individuals, and memory TsDTH cells would be generated. Such immunization would favor the induction of antibody upon subsequent exposure, such as that following natural infection. Such immunization is expected to increase susceptibility of mice belonging to all strains.

Immunization with dose C would induce only a cell-mediated response in mice of strains 1 and 3, and would not immunize mice of strain 2, and

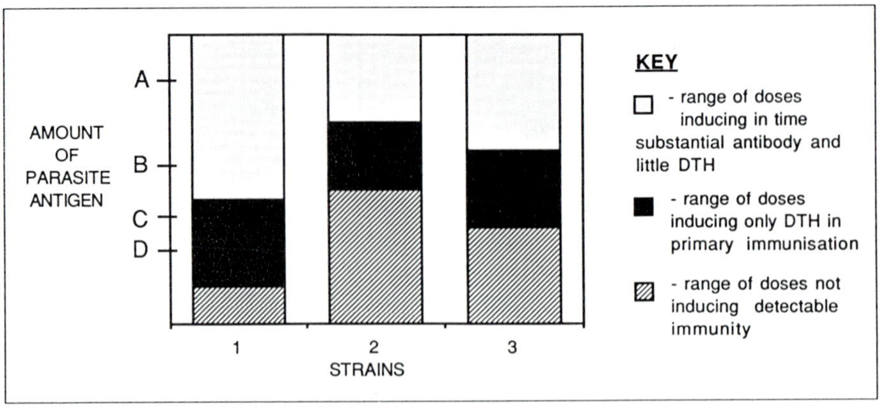

Fig. 3. Illustration of a strategy by which a standard vaccination procedure can be efficacious in a genetically diverse population of individuals. For explanation, see text.

hence make the mice of strains 1 and 3 more resistant and leave mice of strain 2 unaffected. Administration of the dose D would render mice of strain 1 more resistant and not affect mice of strains 2 and 3.

Consider what would happen if we gave a slowly growing parasite, such as BCG, at the dose D. Such a dose would induce cell-mediated immunity in mice of strain 1. As there is no effective immune response in mice of strains 2 and 3, the parasite is expected to grow until it reaches a threshold where it can induce a cell-mediated response. This example illustrates the potential consequences of administering a very small dose that is itself below that able to induce antibody in any member of the population, but which either induces cell-mediated immunity, or is itself below the threshold required to induce such a response; in this case, the parasite is expected to grow until it reaches the threshold, with tl. consequence that it will induce cell-mediated immunity in mice of all strains. We expect, by extrapolation, that a sufficiently low dose will induce a cell-mediated response in all humans independently of their genetic constitution. This may provide a strategy by which a standard vaccination procedure can provide universal protection against those parasites uniquely susceptible to a cell-mediated attack.

References

1. Pearson RD, Wheeler DA, Harrison LH, Kay HD. The immunobiology of leishmaniasis. Rev Infect Dis 1983; 5: 907-927
2. Turk JL, Bryceson ADM. Immunological phenomena in leprosy and related diseases. Adv Immunol 1971; 13: 209-266
3. Ellner JJ et al. Regulation of the immune response to *Mycobacterium tuberculosis.* In: Ayoub EM, Cassel GH, Branche WC, Microbial Determinants of Virulence and Host Response, Washington DC : American Society for Microbiology, 1990: 77-90.
4. Parish CR. The relationship between humoral and cell-mediated immunity. Transplant Rev 1972; 13: 35-66
5. Lagrange PH, MacKaness GB, Miller TE. The influence of dose and route of antigen injection on the immunological induction of T cells. J Exp Med

1974; 139: 528-542

6. Locksley RM, Scott, P. Helper T cell subsets in mouse leishmaniasis: induction, expansion and effector function. In: Ash C, Gallagher RG, Immunoparasitol Today. Cambridge:Elsevier Trends Jounals,1991: A58-A61.
7. Howard JG. Immunological regulation and control of experimental leishmaniasis. Int Rev Exp Pathol 1986; 28: 79-116
8. Blanden RV. T cell responses to bacterial and viral infections. Trans Rev 1974; 19: 56-88
9. Mosmann TR, Coffman RL. Th1 and Th2 cells: different patterns of lymphokine secretion lead to different functional properties. Ann Rev Immunol 1989; 7: 145-73
10. Shearer GM, Clerici M. T helper cell dysfunction in asymptomatic, HIV1-seropositive individuals: the role of Th1-Th2 cross-regulation. In: Fitch, FW, Ishizaka I, Lachman PJ, Chemical Immunology. Basel:Karger S, 1992: 21-43 ; Salk J et al. A strategy for prophylactic vaccination against HIV. Science 1993;260:1270-72
11. Asherson CR, Stone SH. Selective and specific inhibition of 24 hour skin reactions in the guinea pig. I. Immune deviation: description of the phenomenon and the effect of splenectomy. Immunol 1962; 9: 205-217
12. Mitchison NA. Induction of immunological paralysis in two zones of dosage. Proc Roy Soc B 1964; 161: 275-476
13. Weber G, Kolsch E. Transfer of low zone tolerance to normal syngeneic mice by theta positive cells . Eur J Immunol 1973; 13: 767-772
14. Bretscher PA. Hypothesis: On the control between cell-mediated IgM and IgG immunity. Cell Immunol 1974; 13: 171-195
15. Bretscher PA. Significance and mechanisms of the cellular regulation of the immune response. Fed Proc 1981; 40: 1473-78
16. Ramshaw IA, Bretscher PA, Parish CR. Regulation of the immune response. I Suppression of delayed-type hypersensitivity by T cells from mice expressing humoral immunity. Eur J Immunol 1976; 6:674-679
17 Ramshaw IA, Bretscher PA, Mckenzie IFC, Parish CR. Discrimination of suppressor T cells of humoral and cell-mediated immunity by anti-Ly and anti-Ia sera. Cell Immunol 1977; 31: 364-369
18. Bretscher PA. In vitro analysis of the cellular interactions between unprimed lymphocytes responsible for determining the class of response an antigen induces; specific T cells switch a cell-mediated response to a humoral response. J Immunol 1983; 131: 1103-1107
19. Bretscher PA. Regulation of the immune response induced by antigen. I Specific T cells switch the in vivo immune response from a cell-mediated to a humoral mode. Cell Immunol 1983; 81: 345-56
20. Ramshaw IA, Bretscher PA, Parish CR. Regulation of the immune response. II Repressor T cells in cyclophosphamide-induced tolerant mice. Eur J Immunol 1977; 7: 180-185
21. Tuttosi S, Bretscher PA. Antigen-specific CD8+ T cells switch the immune response induced by antigen from an IgG to a cell-mediated mode. J Immunol 1992; 148: 397-403
22. Bretscher PA. The regulatory function of CD4+ and CD8+ T-cell subsets in immune regulation. Res Immunol 1991; 142: 45-49
23. Mosmann TR, Moore KW. The role of IL-10 in cross-regulation of Th1 and Th2 responses. In: Ash C, Gallagher RG, Immunoparasitol Today.

Cambridge:Elsevier Trends Jounals,1991: A49-A53
24. Mosmann TR. Cytokine secretion phenotypes of Th cells:how many subsets, how much regulation? Res in Immunol 1991; 142: 9-13
25. Tucker MJ, Bretscher PA. T cells cooperating in the induction of delayed-type hypersensitivity act via the linked recognition of antigenic determinants. J Exp Med 1982; 155:1037-1049
26. Bretscher PA. A strategy to improve the efficacy of vaccination against tuberculosis and leprosy. Immunol Today 1992; 13: 342-345
27. Bretscher et al. Establishment of stable cell-mediated immunity that makes "susceptible" mice resistant to *Leishmania major*. Science 1992; 257: 539-542
28. Snapper CM, Paul WE. Interferon-g and B cell stimulatory factor-1 reciprocally regulate Ig isotype production. Science 1987; 236: 944-47
29. North RJ. The murine antitumor immune response and its therapeutic manipulation. Adv Immunol 1984; 35: 89-155
30. Preson PM, Behbehani K, Dumonde DC. Experimental cutaneous leishmaniasis VI: anergy and allergy in the cellular immune response during non-healing infection in different strains of mice. J Clin Lab Immunol 1978; 1: 207-219

CHAPTER 8

CD4+ FUNCTIONAL T CELL SUBSETS: THEIR ROLES IN INFECTION AND VACCINE DEVELOPMENT

Gene M. Shearer
Mario Clerici

INTRODUCTION

CD4+ T lymphocytes can be divided into subsets on the basis of their surface markers and functional properties. CD4+ cell markers are commonly detected by monoclonal antibodies and flow cytometry and include subcategories such as CD45RA and CD45RO that distinguish naive from memory cells. Functional distinctions within the CD4 subset can include helpers, effectors and suppressors, although CD4+ cells are often considered to be synonymous with helper cells. A further distinction within CD4+ cells involves the immunoregulatory cytokine profiles produced by this subset. Thus both murine[1] and human[2] CD4+ lymphocytes have been cloned and subdivided into functionally distinct "Th1" and "Th2" phenotypes on the basis of the cytokines they produce. However, due to the lack of antibodies that identify these subgroups, investigators have had to rely exclusively on cytokine expression or production to distinguish between these two types of cells. The present chapter considers some aspects of Th1-like (type 1) and Th2-like (type 2) responses in infection and vaccine development. We summarize our findings of HIV-infected individuals as they apply to type 1 and type 2 cytokine profiles, compare them with other infections and speculate on vaccines designed from the perspective of type 1 and type 2 responses.

Strategies in Vaccine Design edited by Gordon L. Ada, D.Sc.

TH1 VERSUS TH2 CD4+ CELLS AND TYPE 1 VERSUS TYPE 2 RESPONSES

$CD4^+$ T cells can be categorized on the basis of the cytokines they produce, and to some extent, on the types of effector functions that they enhance or suppress. Thus it is well documented that murine T lymphocytes can be cloned so as to produce interferon-γ (IFN-γ) and interleukin 2 (IL-2), produced by Th1 clones or IL-4, IL-5 and IL-10, the products of Th2 clones.[3] Recently human T cells have been cloned to produce similar cytokine profiles.[4] It should be noted however that IL-10 is produced by both human Th1 and Th2 clones.[5] The Th1 versus Th2 issue is further complicated by the identification of less differentiated subgroups termed TH0 and THp.[1,3,6]

Another distinction can be made concerning the Th1 and Th2 cytokine issue that is not based on the cytokines produced by cloned $CD4^+$ cells. This distinction is based rather on the cytokines detected in primary cultures from patients' peripheral blood mononuclear cells (PBMC) that can be produced by $CD4^+$ and/or $CD8^+$ cells and/or by accessory cells. Irrespective of which cell type(s) produce these cytokine, the cytokines can regulate $CD4^+$ T cell responses in a way that resembles the Th1 and Th2 dichotomy. Thus we have adopted the terminology of "type 1" and "type 2" responses to denote certain cytokine profiles expressed and/or produced by unfractionated PBMC. By our definition a type 1 response would exhibit a cytokine profile of high IFN-γ and high IL-2 (the latter to recall antigens) and low IL-4 and IL-10 expression or production. A type 2 response would exhibit a cytokine profile of low IFN-γ and IL-2 (to recall antigens) and high IL-4 or IL-10 (see Table 1).[7-10] Although mitogens are often used to stimulate cytokine production by T cells or PBMC in vitro, mitogen-stimulated IL-2 production does not distinguish between type 1 and type 2 responses in unfractionated PBMC (see below). It is sometimes considered that type 1 responses are associated with enhanced cell-mediated effector immunity and that type 2 responses are associated with humoral effector immunity. Although these generalities may predominate, some of the cytokines characteristic of type 1 responses can help antibody responses (for example IgG_{2A} in mice and IgG_1 in humans).[11] It appears that type 1 responses provide help for opsonizing antibodies that bind Fc receptors, and that type 2 responses help non-opsonizing IgG, IgA and IgE responses.[12] Furthermore, type 1 and type 2 cytokine profiles are not necessarily absolute, as there may be a gradual shift from one profile to the other, with some overlapping in cytokine profiles. Finally the process is likely to be dynamic (see Fig. 1).

Table 1. Immunoregulatory cytokine profiles For type 1 and type 2 responses

Type 1 cytokine profile:	Type 2 cytokine profile:
High IL-2 to recall antigens	Low IL-2 to recall antigens
High IFN-γ	Low IFN-γ
Low IL-4	High IL-4
Low IL-10	High IL-10

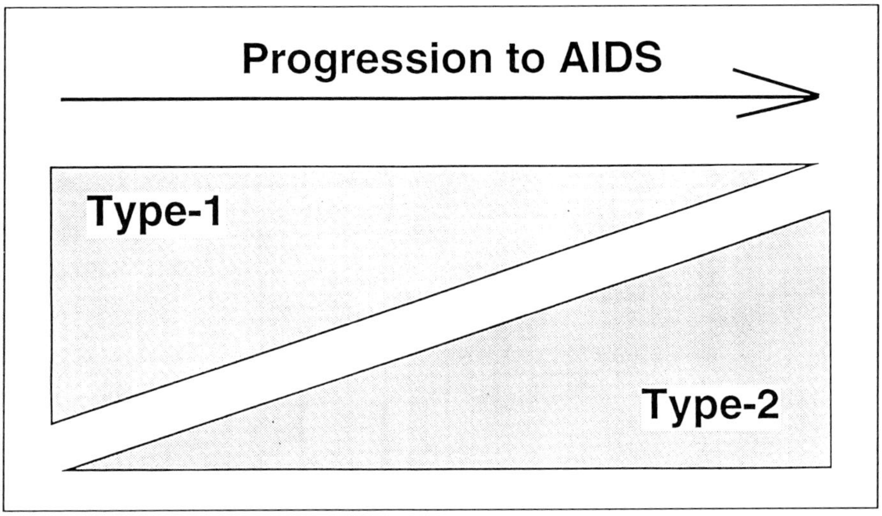

Fig. 1. Illustration of overlapping nature of type 1 and type 2 responses in the progression toward AIDS.

TYPE 1 VERSUS TYPE 2 RESPONSES AND PROTECTION VERSUS SUSCEPTIBILITY

In general immunization against an antigen stimulates both the cellular and humoral effector arms of the immune system, and protective immunity against many infectious agents involves both cell-mediated immunity (CMI), often in the form of cytotoxic T lymphocytes (CTL), and antibody (Ab) production. Typically CMI appears first after immunization, followed by a rise in Ab titer. CMI is frequently observed to decline concomitantly with increasing Ab titers, which can remain elevated for extended periods of time. This does not necessarily mean however that effector CMI is undetectable or insignificant in the presence of Ab. Because of the cross-regulatory nature of certain immunoregulatory cytokines (see Fig. 2),[1] we view this decline in CMI and the increase in Ab as the natural consequence of an increase in type 2 immunoregulatory cytokines such as IL-4 and IL-10. If protective immunity involves both CMI and Ab, such a dynamic change in the effector arms of the immune response would be beneficial. Immunity against influenza A virus is a classical example in which both CTL and Ab contribute to protection and recovery from infection.[13] However, if an infection occurred for which CMI was protective but Ab was either not protective or was considerably less protective than CMI, we could envision a situation in which the classical immune response of strong CMI followed by downregulation of CMI and a concomitant increase in Ab would not be beneficial, provided the initial cellular response did not eliminate or control the infection. From the perspective of type 1 versus type 2 cytokine regulation of immune responses, we perceive that such a situation could and does exist. Furthermore this is not a rare occurrence, as several agents that induce chronic, latent or "smoldering" infections tend to result in CMI followed by Ab responses, the latter of which do not appear to be associated with protection. Some examples include helminth parasitic infections,[14] the lepromatous phase of leprosy,[15] syphilis[16] and asymptomatic period of HIV infection (see below).[10,17]

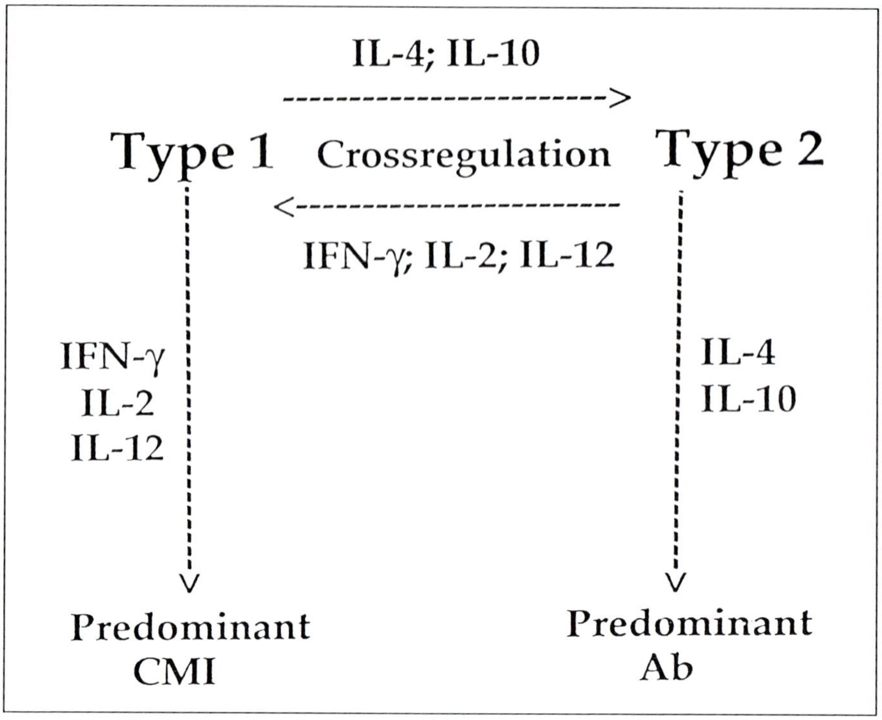

Fig. 2. Schematic diagram of type 1 (Th1-like) and type 2 (Th2-like) cytokine profiles and the effector responses they predominantly regulate.

These infections are also associated with a type 1-to-type 2 switch in the immunoregulatory cytokine profile, such that animals or humans so infected fail to respond or respond poorly by CMI to other unrelated antigens. Instead they can go directly into an Ab production mode. Thus such infections can induce immune dysregulation so as to exert an effect on immune reactivity to other non-crossreacting antigens. A example of this phenomenon was reported in BALB/c mice, which normally respond to sperm whale myoglobin by CMI followed by Ab. Infection of susceptible BALB/c mice with the helminth parasite *Schistisoma mansoni* prior to immunization with myoglobin induced a type 1-to-type 2 switch, which resulted in the production of myoglobin-specific Ab without the usual CMI phase.[18] In a follow-up and related study, immunization with myoglobin was substituted by infection with vaccinia. The parasite-infected animals did not generate a strong anti-vaccinia cellular response and were thereby rendered susceptible to the viral infection.[19] It should also be noted that antigenic stimulation induced by a chronic graft-versus-host reaction, in which the grafted $CD4^+$ cells recognize only class II major histocompatibility antigens of the host, induces a similar condition of loss of CMI to unrelated antigens.[20] Furthermore humans who have systemic lupus erythematosus can present with a pattern of reduced CMI despite being in a state of B cell hyperactivity.[21] Thus it may be that chronic antigenic stimulation irrespective of whether it is induced by an infectious agent can induce a state of prolonged immune dysregulation which is generally skewed toward upregulation of Ab and downregulation of CMI (a type 1-to-type 2 switch).

It should be noted that at least one human virus induces a rapid type 1-to-type 2 switch that results in T cell anergy that can last for two years or more.[22, 23] Thus measles virus infection results in a rapid type 1-to-type 2 shift with a reduction in the production of IL-2 and IFN-γ and increases in IL-4 and IL-10 production.[23] This shift is much more rapid than in HIV infection. Furthermore, measles infection of infants can be associated with increased mortality that is suspected to be due to immune dysfunction and susceptibility to other infections.[22] Similarly, immunization of infants with high titered live attenuated measles vaccine can be associated with T cell anergy and increased mortality.[22] A major difference between measles and HIV infection is that in the anergy associated with HIV infection is more prolonged and infection is not cleared, which ultimately results in CD4± cell depletion.

TYPE 1/TYPE 2 RESPONSES IN HIV INFECTION

The best known immunologic change that occurs as the result of infection with HIV is the dramatic but protracted decline in the number of $CD4^+$ T cells (CD4 count),[24] which has been attributed to the loss of T helper cell function. However other more subtle changes occur, including B cell activation and hypergammaglobulinema,[24] as well as the loss of T helper cell function that occurs prior to a critical decline in CD4 count.[7,25,26] We found this immune dysregulation to be associated with changes in the immunoregulatory cytokine profile such that IL-2 and IFN-γ production were decreased concomitant with an increase in IL-4, which was followed by an increase in IL-10 production.[7-9] These observations led us to postulate that a type 1-to-type 2 cytokine switch occurs in HIV^+ individuals in progression to AIDS, and that a dominant type 1 cytokine profile is protective against progression of HIV^+ individuals to AIDS, as well as against HIV infection.[10, 17] In contrast, we view a dominant type 2 cytokine profile as characteristic of a susceptible condition for both progression and infection.

Some additional points of evidence suggest a role for CMI in protection against HIV infection and AIDS progression. First the acute phase of HIV infection results in viremia, followed by a dramatic decline in virus detected in the blood. This reduction in viral titer occurs simultaneously with the appearance of virus-specific CTL.[27] Second the increase in viral titer near the time of AIDS diagnosis is frequently timed with the loss in CTL activity.[28] Third long-term survivors of HIV infection appear to have stronger CTL responses than individuals who are progressing more rapidly to AIDS.[29] Fourth we have identified numerous individuals who have been exposed to HIV (many of them, multiple times), but who are seronegative.[30-33] Approximately 50% of such individuals exhibit strong HIV-specific CMI without detectable serum antibodies. These CMI responses include HIV-induced proliferation and IL-2 production, as well as HIV-specific CTL in some individuals. Fifth macaques exposed to very low non-infectious doses of simian immunodeficiency virus (SIV), and subsequently challenged with an infectious dose of the homologous virus did not produce antibodies, were PCR-negative, exhibited no signs of an AIDS-like illness, but had strong SIV-specific CMI activity one year after challenge. In contrast, macaques that received the same challenge but that did not get the initial non-infectious inoculum seroconverted, were PCR-positive, developed an

AIDS-like illness, but did not exhibit SIV-specific CMI one year after challenge (M. Clerici et al, manuscript submitted for publication). Although there have been some reports of antibody protection against HIV and SIV infection,[34, 35] it may be that neutralizing antibodies do not play a major role in protection against infection with these retroviruses.[36] It is beginning to appear that despite more than a decade of attempting to develop an AIDS vaccine based on antibody, protective immunity will reside mainly in CMI, and stimulation of a type 1 cytokine profile. This does not mean however that there are no protective antibodies against HIV infection or progression to AIDS, and it may be that antibodies stimulated by a type 1 profile will also contribute to protection.

HIV has recently been considered to be an extraordinary virus in that its integration into host cells is mandatory and that transmission can occur via cell-to-cell interaction.[22] We suggest that another extraordinary characteristic of HIV may reside in the relative lack of protection by antibodies against infection and/or progression to disease. Based on these points we view HIV infection as fitting into the category of those infectious agents noted in the previous section that induce chronic antigenic stimulation. In fact a state of immune activation is characteristic of HIV infection.[37] Thus by inducing a type 1-to-type 2 switch, HIV infection downregulates the very component of the immune system on which it likely depends for protection against progression to AIDS and possibly against successful HIV infection.

TYPE 1/TYPE 2 RESPONSES FOR AN AIDS VACCINE

The objective of this section is to extend our observations of immunologic exposure to HIV in the absence of detectable infection to probe into approaches that we suggest for the redesign of an AIDS vaccine. Assuming that neutralizing antibody is not sufficiently protective to prevent HIV infection, how could or should an effective AIDS vaccine be developed? Because of the type 1-to-type 2 cytokine profile switch detected in the progression to AIDS, we would approach the problem from an immunoregulatory cytokine perspective. As noted above a type 1 cytokine profile can provide help for certain classes of antibodies as well as enhancing CMI. Thus it is possible that a type 1 response would not only provide help for CMI but also for certain types of antibodies. We do not know whether the neutralizing antibody responses that have been used to test for efficient protection against HIV or SIV infection are generated from type 1, type 2 or both types of helper responses. However it is probable that such human antibodies were generated by a type 2 response because the adjuvant used was alum, which is considered to be a type 2 adjuvant.[11] If both CMI and Ab responses can be generated by either type of functional T helper cell, one might expect to be able to achieve the best of both worlds—CMI and Ab. It has been documented that both CMI and Ab responses can co-exist in HIV+ individuals,[38] as well as in uninfected AIDS vaccines.[39] Furthermore HIV+ individuals given the rgp160 vaccine for immune-based therapy can show elevated CMI and Ab responses.[40] Yet protection from infection and progression to disease did not occur in naturally-infected individuals who generated both HIV-specific CMI and Ab responses, and it is too early to know the effect of the immune-based therapy trials. The fact that CMI and/or Ab failed to protect unimmunized naturally-infected individuals is not surprising because the immune systems of naive individuals would not have been primed to HIV. Furthermore the fact that CMI and Ab can be simultaneously detected in the same patient does not tell us whether either or both of the effector responses were optimally stimulated. It is possible that both CMI and Ab would be detected but that the CMI response would be less than maximal when Ab are detected, due to type 2 cytokine-induced downregulation of CMI to below optimal protective levels.

Because of the recent findings that CMI but not Ab appeared to be protective against SIV infection in macaques [M. Clerici et al, manuscript submitted for publication], we suggest that CMI will be the major mechanism for protection against SIV and HIV. Our opinion is also based on the fact (noted above) that many individuals who have been exposed to HIV generate strong HIV-specific CMI responses, but do not produce antibodies detected by standard assays. Although such individuals may have been only exposed to HIV antigens and not infected, 3 of approximately 60 individuals tested were found to contain HIV DNA by the polymerase chain reaction [M. Clerici et al, manuscript submitted for publication]. Furthermore the life styles of some of the individuals were such that they should have frequently encountered infectious virus during the five to seven years that they have been followed and remain seronegative. We interpret these findings to indicate that these individuals first encountered non-infectious or low doses of infectious HIV which resulted in the selective immunization of a CMI response without activating the Ab-producing arm of immunity.[17]

The selective activation of CMI but not Ab by low dose immunization is a well-documented phenomenon in mice,[41,42] and has also been observed in uninfected humans immunized with low doses (40-80 μg) of the rgp160 candidate AIDS vaccine.[43] Thus we view low dose immunization as one component of a vaccine protocol designed primarily to optimize the CMI effector arm, possibly CTL (see Table 2). It may be that certain antibodies will also be elicited by the same protocol, but we would not expect the Ab response to predominate. Based on research performed mainly by Bretscher[44] (see Chapter 7), it may be possible by low dose immunization to "lock in" a type 1 response and prevent its decline by the activation of type 2 cytokines.[17] This could be an advantage if CMI is more protective against HIV infection than Ab. Figure 3 illustrates a comparison of the effects of immunization under conditions that would induce the more traditional response of CMI followed by Ab (upper panel) compared to conditions that would induce predominantly CMI (lower panel). Type 1 and type 2 cytokines could contribute to the change from CMI to Ab predominance in the upper panel. If persistent CMI is more protective than a wave of strong CMI, followed by a decline in CMI concomitant with increasing Ab titer, then the immune response profile shown in the lower panel will be more protective than that in the upper panel. This is our view of the immune response to HIV and the AIDS vaccine issue. A primary immune response to a successful infection with HIV should appear similar to the upper panel, because a relatively high dose of HIV will overwhelm an unprimed immune system, and due to the higher dose, will induce a traditional response of CMI followed by Ab. In contrast the response to a limited infection or to HIV antigen only should appear as in the lower panel because the dose will be too low to activate an Ab response[17] and a cell-mediated effector response will not only be dominant but will also be persistent.

Table 2. Immune response patterns in HIV-individuals immunized with rgp160

Immunizing dose (mg)	Type of response CMI	Ab
40 or 80	+	-
160	+	+
>160	+	+

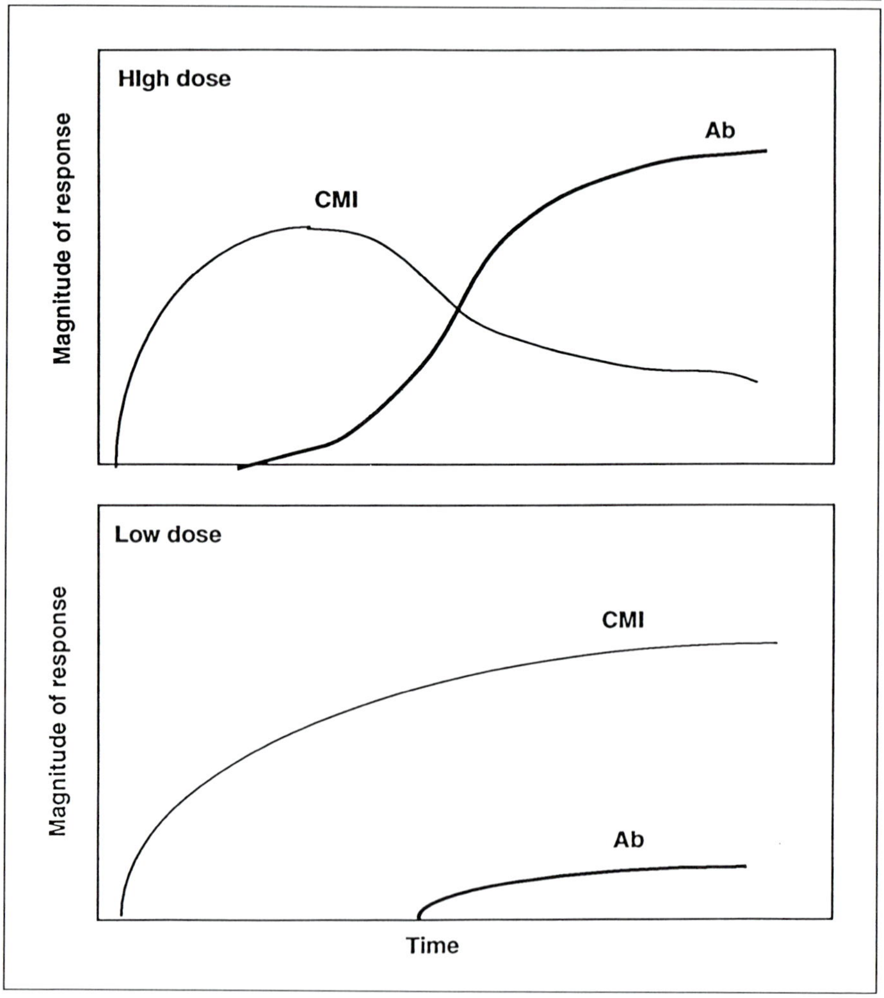

Fig. 3. Model of kinetics of CMI and Ab production at relatively high and low doses of antigen.

The above suggestions are focused on a prophylactic vaccine, and do not necessarily apply to immune-based therapy. It is unclear whether neutralizing antibodies provide protection for individuals already infected with HIV. However because the switch from a type 1 to a type 2 cytokine profile is associated with progression to AIDS,[7-10,45] it is likely that CMI will provide a major component of protective immunity against progression of disease. We suggest therefore that immune-based therapy consider the type 1 and type 2 cytokine profiles of HIV+ individuals as part of the protocol. In particular, patients would first be classified as to their cytokine profiles. If they exhibit a predominant type 2 greater than type 1 profile, consideration should be given to cytokine-based therapy designed to reverse this profile to a type 1 greater than type 2 profile. This reversal might be achieved by administering cross-regulatory cytokines such as IL-2, IFN-γ or IL-12.[46] If needed, immunization with an AIDS vaccine might then be given to boost CMI.

An alternate possibility is the use of adjuvants to induce a type 1-to-type 2 switch. It has been noted that immunization with BCG can protect against leprosy, a disease that involves a type 1-to-type 2 switch.[15] Thus this type 1 adjuvant[11] may have induced or maintained a protective dominant type 1 cytokine profile. In this context it is noteworthy that a recent preliminary study suggests that immunization of HIV+ individuals with *M. vaccae* results in lack of progression of HIV infection and loss of AIDS-like symptoms.[47] Is it possible to effect immune-based therapy against AIDS simply by immunizing with type 1-promoting adjuvants? Such an approach would be inexpensive and would not introduce many of the potential risks now associated with HIV vaccines.

Factors that need to be considered in the design of any vaccine protocol aimed at selectively taking advantage of one effector arm or the other will need to include antigen dose, the adjuvant, route of immunization, and possibly even the antigenic determinants. One should also be aware that type 1 and type 2 cytokine profiles and the effector responses that they regulate may be compartmentalized such that lymphoid tissues in different parts of the body may exhibit different immune profiles. These differences may be the result of localized immunologic stimuli, infections or inflammatory reactions.[48]

CONCLUSIONS

We have developed an infectious model based partly on fact and partly on hypothesis for protection and susceptibility to HIV infection and AIDS progression. It has been the general experience of viral immunologists to conclude that both CMI and Ab contribute to protection. What has not been considered until now is the possibility that we may not have the option of maximizing both arms of the immune system simultaneously, due to cytokine cross-regulation. On the basis of available data it appears that the cell-mediated arm of immunity is going to be more protective than antibody in HIV infection, and possibly could be the only protective component. The issue here may be that type 1 and type 2 cross-regulatory cytokines will govern the relative strengths of these two components of immunity, and that we may have to go with the component that proves to work best. It would be of interest to question whether there have been "failed" vaccine attempts for other infectious agents for which the immunologic readout was neutralizing antibodies. If such examples exist, perhaps these failures should be re-evaluated and new vaccine attempts based on CMI should be considered and tested as an alternative possibility. Thus we suggest that vaccine trials based only on the humoral (or only the cell-mediated) arm of the immune system are inadequate to determine the efficacy of candidate vaccines. Both arms of the immune system need to be examined—in concert and individually.

References

1. Mossman TR, Coffman RL. Th1 and Th2 cells: Different patterns of lymphokine secretion lead to different functional properties. Ann Rev Immunol 1989; 7: 145-173.
2. Romagnani S. Human Th1 and Th2 subsets: doubt no more. Immunol Today. 1991; 12: 256-257.
3. Swain SL, Bradley LM, Croft M, et al. Helper T-cell subsets: phenotype, function and the role of lymphokines in regulating their development. Immunol Rev. 1991; 123: 115-144.
4. Del Prete GF, De Carli M, Mastromauri C, et al. Purified protein derivative of *Mycobacterium tuberculosis* and excretory-secretory antigen(s) of *Toxocara canis* expand in vitro human T cells with stable and opposite (type 1 T helper of type 2 T helper) profile of cytokine production. J Clin Invest. 1991; 88: 346-350.
5. Del Prete GF, De Carli M, Almerigogna F, et al. Human IL-10 is produced by both type 1 helper T clones and type 2 helper T clones and inhibits their antigen-specific proliferation and cytokine production. J Immunol. 1993; 150: 353-360.
6. Mossman TR and Coffman RL. Heterogeneity of cytokine secretion patterns and functions of helper T cells. Adv Immunol 1989; 46: 111-147.
7. Clerici M, Stocks NI, Zajac RA, et al. Detection of three distinct patterns of T helper cell dysfunction in asymptomatic, human immunodeficiency virus-seropositive patients: independence of CD4 cell number and clinical staging. 1989; 84: 1892-1899.
8. Clerici M, Hakim FT, Venzon DJ et al. Changes in interleukin 2 and interleukin 4 production in asymptomatic, HIV-seropositive individuals. J Clin Invest. 1993; 91: 759-765.
9. Clerici M, Role of interleukin-10 (IL-10) in T helper cell dysfunction in asymptomatic individuals infected with the human immunodeficiency virus (HIV-1). J Clin Invest. in press.
10. Clerici M, Shearer GM. A Th1—>Th2 switch is a critical step in the etiology of HIV infection. Immunol Today. 1993; 14: 107-111.
11. Allison AC, Byars NE. Immunological Adjuvants: Desirable properties and side-effects. 1991; 28: 279-284.
12. Lanzavecchia A. Identifying strategies for immune intervention. Science. 1993; 260: 937-944.
13. Ada GL, Jones PD. The immune response to influenza virus. Curr Topics Microbiol Immunol. 1986; 128:1-54.
14. Sher A, Coffman RL. Regulation of immunity to parasites by T cells and T cell-derived cytokines. Advanc Immunol. 1992; 10: 385-409.
15. Yamamura M, Uyemura K, Deans RJ, et al. Defining protective responses to pathogens: cytokine profiles in leprosy lesions. Science. 1991; 254: 277-279.
16. Fitzgerald TS. The Th1/Th2 switch in syphilitic infection: Is it detrimental? Infect Immun 1992; 60: 3475- 3479.
17. Salk J, Bretscher PA, Salk PL, Clerici M, Shearer GM. A strategy for prophylactic vaccination against HIV. Science. 1993; 260: 1270-1272.
18. Kulberg MC, Pearce EJ, Hieny SE, Sher A, Berzofsky JA. Infection with *Schistisoma mansoni* alters Th1/Th2 cytokine responses to a non-parasite antigen. J immunol. 1992; 148: 3246-3270.

19. Actor JKD, Shiari M, Kulberg MC, et al. Helminth infection results in decreased virus-specific CD8+ cytotoxic T-cell and Th1 cytokine responses as well as delayed virus clearance. Proc Natl Acad Sci USA. 1993; 90: 948-952.
20. Via CS, Shearer GM. T-cell interactions in autoimmunity: insights from a murine model of graft-versus-host disease. Immunol Today. 1988; 9: 207-213.
21. Via CS, Tsokos, GC, Bermas B, et al. T cell-antigen-presenting cell interactions in human systemic lupus erythematosus: evidence for heterogenous expression of multiple defects. J Immunol. 1993; 151: 3914-3922.
22. Hilleman MR. The dilemma of AIDS vaccine and therapy. Possible clues from comparative pathogenesis with measles. AIDS Res Hum Retrovir. 1992; 8: 1743-1747.
23. Griffin DE, Ward BJ. Differential CD4 cell activation in measles. J Infect Dis. 1993; 168: 275-281.
24. Fauci AS. The human immunodeficiency virus: infectivity and mechanisms of pathogenesis. Science. 1988; 239: 617-623.
25. Shearer GM, Bernstein DC, Tung KS, et al. A model for the selective loss of major histocompatibility self-restricted T-cell immune responses during the development of acquired immune deficiency syndrome (AIDS) J Immunol 1986; 137: 2514-2521.
26. Miedema F, Chantal-Petie AJ, Terpstra FG, et al. Immunological abnormalities in human immunodeficiency virus (HIV)-infected asymptomatic homosexual men: HIV affects the immune system before CD4+ T cell depletion occurs. J Clin Invest. 1988; 82: 1908-1914.
27. Yasutomi Y, Reimann KA, Lord CI, et al. Simian immunodeficiency virus-specific CD8+ lymphocyte response in acutely infected rhesus monkeys. J Virol. 1993; 67: 1707-1711.
28. Greenough T, Brettler D, McManus M, et al. Low levels of HIV-1 specific T-lymphocyte activity and high viral load are associated with rapid disease progression in infected males with hemophilia. IX Inter Conf AIDS. Berlin 6-11 June 1993. (Abstract #PO-B01-1419) p288.
29. Harrer E, Harrer T, Buchbinder S, et al. HIV-specific CTL response in healthy long-term seropositive persons. IX Inter Conf AIDS. Berlin. 6-11 June 1993 (Abstract #PO-A22-0484) p 215.
30. Clerici M, Berzofsky JA, Shearer GM, Tacket CO. Exposure to human immunodeficiency virus type 1 indicated by HIV-specific T helper cell responses before detection of infection by polymerase chain reaction and serum antibodies. J Infect Dis. 1991; 164: 178-182.
31. Clerici M, Giorgi JV, Chou C-C, et al. Cell-mediated immune response to human immunodeficiency virus type I (HIV-1) in seronegative homosexual men with recent sexual exposure to HIV-1. J Infect Dis. 1992; 165: 1012-1019.
32. Clerici M, Sison AV, Berzofsky JA, et al. Cellular immune factors associated with mother-to-infant transmission of HIV. AIDS . 1993; in press.
33. Clerici M, Levin JM, Kessler HA, et al. Human immunodeficiency virus (HIV)-specific T helper cell activity in HIV seronegative health care workers accidentally exposed to HIV-contaminated blood. J Amer Med Assoc. in press.
34. Emini EA, Schleif WA, Nunberg JH, et al. Prevention of HIV-1 infection in chimpanzees by gp120 V3 dominant-specific monoclonal antibody. Nature. 1992; 355: 728-730.

35. Prince AM , Reesink H, Pascual D, et al. Prevention of HIV infection by passive immunization with HIV immunoglobulin. AIDS Res Hum Retrovir. 1991; 7: 971-973.
36. Prince AM, Horowitz B, Baker L, et al. Failure of a human immunodeficiency virus (HIV) immune globulin o protect chimpanzees against experimental challenge with HIV. Proc Natl Acad Sci USA. 1988; 85: 5200-5204.
37. Fuchs D, Hausen A, Hengster G, et al. Neoptrin as a marker for activated cell-mediated immunity: application in HIV infection. Immunol Today. 1988; 9: 150-152.
38. Walker BD, Chakrabarti S, Moss B, et al. HIV-specific cytotoxic T lymphocytes in seropositive individuals. Nature. 1987; 328: 345-351.
39. Dolin R, Graham BS, Greenberg SB, et al. The safety and immunogenicity of a human immunodeficiency virus type 1 (HIV-1) recombinant gp160 candidate vaccine in humans. Ann Inter Med. 1991; 114: 119-127.
40. Cooney EL, McElrath MJ, Corey L, et al. Enhanced immunity to human immunodeficiency virus (HIV) envelope elicited by a combined vaccine regimen consisting of priming with a vaccinia recombinant expressing HIV envelope and boosting with gp160 protein. Proc Nal Acad Sci USA 1993; 90: 1882-1886.
41. Parish CR, Liew FY. Immune response to chemically modified flagellin. III. Enhanced cell-mediated immunity during high and low zone antibody tolerance to flagellin. J Exp Med 1972; 135: 298-311.
42. Bretscher PA. Regulation of the immune response by antigen. I. Specific T cells switch the in vivo response from a cell-mediated to a humoral mode. Cell Immunol. 1983; 81: 345-352.
43. Clerici M, Tacket CO, Via CS, et al. Immunization with subunit human immunodeficiency virus vaccine generates stronger T helper cell immunity than natural infection. Eur J Immunol. 1991; 21: 1345-1349.
44. Bretscher PA, Wei G Menon JN, Bielefeldt-Ohmann H. Establishment of stable, cell-mediated immunity that makes "susceptible" mice resistant to *Leishmania major.* Science. 1992; 2757: 539-542.
45. Mayaard L, Otto SA, de Jong R, Miedema F. Preferential outgrowth of Th2 cells after HIV infection. IX Inter Conf AIDS. Berlin 6-11 June 1993 (Abstract # WS-A16-3) p 32.
46. Clerici M, Restoration of HIV-specific cell-mediated immune responses by interleukin-12 in vitro. Science. 1993; 262:1721-1724.
47. Stanford J, Onyebujoh PC, Rook GAW, et al. Old plague, new plague, and treatment for both? AIDS. 1993; 7: 1275-1277.
48. Urnovitz HB, Clerici M, Shearer GM , et al. HIV-1 antibody serum negativity with urine positivity. Lancet. in press.

CHAPTER 9

The Selective Induction of Different Immune Responses by Vaccine Adjuvants

Peter D. Cooper

After some half-century of accepting existing killed or partly purified vaccines we are now intensively developing new ones and reformulating old ones. This change over the last decade has of course been propelled by the new recombinant DNA, peptide synthesis and protein isolation technologies, and arose from concerns about efficacy and impurities and the need to cover more human and veterinary diseases.

Vaccine adjuvants (in the original sense of 'helpers') have developed in parallel, with a dormant period and busy recent growth.[1-8] The new, more pure and more specifically targeted vaccine immunogens unfortunately induce responses that are too small or of the wrong type. Indeed, many of the unwanted impurities were natural immune stimulants or enhancing carrier particles. The new-generation vaccines usually need a suitable adjuvant, and there is now a large list of fairly simple substances with adjuvant activity of which a few combinations are being seriously tested for commercial vaccines.

Adjuvants increase the immune response, but an intriguing and useful property is often to alter the type of response. The immunoglobulin (Ig) isotypes and subclasses are usually changed from those of the immunogen alone, and cell-mediated immunity (CMI, used in a general sense for any response in which antibody is subordinate) may be induced if absent. The changes may still not apply well to the disease process targeted, and what suits one disease may not suit all. Thus different vaccines may need different individually tailored adjuvants and so some choice is desirable, together with some idea of how they work and of the relevant disease process.

Our focus here is the way in which adjuvants modify responses to various immunogens (including adverse or toxic reactions as a type of

Strategies in Vaccine Design, edited by Gordon L. Ada, D.Sc..

altered response), mainly those adjuvants of current interest for human use although some others are included for comparison. It will be clear that our understanding of adjuvant action in terms of basic immunology is quite sketchy, especially as information on the crucial early processing of immunogens carried by particulate adjuvants in both primary and secondary responses is glaringly missing. In this chapter it has sometimes been possible to include some speculative suggesions.

1. WHAT MAKES A GOOD VACCINE ADJUVANT?

It is worthwhile to summarize aspects of a rational design of adjuvants for human vaccines[9] as they constrain the choices available.

Since most vaccines are prophylactics for large numbers of healthy people, safety will have absolute priority in the trade-off with efficacy. Possible exceptions are therapeutics for pre-existing disease such as HIV and herpes type II infections and melanoma or other cancers. The improvement by the adjuvant must be balanced against comparative risks (from adjuvant toxicity or the disease itself) of the improved versus the unimproved vaccine. Any risks in a normal vaccine must nowadays be vanishingly small.

Ideally, a low-risk/high-benefit adjuvant will interact specifically with a limited subset of leukocytes to produce only the desired immune response. Other, excessive or nonspecific responses have more risk of adverse effects such as granulomas, local necrosis, hypersensitivity, fever or autoimmune disease. Interaction with cells other than leukocytes seems undesirable. Myers and Gustafson[9] warn that most adjuvant signals may be transduced via membrane phospholipase activation, and that nonspecific perturbation of membrane structure by surfactants, oily or fatty droplets could cause broad and nonspecific patterns of cell activation. Thus the adjuvant should be targeted to specific immune cells, preferably via specific receptors on leukocyte surfaces. Adjuvants for which specific receptors are not identified may not prove attractive. Many adjuvants are derived from natural pathogens and it is also arguable that the body has evolved to cope with these natural stimulants which are preferable to 'unnatural' ones.

The adjuvant should be biodegradable with a short half-life, be nonantigenic and not immunologically cross-reactive with host tissue antigens (probably ruling out protein adjuvants). It must not be carcinogenic, teratogenic or abortogenic, but be stable, cheap and simple to manufacture reproducibly, and have good storage life preferably without refrigeration. A minimal make-up and simple, known chemical structure are desirable. A customized synthesis for each adjuvant-immunogen batch is harder to reproduce than simple mixing and is undesirable.

Rules for the best design of an effective adjuvant are emerging. A granulomatous depot at the injection site once seemed desirable,[7] but excision of the site 14 days (alum)[10] or one day (Incomplete Freund's Adjuvant: IFA)[11] after injection did not decrease the response and the presumed advantage of slow release was not reproduced by multiple small injections.[12] Overt granulomas will trap immunogen and adjuvant and are probably best avoided. Any depot or slow release effect is now thought likely to be due to antigen retention on dendritic cells in the lymph node follicle,[13] for which complement activation is essential in B cell triggering and selection.[14]

The adjuvant really has to mimic and possibly exaggerate the invasive process in a non-toxic way, carrying and presenting the immunogen correctly and triggering the right T cell subset to appropriate responses. In 'natural' disease most immunogens enter the body via internal or external epithelial surfaces and encounter the immune system as particles (bacterial, fungal, protozoan or worm parasite cells, viruses, pollen grains, dust particles, etc.) which also contain or produce other substances capable of reacting with trigger cells or other leukocytes that influence the size and type of response (see below and ref. 31). It is not surprising therefore that the most effective adjuvants present immunogens in particulate form in association with such trigger substances, which may be referred to as immune stimulants (or modulators or response modifiers). Route of dosage affects the type of response and must be defined for each vaccine, in practice for humans limited to intramuscular (i.m.), subcutaneous (SC) or oral; again not surprisingly, intradermal injection can give highest responses[14a] but SC may often be the route of choice.

Soluble antigens or immune stimulants are likely to diffuse through the body: best results are obtained with immunogen and stimulant immobilized on the one particle, forcing their concentration in the draining lymph node. This usually requires design of carrier particles that can bind both soluble immunogen and stimulant, which then activates and promotes trapping of leukocytes close to the antigen. Such simultaneous delivery to a lymph node is desirable as cytokine action is often short-range and leukocyte activation may not last long. Adjuvant and immunogen should be mixed in such a way that each particle gets a similar antigen load, and the two must be shown to be compatible in at least one model system. Immunogen on particle surfaces can present a multimeric array that improves responses. 'Particles' may be solid or oil droplets emulsified in water, or be liposomes, micelles or ISCOMs (see below). Their best diameter for dispersion and easy transfer to lymph nodes, in larger animals as opposed to rodents,[15] is < 1 µm. Because they may interact with different cells, easy dissociation of components is preferred to covalent bonding.

Naturally, type of response should be tailored to targeted disease (see below).

2. WHAT MAKES AN IMMUNE STIMULANT?

Immune responses begin when an exposed portion (B cell epitope) of an injected immunogen finds an antibody-producing B lymphocyte whose naturally occurring membrane-bound surface Ig (sIg) receptors, either sIgM or IgD, have the specificity to react with it.[16] This epitope may be represented by a linear oligopeptide or by those non-contiguous amino acids that form a conformational recognition site on the surface of the immunogen molecule. The immunogen is internalized and broken down into peptides, some of which (T cell epitopes, linear oligopeptides usually different from the B cell epitopes) are re-presented at the B cell surface in association with class II major histocompatibility complex (MHC) molecules, the second of two main classes of the MHC. The B cell then acts as an antigen-presenting cell (APC). The peptide-MHC complex is recognized by an antigen-specific receptor on an MHC class II T lymphocyte,[17,18] forming a physical B-T cell conjugate. This recognition is proposed[18a] to trigger the T cell to express a new cell surface protein (T cell-induced cell-contact ligand, TICCL), together with several lymphokines. TICCL reacts with a constitutive receptor (CD40) on the B cell surface to initiate activation and proliferation of that B cell, which is induced to differentiate by the lymphokines, leading to Ig secretion and isotype switching. Immunogen specificity is maintained by these interactions, probably aided by a short life for the TICCL and "focusing" of the lymphokines towards the specific B cell. Thus the reaction selects for and stimulates clonal proliferation and differentiation of that B cell, keeping antigen specificity, and induces it to produce the specific Ig as a secretable molecule.

The secondary immune stimulus, essential for good long-term immunity, must be delayed for some weeks to allow clonal amplification and maturation of high affinity memory B and T cells. The B cells now proliferate in germinal centers formed around follicular dendritic cells (FDC), and B cell maturation depends on long-term retention of antigen-antibody complexes on these FDCs to allow selection of B cell clones secreting high affinity antibodies produced by somatic hypermutation after Ig class-switching.

Macrophages and dendritic cells (among which Langerhans cells may be particularly important for vaccines) can also bind and internalize antigens and then act as APCs, presenting peptides in association with MHC of either class I or class II. These cells may play a role in initial processing of the particulate immunogens encountered in normal disease or in adjuvanted vaccines. Cell-surface adhesion and internalization is improved if the immunogen is opsonized either by attached Ig or complement (C3 fragments), or both, which ligate specific receptors on the APC.

MHC class I plus peptide on the APC is recognized by and activates $CD8^+$ antigen-specific Ts (suppressor T) or Tc (cytotoxic T) cell precursors. MHC class II plus peptide on the APC is recognized by and activates $CD4^+$ antigen-specific Th (helper T) cells, Td (DTH or delayed (type IV) hypersensitivity T) cells and other kinds of Ts cells. These T cells are selected and stimulated to proliferate, differentiate and release soluble factors (lymphokines) by that interaction. Other cytokines (e.g., IL-1) are released by the APCs that promote specific responses (proliferation, differentiation, cytokine release) by the T cells. Certain lymphokines (e.g., INF-γ) feed back to amplify the original and other APCs while others stimulate and influence the Ig isotype of the clones of specific-antibody-secreting B cells, or amplify other T cell functions.

This (very) simplified scheme for the immune response represents an amplification cascade network in which a small trigger eventually produces a large, varied and remembered response while keeping specificity.

Immune stimulants or their effector products may intervene in a variety of ways and at many points in this complex process, probably inducing their own leukocyte-cytokine cascade. Aspects of some examples are detailed in Section 6. Their effect is both quantitative and (usually) qualitative, enhancing humoral and cellular responses and changing their nature (selecting for or switching Ig isotype and cell type). Both activities are of key importance for vaccines and presumably result from changed cytokine patterns at critical steps. Immune stimulants can even directly affect the DNA recombinational events leading to isotype switching,[19] but direct evidence for this is usually lacking.

In addition, other important cell surface molecules (MHC complexes, cytokine, Fc or complement receptors) may be up- or downregulated by immune stimulants. Other secreted substances (proteases, mitogens, arachidonic acid metabolites)[20] may also enhance or suppress responses. Immune signals may depend on receptor-mediated transduction processes involving G proteins[21,22] or activation of membrane phospholipases.[23] Since the effects of different stimulants are usually not the same, their initial signals and point(s) of interaction and the induced cascades must also differ. A given stimulant could induce more than one cascade, not always the same in all animal species. Most of our data relates to mice while our main concern is for humans, but the nature and components of the cascades from any immune stimulant are not well understood in any species.

Several immune stimulants of current interest come from foreign natural substances derived from microbial pathogens. Vertebrates have clearly long contended with microbes and their immune system has evolved specific responses. As a cell-mediated defense, vertebrate leukocytes have developed surface receptors specific for conserved sequences of microbial cell-wall components such as β-glucan, peptidoglycan and lipopolysaccharide (LPS) or their subfractions as enlarged upon below. Ligation of these receptors provokes particular responses and the specificity of receptor and response gives some confidence that the responses are important in defense against the particular parasite involved.

Vertebrates have also evolved a humoral immune surveillance to detect and interact with foreign substances, especially polysaccharide or glycoprotein surfaces. This comprises the enzymic cascade known as the alternative complement pathway (ACP), based on the multifunctional complement protein C3.[24] Nonself materials activate the ACP to cleave C3 to fragments that bond covalently with hydroxyl or amino groups on surfaces or large molecules, 'opsonizing' them for several types of specific complement receptor (CR) on a wide range of leukocytes.[25] Substances that activate the ACP are highly effective and specific immune stimulants.[26]

3. DIFFERENT LEUKOCYTE-CYTOKINE CASCADES LEAD TO DIFFERENT IMMUNE RESPONSES

In vitro cloning of T cells showed that there were two types of murine $CD4^+$ T helper cells.[27] On stimulation, one subset (Th1) secreted INF-γ and IL-2, while the other (Th2) secreted IL-4 and IL-5. No subset secreted both IL-4 and INF-γ. These findings are most important for vaccine design.

Later work showed that some $CD4^+$ T cells produced both IL-4 and IFN-γ,[28] and these cells (Th0) are now suggested as precursors to Th1 and Th2 cells whose differentiation is respectively directed by traces of the switch factors[29] INF-γ or IL-4 in their early environment,[30] possibly by initial stimulation of natural killer (NK) or basophil/mast cells.[31] Thus the very first cytokine pattern seen by a local Th0 population may determine its overall later nature. Th1 and Th2 subsets also occur in vivo[32] although the situation is less clear-cut[33] and may relate only to long-established antigen-committed clones in sites located away from peripheral blood.

Figure 1 summarizes these findings, with some additions suggested by the data presented below. (The subset designation has been extended to

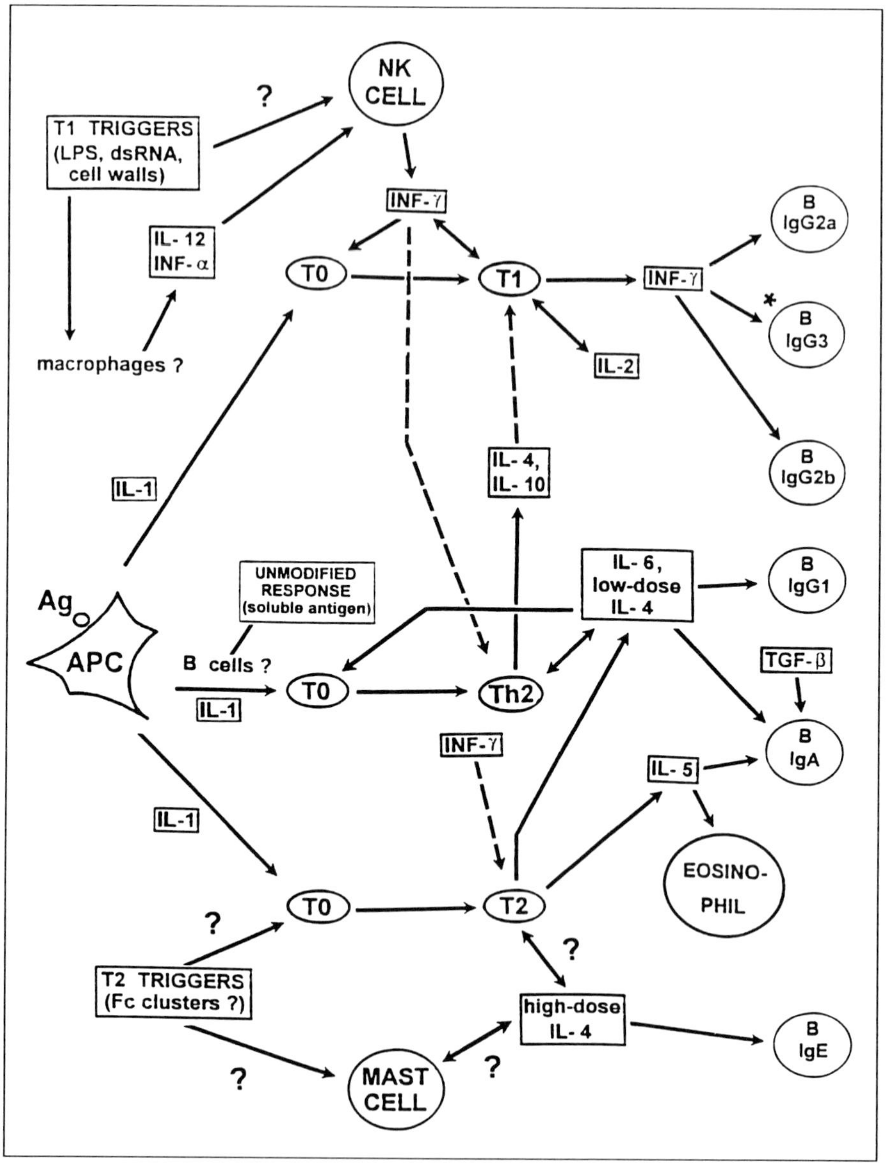

Fig. 1. Suggested outline of some murine leukocyte-cytokine interactions relevant to vaccine design. Broken arrows indicate suppressive action.

T1 = Th ($CD4^+$), Tc ($CD8^+$), Td ($CD4^+$) or Ts ($CD4^+$ or $CD8^+$) cells.

T2 = Th ($CD4^+$) or Ts ($CD8^+$) cells.

Ag = antigen; APC = antigen-presenting cell; NK = natural killer.

**Only via Fc cooperative binding?*

$CD8^+$ T cells and the useful suggestion made simply to refer to T1 and T2 subsets for helper, cytotoxic and suppressor functions,[34] but we will retain the older convention for the present). The Th1 and Th2 pathways are mutually suppressive. In the Th2 pathway, induction of IgE appears to need a higher dose of IL-4 than does IgG_1 which is suppressed at higher IL-4 levels,[35] suggesting two functional pathways within the Th2 subset (Fig. 1).

A localized focus of 'high dose' IL-4 production will be surrounded by an outer zone of 'low dose' IL-4 and so IgE induction can be expected to be accompanied by IgG_1.

Most natural immunogens also contain or produce other substances capable of reacting with 'trigger' cells such as NK or basophil/mast cells,[31] that may be able to direct T cell differentiation to Th1 or Th2 pathways, respectively. The Th1 pathway defends *inter alia* against and is stimulated by intracellular parasites that express cell-surface antigens (e.g. influenza virus), enhancing IgG_{2a} (and perhaps IgG_3), Tc and Td effector T cells. The Th2 pathway defends against and is stimulated by worm parasites and soluble immunogen, enhancing IgG_1, IgG_{2b}, IgA, IgE and eosinophil and basophil/mast cell and antigen-specific Ts cell responses. Soluble antigen alone elicits an 'unmodified' response that appears to follow the 'low-dose IL-4' portion of the Th2 pathway, probably because it is recognized by sIg on B cells, which if then acting as APCs express MHC class II and preferentially enhance Th2 $CD4^+$ cells.[34]

After initial difficulty[36] most but not all human $CD4^+$ T cell clones from particular body locations in various disease states were shown[31,37] to produce either IL-4 plus IL-5 or INF-γ plus IL-2. Later studies showed that T cell clones from healthy human donors exhibited stable Th1 or Th2 patterns and that their expression relates to the antigens or conditions of immunization. Isotype patterns of human and murine $CD4^+$ T help were quite analogous, human Th2 clones inducing specific IgM, IgG, IgA and IgE synthesis, while human Th1 clones induced specific IgM, IgG and IgA only. The make-up of the human IgG subclasses may be useful further data.

4. WHAT ARE THE IMMUNE RESPONSES TO AIM FOR IN A VACCINE?

"No one cytokine response gives the best protection against all parasites", and "it is incumbent upon the host immune system to match the response to a particular parasite".[38] It is also incumbent upon a vaccine designer to match response to targeted disease. The vaccine may need more than one immunogen, which should contain conserved parasite sequences crucial to its invasive process preferably as highly immunogenic B and T cell epitopes. Humoral responses should be high in neutralizing antibodies and the immunogen(s) may also have to elicit a fitting CMI response.

What exactly are appropriate responses? We do not know enough to answer this properly, but host responses to the natural disease in question are revealing, particularly challenge-protection tests in relevant models.

For example, a prominence of IgG_{2a} was implied for clearance of mouse infections in vivo.[39-43] Murine humoral responses to most viral infections and intracellular parasites generally favor specific IgG_{2a} (even though in particular mouse strains this is not the dominant isotype[41]), suggesting that IgG_{2a} is the most protective isotype. While this may be so, in these diseases infected cells present surface antigens that stimulate Tc cells in the Th1 pathway (Fig. 1), which happens also to enhance IgG_{2a} B cells. It is thus not clear whether the Tc cell or the IgG_{2a} is the primary protective function, and in vivo the IgG_1 response still predominates. IgG_{2a} effects macrophage antibody-dependent cell-mediated cytotoxicity (ADCC),[44,45] and IgG_{2a} better protects against murine tumors[46,47] and parasites.[48] IgG_{2a} strongly binds

C1q of the classical complement pathway (relative affinities are IgG_{2a}=IgG_{2b}>IgG_1),[49] which opsonizes cells or antibody clusters with C3 fragments. Ligation of Fcγ2aR or Fcγ1/2bR on macrophage activation factor– (MAF)-primed macrophages respectively raise intracellular cAMP or arachidonic acid release,[50] suggesting a difference in their response to $IgG_1/_{2b}$ and IgG_{2a}. There is no subclass distinction in their phagocytosis.[51]

Murine IgG_1 is often held not to fix complement (and thus to be less desirable) but this may not be so: mouse IgG_1 does indeed fix complement although less strongly,[49,52] but because it is aggregated IgG that fixes C1q in vivo, the predominance of specific IgG_1 means that its total effect may be similar to that of the less numerous IgG_{2a} molecules.

Antigen-specific murine IgG_3 may be most useful against, and is possibly selectively enhanced by, multivalent antigens such as polysaccharides because IgG_3 Fc regions can aggregate noncovalently to produce cooperative, more powerful binding.[53] However, cooperative aggregates have not yet been found among human Igs although it is known that polysaccharide antigens in humans induce mainly specific IgG2.[54]

As specific IgM-producing B cells are not normally present in immunological memory their induction may seem irrelevant for a vaccine, but possible polyclonal enhancement of some IgM B cells *before* DNA commitment by isotype switching[55] may later increase other isotypes. Some IgM enhancement may be the price to pay for those isotypes entering memory.

For many infections the presence of specific IgA, especially mucosal IgA, is highly desirable. Some adjuvants enhance IgA but it is usually difficult to do so.

In contrast to intracellular parasites, most worm infestations induce mainly specific IgG_1 and IgE and these are the protective isotypes in these diseases,[38] both for example mediating eosinophil ADCC and degranulating mast cells. In vaccination against murine *Schistosoma mansoni*, alum (inducing specific IgE) but not Complete Freund's Adjuvant (CFA) (not inducing specific IgE) protected against challenge.[56]

Other antibody responses favorable for a vaccine, such as specificity for native rather than to denatured antigen, a high affinity for antigen and ability to neutralize an active site, can be affected by adjuvants.[57] Some relation here between high affinity and high titer suggests that a strong adjuvant allows more opportunity for affinity maturation. A denaturing adjuvant such as CFA gave a higher ratio of responses to denatured:native human serum albumin (HSA) than did, e.g., Quil A and Ribi adjuvant system (Section 6G). Perhaps because of denaturation by CFA, the oil-in water system SAF-1 (Section 6D) was more effective than CFA in inducing neutralizing antibodies for IL-1α, but in mice immunized with a nonreplicating antigen (purified influenza virus hemagglutinin) no isolated IgG subclass was outstandingly able to inhibit hemagglutination or neutralize infectivity.[41]

CMI is a crucial component of many immune responses and its induction is markedly influenced by adjuvants, which possibly directly activate antigen-presenting dendritic cells; these cells express copious MHC class I as well as class II.[58] Tc and Td cell responses are part of the Th1 pathway (Fig. 1) and although Td cells may only afford protection in certain diseases (not influenza), Th1 CMI is often measured by the easier DTH assay.

Induction of eosinophilia and mucosal mastocytosis (Th2 CMI?) are equally important components of the response to helminth parasites and are characteristic of the Th2 pathway.

What information relevant to human vaccines can be gained from mouse isotype studies? IgG subclasses differentiated after the evolutionary divergence of mouse and human ancestors[29] and so an analogy of function, if any, results from convergent evolution driven by particular purposes. The nature of these purposes, again if any, would be valuable information. IgG subclasses differ only in the Fc portion which interacts with other effector systems such as cell receptors or C1q. All human IgGs bind C1q (IgG_3>IgG_1>IgG_2>IgG_4)[59] and the affinity constants vary only over a six-fold range (two-fold for IgG_3 and IgG_1), implying no great advantage for any one subclass. The human macrophage Fc receptor for ADCC is probably the high affinity FcγRI,[60] which also binds all subclasses (IgG_1>IgG_3>IgG_4>>IgG_2).[61] Diphtheria and tetanus toxoids adjuvanted with alum give excellent long-memory protection and in the natural disease these antigens are soluble rather than cell-associated. Both aspects suggest that the Th2 pathway is mainly involved, but in fact human anti-tetanus toxoid antibodies are distributed among IgG_1, $_2$, $_3$ and $_4$ subclasses,[62] although IgG_1 predominates.[63] Antibodies to polysaccharides are restricted to IgG_2, in polio, rubella and herpes simplex the antibodies are restricted to IgG_3 but in some chronic diseases they are IgG_4. In switching from IgM to IgG, early IgG is IgG_3 followed by IgG_1 in some diseases while in others all subclasses are represented.[63] Different human subclasses develop at different stages of childhood.[63] More work on human IgG subclass function is needed.

Altogether our ideas on murine protective IgG subclasses do not seem to correspond much with the human situation (a similar conclusion was reached from cytokine-subclass relationships[29]) and at present adjuvant effects on murine IgG subclasses seem irrelevant to human vaccines. On the other hand, analogies between murine and human Th1 and Th2 subsets[37] and IgA, IgE and IgM isotype relationships[29] seem valid, for example alum also enhanced anti-diphtheria toxoid IgE in humans,[63a] and human $CD4^+$ clones specific to tetanus toxoid (alum-adjuvanted?) produce IL-4 and IL-5 but little INF-γ.[64]

5. 'INERT' CARRIER PARTICLES

Unadjuvanted (soluble) antigens usually elicit in mice IgM and IgG_1 with some IgG_{2b} and little CMI.[65-67] Some adjuvants enhance immune responses without changing their nature and thus may be considered immunologically inert. If they truly are so they illustrate the usefulness of carrier particles that simply concentrate the immunogen in the draining lymph node. They are not highly potent without added immune stimulants and they lack specific receptor targeting, presumably interacting nonspecifically with leukocytes perhaps via lipid adhesions and cell surface fusion or phagocytosis.

IFA is a light mineral oil plus a surfactant emulsifier (Arlacel A, mannide monooleate). It is homogenized with an equal volume of aqueous immunogen to produce a suspension of finely dispersed water droplets (water-in-oil emulsion). Metabolizable oils and other emulsifiers have also been examined.[1]

Adverse injection-site reactions were not severe in humans[68] but are nevertheless discouraging.[2] The bolus attracts macrophages and monocytes, and oil droplets later turn up in lymph nodes.[128] IFA-enhanced isotype patterns were unchanged from controls with IgG, IgA and IgM all increased equally,[65] and DTH was only slightly increased.[69,70]

Fine (200 nm) oil-in-water emulsions are more easily tolerated and suitable oils and emulsifiers have been extensively studied.[1] The oil droplets adsorb and present proteins on their surface, normally aided by the emulsifier but better if the antigens have hydrophobic regions.[71] The small particles diffuse readily from the injection site but have no inherent immunomodulation.[72,73]

Liposomes are water droplets (20 nm to 3 μm) enclosed by single or multiple-concentric phospholipid bilayers perhaps also including cholesterol and surfactants. Preparation and associated parameters are complex[1,9,74] and antigen inclusion is customized. Antigens may be carried inside or on the outer surface, as may immune stimulants,[74] which however could lead to autoimmunity against membrane phospholipid or cholesterol.[75,76] Liposomes do not cause granulomas and are biodegradable but macrophages are nonspecifically attracted to them. They do not react with specific cell receptors and may cause nonspecific side reactions by disturbing membrane transduction systems,[9] although inclusion of mannosylated albumin allowed targeting to a specific macrophage receptor and enhanced adjuvanticity.[77] Liposomes injected in a site distant from antigen do not enhance responses,[78] and the isotype response is unchanged[79] although DTH can be induced if hydrophobic antigenic domains are presented.[74]

Calcium phosphate is a moderately effective adsorptive adjuvant.[80,81] As a natural body component it is unlikely to be an immune stimulant (particularly for CMI), for which the main published evidence is its lack of IgE induction compared with that of alum.[82]

6. HOW IMMUNE STIMULANTS CAN MODIFY IMMUNE RESPONSES

A. Gamma Inulin

Background. Inulin is a neutral, edible storage carbohydrate of *Compositae*, of completely known structure (unbranched β-D-(2-1)polyfructofuranosyl α-D-glucose, with a range of degrees of polymerization). It was long known to activate complement to exhaustion, and was shown to do so[83] by an enzymic cascade (the ACP) that was alternative to the 'classical' one known at that time. This humoral defense has not been exploited for vaccines before although its components and processes are well understood[24,84] and the multiple effects of its activation are of current research interest.[25,85-88] The key to its vaccine use was gamma inulin (γ-IN),[89] the most recent new-generation commercial immune stimulant. At 37°C inulin suspensions pass through several polymorphic forms of decreasing solubility to γ-IN, a new polymorph virtually insoluble at 37°C and apparently responsible for ACP activation. Gamma inulin is 100-fold more active than shelf inulin[90] and is formulated as a suspension of quasi-crystalline 1 μm ovoids activating the ACP of many animal species including humans at low doses.

Immune responses. Gamma inulin increased secondary total IgG responses to keyhole limpet hemocyanin (KLH) up to 28-fold in mice, inducing immunological memory and memory recall.[66] Specific IgG_{2a}, IgG_{2b} and IgG_3 were boosted several hundred-fold, IgG_1 ten-fold and IgM, IgA and IgE four- to six-fold. The large enhancement of IgG_3 may reflect the highly multimeric and hence multivalent[53] nature of KLH, as for other antigens IgG_3 was not enhanced (unpublished). Th1 CMI is enhanced, as sheep red blood cell (SRBC) doses required to prime for given DTH responses were decreased ten-fold, and Tc cell responses (inferred from cross-serotype protection in a lethal influenza virus model) were also boosted. Gamma inulin has an antitumor effect in mice[91] and some domestic animals[26] that is probably cell-mediated. Since γ–IN is effective if given *before* antigen in the anti-tumor, DTH and IgG models[26,66,92] it is an immune stimulant. Gamma inulin enhances both Th1 and Th2 characters, with emphasis on Th1.

Leukocyte-cytokine interactions. In vitro antigen-specific IL-2 and INF-γ secretion and lymphocyte proliferation by sheep peripheral blood lymphocytes were more enhanced by γ–IN than by CFA in vivo, using a recombinant *Taenia ovis* antigen[93] (IgG is not enhanced by γ–IN in sheep). Human peripheral blood leukocytes secreted IL-2 but not IL-1 in response to γ–IN plus tetanus toxoid in vitro (J. Hamilton, unpublished). Gamma inulin behaved as, or generated, a 'priming' MAF in vivo not a fully activating 'second signal', as adherent peritoneal exudate cells (PEC) isolated by D. George and M.J. Weidemann (unpublished) 5-10 days after intraperitoneal (i.p.) γ–IN did not produce a respiratory burst in vitro unless triggered with phorbol ester. Saline controls were not so primed. By 15-20 days after γ–IN, PEC macrophages developed cytotoxicity for L929 cells (G.S. Sraml and M.J. Weidemann, unpublished). Gamma inulin's lack of pyrogenicity implies little secretion of IL-1, TNF and INF-α, all activated-macrophage products causing fever,[94] and γ–IN priming failed to enhance LPS toxicity,[26] an activated-macrophage TNF response primed by *C. parvum*.[95] In other systems, C3 opsonization has MAF activity as it allows binding to monocytes, macrophages or neutrophils, which however need a second signal for phagocytosis[26] that is provided to macrophage receptors by the polyglucose of zymosan or lentinan but not by the polyfructose of γ–IN. PEC macrophage numbers did not change after i.p. γ–IN,[26] but lymphocytes increased eight-fold ($p<0.004$) five days after injection and neutrophils were massively (1000-fold) recruited by five hours.

Cytokines play secondary roles in immune stimulation by ACP activation, as C3 cleavage products, especially immobilized C3b, iC3b, C3c, C3d or C3dg, are direct and sometimes crucial primary effectors via complement receptors (CR) in the acquired immune response.[85] Immediately on injection, some surface hydroxyl groups on γ–IN particles will covalently bond (via the thiolester) traces of C3b always present,[96] which then forms the C3 convertase C3b,Bb. This enzyme is (sterically?) protected from serum inactivators and the particle now becomes a stable, mobile C3 convertase unit, self-amplifying by a chain reaction to create surface arrays of C3 pieces, on itself or on adjacent antibody or antigen molecules and APC, T or B cell surfaces.

These C3 'tags' specifically ligate several types of CR on many leukocyte surfaces, with many stimulatory effects.

1. Crosslinking CR1 or CR2 on B cells induces mitosis in absence of macrophage-derived growth factors.[97]
2. B cell CR1 and CR2 seem important in enhancing primary antibody responses to many T-dependent and T-independent antigens.[98]
3. C3 arrays (aggregated C3 or C3b) plus IL-2 costimulate Th cell clones.[99,100]
4. Proliferation of antigen-specific T cells is enhanced by immune complex-bound C3b during antigen presentation, and CR1 and CR2 focus opsonized antigen on APC surfaces.[101]
5. Macrophage-bound C3 fragments influence growth and differentiation into plasma cells of pre-activated germinal center B cells[85] and interact with CR1 and CR2 on activated T cells[102,103] to promote cell-cell adhesion.
6. Follicular trapping of antigen is absolutely C3 dependent.[14]

These factors suggest that pre-antigen priming by γ-IN may result frompolyclonal activation and proliferation of B and T cells.

Adverse effects. Like other ACP activators including cellulosic hemodialysis membranes,[26] γ–IN is nonpyrogenic and has very low toxicity at vaccine-equivalent doses. It is not antigenic, when dissolved has no physiological effect and when particulate is probably digested inside phagocytes.[26,104] Unlike CFA, γ–IN did not induce autoimmune disease in experimental autoimmune encephalomyelitis in rats and granulomas were difficult to obtain.[26]

B. Alum

Background. Alum (hydrated aluminum oxide gel) is at neutral pH a positively charged polyelectrolyte with avid salt-like binding for negatively charged molecules such as most proteins and polysaccharides. Heavy floccules form at certain alum:protein ratios, and this crosslinking ratio has been a criterion for vaccine preparation[105] with little evidence that the result is optimal. Of many different crystalline and amorphous forms of alum,[106] some are unstable and some do not adsorb antigens at all. Some vaccines are prepared by coprecipitation of alum and antigen but made in this way its adsorptive capacity decays in weeks and because of likely variability in response such preparation seems better avoided. The character of the alum at time of use is rarely defined in research papers. The proprietary Alhydrogel is stable and reproducible, has a long, reliable record and is a recommended standard.[107]

Immune responses. Alum alone is not immunologically inert, since (unlike IFA and liposomes) it alters the pattern of the response to increase the IgE:IgG ratio in mice (Fig. 2) and probably in humans.[63a] It thus has an immune stimulant effect. It is not highly potent but is best for humoral responses to weak antigens,[109] increasing for example total IgG responses to KLH up to 100-fold in proportion to dose and to levels similar to IFA.[67,110] It may only enhance the primary response in some cases.[108] The 'most improved' isotypes are usually IgE and IgG_1 then IgG_{2b},[110-112] alum being better than CFA for IgE.[111] Alum is a poor adjuvant for DTH responses[70] but may be good for Th2 CMI (especially eosinophils) and this deserves direct study. Alum is thus a Th2 adjuvant, but it can also act as a carrier particle and is much more effective if the alum-antigen particles also carry attached immune stimulants such as γ-IN[110] (Section 6C), [Thr[1]]MDP[57] (Section 6E) or MPL (Section 6G). Gamma inulin, MDP and probably MPL then alter the response towards a Th1 type.

Leukocyte-cytokine interactions. Alum's adsorptive capacity is a hitherto unconsidered factor in its immune stimulant effect. After alum is mixed with serum the centrifuged pellet is several-fold larger than the starting material: there is massive protein uptake. In fact it is exceedingly unlikely that free alum can exist for long in vivo. Upon injection, alum with the usual nonsaturating dose of antigen will be immediately saturated with soluble lymph proteins, over 10% of which will be Ig (alternative pathway complement is reportedly destroyed by alum[112a] but probably not via C3 activation, so that alum will not carry much opsonically recognizable C3). This is likely to have two effects: 1) at higher or more concentrated alum doses the particles may crosslink with lymph proteins and become 'fixed' in situ, creating a granuloma impenetrable by phagocytes, and 2) at lower or more dilute alum doses the particles will be fully coated with proteins including Ig. Some protruding Fc moieties will present an Fc opsonized surface binding to leukocyte receptors particularly FcγR, thus specifically targeting alum particles for leukocyte surfaces. This idea is supported by the increase in adjuvanticity with increase of antigen-free alum,[108,110] and particularly by

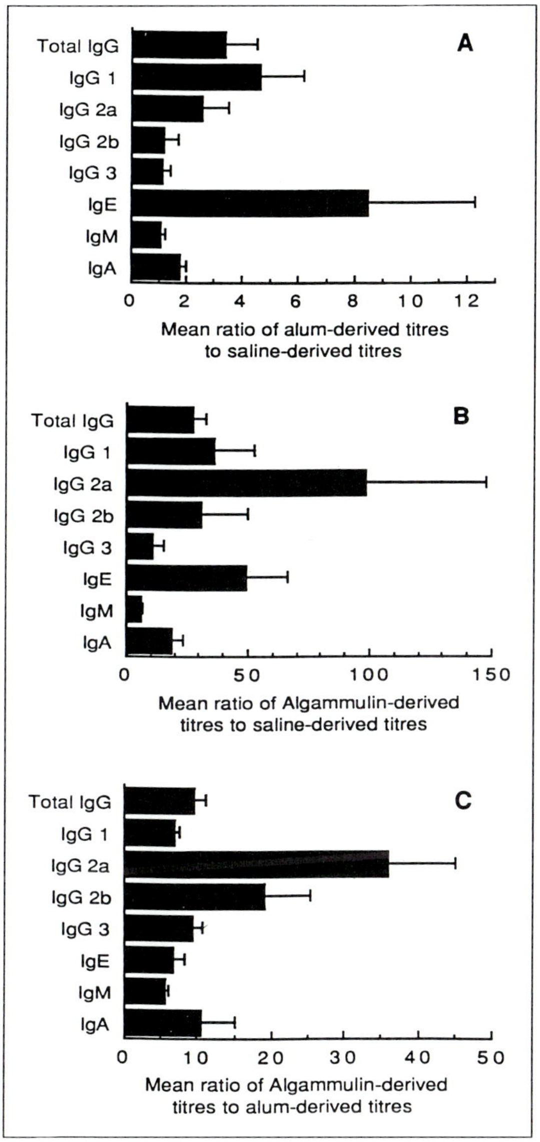

Fig. 2. Isotype and subclass distribution of secondary specific responses to 1 μg keyhole limpet hemocyanin in saline or adsorbed to high-alum Algammulin or equivalent doses of alum. (Reprinted by permission of the publishers Butterworth-Heinemann Ltd., from ref. 110).

the abrogation of this increase by saturating free alum with bovine serum albumin.[108] Alum's adjuvanticity may be due as much to this targeting as to its carrier particle ability, one result being the stimulation of antigen uptake and phagocytosis by APCs observed by Mannhalter et al.[113]

Alum attracts eosinophils to the injection site via a T cell-dependent mechanism[114,115] and elicits a carrier-specific helper-cell population for IgE responses (in current terms Th2 cells?).[116] Anticytokine monoclonal antibodies (mAbs) show that alum-induced Th responses depend on IL-1 and IL-4.[117] An explanation for alum's switch to Th2 responses could be that some of the Fc-opsonized alum particles may react with mast cell or Th cell FcR. Crosslinking of FcR on mast cells liberates several Th2 cytokines[118,119] including the Th2 switch factor IL-4, and mast cells/basophils have been implicated as primary 'natural immunity' triggers for Th2 responses.[31] FcγR molecules on mouse T cells include the Ly-17 locus[120,121] to which the Mls locus is tightly linked.[122] Disturbances at Mls trigger strong mixed-lymphocyte-reaction mitogenic responses but do not generate Tc cells,[60] suggesting an emphasis on Th2 pathways. With a different approach, Urban et al[38] considered proteolytic enzymes as helminth Th2 trigger factors analogous to LPS and polyribonucleotides as Th1 triggers and found that injected papain induced IgE and IgG_1 but not IgG_{2a}. Body proteolytic products seem more likely than the enzymes per se to be specifically recognized, so again Fc fragments are good candidates for induction of Th2 responses. The role of multiple Fc ligation in Th2 induction deserves direct study.

Adverse effects. Alum has a long safety record but local granulomas at adjuvant doses in humans are sometimes reported. Higher doses will regularly yield granulomas in animals. Alum is not pyrogenic or antigenic. Allergic reactions are not usually a clinical problem for alum[4] even in high IgE-responder allergic patients[123] although its enhancement of IgE has raised disquiet.[80,81]

C. Algammulin

Background. Co-crystallization of γ–IN with alum (Alhydrogel) yields 2-3 μm particles of γ–IN containing alum ('Algammulin') that bind antigen and still activate complement.[90] Formulation in different particle sizes and alum:inulin ratios influences the response.

Immune responses. Total specific IgG responses were increased almost 200-fold by Algammulin to the same levels as CFA, against KLH[110] and malaria peptide-diphtheria toxoid conjugate.[124] In this malaria model, a protective response against *Plasmodium chabaudi* challenge was also obtained,[125] for which a Th2 adjuvant (alum), a Th1/Th2 adjuvant (high-alum Algammulin) and a Th1 adjuvant (CFA) gave equally good protection correlated with antibody titer. It would be interesting to measure Th1 and Th2 CMI in this model. Hepatitis B surface antigen was boosted more by Algammulin than by alum.[126] At the high-alum ratio used (alum:inulin = 1:10), the KLH-specific isotype pattern was intermediate between those from alum and γ–IN, although IgG_{2a} was still the most increased isotype (Fig. 2). The IgE:IgG ratio was half that from alum, while IgA and total IgG were increased 10-fold. Lower alum:inulin ratios (e.g., 1:30) can decrease the IgE:IgG ratio still further. Sonication reduces Algammulin particle sizes and at 0.5 μm its activity was increased five-fold w/w.[90] Increasing the dose of Algammulin particles carrying a small antigen load (five molecules/particle) gave a better response than increasing the antigen load per particle. As with γ-IN, immunological memory and memory recall were induced. Algammulin is both a strong Th1 and a Th2 adjuvant, high-alum Algammulin emphasizing Th2 and low-alum Algammulin Th1.

Leukocyte-cytokine interactions. As with γ-IN, antigen-specific IL-2 and INF-γ secretion and lymphocyte proliferation by sheep peripheral blood lymphocytes were strongly enhanced in vitro after in vivo inoculation with KLH or a recombinant *Taenia ovis* protein plus Algammulin, compared with immunogen alone, although again sheep IgG responses were unchanged.[93,127] The Algammulin cytokine responses equaled or exceeded those from CFA or Montanide ISA 50. High-alum Algammulin particles can be flocculated by protein and so some free alum remains uncovered by inulin, and this Algammulin, like alum itself (Section 6B), may also present an Fc array to react with Th2 trigger cells. The available alum surface is smaller at lower alum:inulin ratios, so by adjusting the ratio the response pattern can also be adjusted between that of alum (IgG_1 and IgE emphasized) and that of γ-IN (IgG_{2a}, IgG_{2b} and IgA emphasized). When the Algammulin C3 array also includes antigen, its interaction with B cell sIg should confer specificity on the proliferative response to C3. The C3 array should also enhance follicular trapping of Algammulin-borne antigen,[14] as should the Ig array via FcR, to promote immunological memory.[13]

Adverse effects. Like its components, Algammulin is nonpyrogenic and non-toxic. Local-site reactions of Algammulin are intermediate between those of γ-IN and alum and depend on alum:inulin ratio. Use of the ultrasonicated 'fine formulation' reduces the dose for a given response five-fold.

D. Complete Freund's adjuvant

Background. CFA is IFA with the addition to the oil phase of dried *Mycobacterium tuberculosis* as immune stimulant.[128] As with IFA, it is homogenized with an equal volume of aqueous antigen to form a water-in-oil emulsion before injection. It is too toxic for vaccines but is extremely potent and is a popular benchmark for adjuvant comparisons. It is curiously ineffective for some antigens and subclasses.

Immune responses. CFA strongly enhanced Ig plaque-forming cells (PFCs) for IgM, IgG_1 and IgA, less so for IgG_{2a} and not at all for IgG_3 and IgG_{2b}.[65] In assays for soluble Ig, CFA strongly enhanced IgG_1 and IgG_{2a},[57,67,110,] equally or less so for IgG_{2b},[57,67,129] and not at all for IgG_3 with HSA[57] but was strongly enhanced with KLH.[110] IgA was promoted slightly,[129] IgE was[110] or was not[116,130] promoted, while DTH[70] and CMI[131] were promoted strongly. CFA is a potent Th1 adjuvant.

Leukocyte-cytokine interactions. Increasing sophistication in immune cell analysis has paralleled fading research interest in CFA, and in the few modern studies the stimulatory effects are too universal to be illuminating.

Adverse effects. Severe injection-site granulomas and necrosis resembling DTH reactions are common. CFA induces chronic inflammatory arthritis in one strain of rats[132] and with certain antigens induces various autoimmune diseases.[133]

E. Muramyl peptides

Background. A muramyl tripeptide was chemically the simplest isolate with adjuvant activity from systematic fractionation of *M. tuberculosis*,[134] the immune stimulant of CFA. The tubercle bacillus offers multiple immune signals and several active fractions were found. A synthetic dipeptide analogue (N-acetylmuramyl-L-alanyl-D-isoglutamine, MDP) was equally effective. It is water-soluble and needs a carrier particle to persist effectively in vivo, but added lipid tails help association with oil droplets or liposomes.[6,15,135] MDP itself is pyrogenic but of many nonpyrogenic analogues[136,137] some are incorporated in oil-in-water emulsions for human vaccines ([Thr^1]MDP in SAF-1;[138] MTP-PE in MF59[15]).

Immune responses. MDP (10 μg) in IFA induced specific antibody and DTH responses comparable to CFA in guinea pigs[139] and suppressed IgE in the mouse.[140] MDP in saline was less effective,[139] boosting specific IgG_1,[141] IgE[142] and IgA[142a] and enhancing antigen-specific T-suppressor cells[142b,c] but not specific IgG_2 or IgM[129,141] or DTH[70] in the mouse. Making the MDP lipophilic by coupling with glycerol mycolate gave it CMI capability without oil.[143] The antibody levels induced by MF59 against herpes II gp120 antigen were two- to four-fold above IFA values in primates.[15] SAF-1 gave equal enhancement of IgG_{2a} and IgG1 with some IgG_{2b} in mice but total specific IgG was only 5% of CFA values.[57,124] Thus free MDP enhanced Th2 characters while MDP in a lipid microenvironment is a strong Th1 adjuvant.

Leukocyte-cytokine interactions. Muramyl peptides act directly on lymphocytes and macrophages, although searches for specific surface receptors were not successful.[6] MDP fully activated macrophages to phagocytosis and liberated IL-1,[144] itself a direct adjuvant. Direct contact of macrophage membrane-bound IL-1 with Th cells may be sufficient for MDP's action[145] and high levels of macrophage membrane-bound IL-1 were invariably correlated with adjuvanticity of MDP analogues[137] while pyrogenicity was not. Some difference between the macrophage uptake mechanisms of pyrogenic and nonpyrogenic MDP analogues seems likely. MDP is mitogenic for B cells[146] and induces primary immune responses in T cell-depleted spleen cultures.[147] MDP induces T cells to release the switch factor INF-γ,[148] possibly explaining the Th1 emphasis when in lipid association which itself presumably enhances its influence on T cells.

Adverse effects. IL-1 has highly pleiotropic and sometimes hormone-like activities in vivo[149] and its site for fever- and sleep-inducing actions lies in the CNS. Thus the nonpyrogenic muramyl peptides may induce membrane-bound IL-1 but too little IL-1 secretion to affect the CNS. MDP also has other toxic effects, inducing chronic inflammatory arthritis in rats[150] and increasing vascular permeability with eye inflammation (uveitis) in several species. CFA is a favored adjuvant for eliciting autoimmune disease with the right antigen,[133] and as its subfraction MDP can itself also induce autoimmune diseases[151] it could possibly cause autoimmunity with self-antigens. Although nonpyrogenic MDP analogues are only weakly active in these properties,[152] the chance of such reactions in a genetically predisposed human minority 'seems difficult to exclude'.[153] Conjugated MDP can induce an anti-MDP response.[154]

F. Lipopolysaccharide and Lipid A

Background. Bacterial endotoxin or LPS, the outermost component of Gram-negative bacterial cell walls, is a powerful immune stimulant and is itself antigenic. It is a strong adjuvant but as it is pyrogenic and can lead to toxic shock and death it is useful only for comparison. LPS comprises a large antigenic polysaccharide linked by an oligosaccharide containing heptoses to lipid A, mainly responsible for its toxicity and immune stimulation.[155] ACP activation may cause some effects but is polysaccharide- rather than lipid A-mediated[156] and at low doses will have little effect compared with lipid A. Lipid A (or diphosphoryl lipid A, DPL) has a diglucosamine backbone linked to four long-chain (C12-C16) beta-hydroxy fatty acids; two beta-hydroxy groups are acylated with other long-chain fatty acids, and the diglucosamine has a free phosphate group at each end.

Immune responses. LPS as antigen, like other polysaccharides, elicits in the mouse some IgG_{2b} but mainly IgG_3, which may result in some way from cooperative binding of Fc-aggregating IgG.[53] Enhancements of IgM, IgA and total IgG PFCs were of similar size.[65,157] Primary B cell responses to LPS were IgM while secondary responses included IgG and IgA.[55] If the primary LPS-induced IgM B cells were restimulated by Th cells, IgG1 was produced and IgG_3 was suppressed;[157,158] if restimulated by cytokines, IL-4 caused a switch to Th2 Ig (IgG1, IgE)[35] and INF-γ to Th1 Ig (IgG_{2a}).[159] As an adjuvant LPS can induce similar responses to other antigens, namely mostly specific IgG_3 with IgM and IgG_{2b},[65] but this finding requires additional assumptions if it is to be reconciled with enhancement of IgG_3 by cooperative Fc binding.[53] DTH is enhanced by LPS.[160] LPS is a strong Th1 adjuvant with another variable (IgG_3 enhancement) superimposed.

Leukocyte-cytokine interactions. After some difficulty good evidence is now available for many specific (saturable) LPS and lipid A receptors on splenic B cells and macrophages, and for their action by ligating these receptors.[161] However, LPS also binds to cell membranes in nonspecific (nonsaturable) ways that could give nonspecific responses. The transduction signal of LPS induces biochemical cascades in macrophages,[23] upregulating particularly membrane phospholipase C and protein kinase C. The main cause of LPS toxicity is probably induction of IL-1 and TNF-α from macrophages, which also release IL-6, IL-8, colony-stimulating factors (CSFs) and TGF-β. Neutrophils, endothelial and epithelial cells and platelets are stimulated as well.[161] LPS receptors on T cells are not reported.[161] LPS and lipid A behave as 'second signals' to activate macrophages[162,163] for phagocytosis and tumoricidal activity, requiring priming by a MAF[164] notably INF-γ.[165] INF-γ upregulates MHC expression[166] but LPS suppresses antigen presentation by macrophages.[23] LPS is a T cell-independent, polyclonal B cell mitogen.[167]

Adverse effects. Clinical syndrome of Gram-negative bacterial septicemia.

G. Monophosphoryl lipid A

Background. Acid hydrolysis of LPS from heptose-less mutant bacteria releases 4'-monophosphoryl lipid A (MPL), which is lipid A (DPL) lacking the 1' terminal phosphate.[168] MPL is often tested using a trehalose dimycolate/oil-in-water carrier emulsion (Ribi adjuvant system: RAS).

Immune responses. MPL and DPL enhanced antibodies to ovalbumin and a bacterial antigen[169] equally and PFCs to SRBC as antigen.[170] RAS and CFA both enhanced secondary murine total IgG responses to cytochrome b_5 some 1000-fold.[67] IgG1, IgG_{2a} and IgG_{2b} were equally represented but, in contrast to LPS, IgG_3 was absent. IgE was not detectable but it was not found for alum either in this study. RAS only enhanced primary murine total IgG responses to HSA to 3% of CFA levels,[57] mainly IgG1 and IgG_{2a} but some IgG_{2b} and no IgG_3. In a guinea pig challenge model, an MPL derivative (3-deacyl-monophosphoryl lipid A, with a herpes simplex II gp-D antigen in an oil-in-water emulsion or adsorbed on alum; Francotte M, Hermand Ph, Fabry L et al, personal communication) gave protection and improved DTH and neutralizing antibody responses. Like LPS, MPL is a Th1 adjuvant but lacks ACP activation and antigenicity.

Leukocyte-cytokine interactions. As it is less toxic than LPS or lipid A, MPL interacts with the body at fewer points but nevertheless duplicates several LPS effects. MPL in water forms micelles which, like LPS and lipid A, are potent B cell mitogens, stimulate phagocytosis by mouse PEC macrophages and stimulate production of IL-1 by mouse or human monocytes.[169] MPL generates CSF in mice and inactivates suppressor T cells.[171] Like the nonpyrogenic muramyl peptides, MPL was less effective than LPS at inducing *released* IL-1[169] and induction of TNF secretion was not reported, both perhaps accounting for its lower toxicity. Unlike LPS and CFA, MPL enhanced T cell dependent help and an anamnestic response to the T-independent type III pneumococcal polysaccharide as antigen.[171]

Adverse effects. Although as adjuvant-active, MPL is at least 1000-fold less lethal than LPS in several animal species[169] and 200-fold less active in the dermal Schwartzman test,[172] a measure of LPS-caused blood clotting disturbances. It passed the pyrogenicity test at 10 µg/kg i.v. in rabbits and in proprietary mixtures for human anticancer trials it had only minor adverse effect.[173,174] Antibodies to MPL are found in synovial fluid of some arthritis patients.[174a]

H. Saponin, Quil A, QS-21 and ISCOMs

Background. Saponins are steroid/triterpenoid glycosides and surface active. 'Saponin' is a crude extract of the soap bark tree *Quillaja saponaria;* Quil A[175] is a semi-purified fraction containing over 20 components;[67] QS-21 is one purified component of high adjuvanticity:toxicity ratio;[67] and ISCOMs (immune stimulating complexes[176]) are 35 nm clathrate bodies like micelles made of Quil A, cholesterol, phosphatidyl choline and antigen. The surface activity of saponins suggests a carrier particle function in which antigen is presented in micelle-like structures which attach nonspecifically to cell surfaces. Antigens with accessible hydrophobic regions (e.g., virus membrane proteins) are custom-built into the ISCOM.

Immune responses. Saponins are active in many animal species.[177] Quil A (300 µg) gave the same enhancement of total IgG PFC as 20 µg alum[65] and 10 µg of Quil A gave 10% of the total IgG enhancement of 50 µg alum.[57] Quil A elicited mainly IgG_1 with some IgG_{2a} and enhancements of IgM and IgA were much less than alum.[65] Quil A enhanced IgM and IgG responses to T-independent antigens in athymic nude mice,[178] and is an immune stimulant as it is active in a site distant from antigen.[179,180] Four purified saponins (20 µg each of QS-7, -17, -18, -21) gave enhancements of total IgG against cytochrome b_5 equivalent to that from CFA (1000-fold[67]). QS-7 gave equal enhancement of IgG_1, IgG_{2a} and IgG_{2b}, QS-17 and QS-21 emphasized IgG_{2a} and IgG_{2b} and QS-18 mainly IgG_{2a}, suggesting some differences in action. Although the purified saponins were stated not to enhance IgE,[67] alum (a known IgE enhancer) did not do so either in these tests. Influenza virus ISCOMs induced similar levels of $IgG_{1, 2a, 2b}$ and $_3$ in the mouse[181] and enhanced IgA[182] and antigen-specific IL-2 in vitro.[183] Saponin promoted moderate DTH reactions,[70] but *Toxoplasma* ISCOMs induced DTH reactions[184] and influenza[182] and HIV[185] ISCOMs induced Tc cell responses. Saponins, crude or as Quil A, may be inert or low-grade Th1 adjuvants but purified or in ISCOMs are strong Th1 adjuvants.

Leukocyte-cytokine interactions. Little information is available and the immune stimulant mechanism of saponin is unknown. Saponins seem not to react with specific cell receptors but have high affinity for cholesterol and may intercalate nonspecifically into cell membranes. Quil A induced T cell proliferation.[178]

Adverse effects. Toxicity is a major problem but a given dose of Quil A is more active if in an ISCOM, allowing use of subtoxic doses for the same response. Some components have relatively low lethality:adjuvanticity ratios (especially QS-7 and QS-21[67]), although QS-21 has a 50% SRBC hemolytic concentration (7 μg/ml) much lower than the concentration needed for adjuvant activity (100 μg/ml)[67] so that some local reaction is to be expected. Saponin's nonspecific cellular reactivity allows the chance of autoimmunity against membrane phospholipid or cholesterol[75,76] and of nonspecific side reactions by disturbing membrane transduction systems.[9] HLA antigens in ISCOMs have enhanced immunogenicity[186] but autoimmune reactions with other cell membrane proteins are not reported.

7. ARE ALL ADJUVANTS POLYCLONAL ACTIVATORS?

LPS causes nonspecific polyclonal, T-independent B cell activation and proliferation.[167] MPL is as mitogenic for B cells as is LPS[169] and increases the number of nonspecific IgM-secreting cells polyclonally.[171] IgD on the surface of B cells acts as a nonspecific trigger for clonal expansion when ligated by a recognized antigen and B cells can be induced to proliferate polyclonally by injection of anti-IgD antibody.[32] CFA is reported to induce polyclonal hypergammaglobulinemia.[187] Injection of γ-IN several days *before* the trigger antigen was at least as effective as simultaneous injection for anti-tumor, DTH and IgG responses,[26,66,92] and the IgG responses were three- to five-fold greater if γ-IN was given two to three days before antigen. Mice behaved as if a leukocyte population was nonspecifically (polyclonally) primed by γ-IN to receive a range of antigens. Zymosan and lentinan were also effective adjuvants if given before antigen,[26] but as they both activate the ACP they probably act like γ-IN. Pretreatment with MDP in saline induced Ts cells specific to subsequent antigen.[142c]

More direct evidence comes from PFC assays for total cells secreting Ig of various isotypes regardless of antigen specificity.[65] Injection of all adjuvants tested (IFA, CFA, LPS, alum, Be^{++}, Li^+, Quil A, poly I:C, poly A:U) *without antigen* gave a two- to ten-fold increase (39-fold for LPS) of total PFC number compared with untreated BALBc and Parkes but not CBA mice. The isotype profile differed from the controls: some adjuvants (IFA, Be^{++}, poly I:C, poly A:U) emphasized IgM at the expense of IgA and IgG, while others (CFA, LPS, alum, Li^+, Quil A) did the reverse. Also, background anti-SRBC PFCs in mouse spleen cells cultured in MDP were enhanced in absence of antigenic stimulation.[188,189]

Thus all these adjuvants seem to cause a polyclonal, nonspecific proliferative response of B cells in absence of antigen (in most mouse strains) that is probably systemic. Adjuvants are rarely given before antigen and it is not known whether all immune stimulants cause nonspecific *priming* as does γ–IN, although since most can stimulate from a site distant from antigen this is probably so. It seems important to confirm this. Fortunately, nonspecific priming in human vaccination, giving an unwanted chance of response to any foreign antigen encountered, is probably restricted to the draining lymph node.

8. VACCINE DEVELOPMENT

The immunogen should preferably be developed in conjunction with an adjuvant of the general type expected to be suitable for the targeted disease. Injection of soluble antigen alone, especially i.p., is usually deposited in the body away from the immune cells it would meet in 'natural' disease and is in non-particulate form without accessory trigger factors; except for venoms and toxins it may not be relevant to most disease processes.

Unlike alum and IFA, most new-generation immune stimulants enhance Th1 CMI responses, probably by generating INF-γ early in the process. INF-γ suppresses Th2 responses, including antigen-specific Ts cells which are undesirable factors in several diseases for example melanoma and leprosy. On the other hand, strong reversal of such suppressor cells might also undesirably block aspects of immune self-tolerance[34] possibly leading to autoimmune disease, and this may explain why strong Th1 adjuvants such as CFA and MDP are such good inducers of autoimmunity. Thus subset switching might best be restricted to the local lymph node, or might use immune stimulants such as gamma inulin that enhance both Th1 and Th2 subsets. Following from this, one wonders whether Th2 adjuvants could be used to reverse autoimmune disease.

Future vaccines may include Th1 CMI-enhancing adjuvants with, e.g., the nucleoprotein antigen for influenza to give cross-serotype protection,[190] with appropriate antigens for malaria,[191] with the existing vaccine for hepatitis B but substituting a Th1-CMI adjuvant for alum[126] and with the gD antigen for the therapeutic as well as prophylactic use of herpes type II vaccines (Section 6G). However, IgA induction is desirable for many such vaccines, for which a Th1/Th2 adjuvant such as Algammulin may be preferable. Th2 CMI-enhancing adjuvants such as high-alum Algammulin may be used against parasites not involving humoral defenses (e.g. liver fluke in domestic animals). In certain intracellular viral diseases such as poliomyelitis and hepatitis A, infected cells do not present surface antigens; responses are probably unmodified or Th2 and Salk-like inactivated vaccines may do well if responses can be increased perhaps by adsorption on high-alum Algammulin as a strong but balanced Th2 adjuvant.

Th1 adjuvants are a rational choice for switching away from reaginic responses to desensitizing allergen vaccines and should dramatically reduce the number of inoculations needed.

Responses to polysaccharide immunogens are T-independent and comprise in mice and humans initially IgM, switching mainly to IgG_3 in mice[192] via the switch factor INF-γ[193] and in humans to IgG_2.[54] Protein conjugation such as in the *Haemophilus influenzae* type b vaccines can provide T cell help and an anamnestic response,[194] although as at least one of these vaccines is adjuvanted with alum Th1 CMI may not be available. MPL enhanced T cell help for unconjugated type III pneumococcal polysaccharide,[171] and ligation of CR on B cells enhanced primary antibody responses to T-independent antigens,[98] and so MPL or γ–IN may help polysaccharide vaccines, especially for CMI responses.

IL-1,[144,195] IL-2[196] and INF-γ[197,198] are direct adjuvants with isotype promotion as expected, and probably most cytokines will do as well. A difficulty lies in giving them in the right place, time, duration and dose in relation to antigen. Even a partial synthesis of the immune response is daunting because of potential toxic and suppression effects and timing problems. The 'natural' immune stimulants ligating identified receptors seem preferable for now, selecting for Th1 or Th2 pathways as required and allowing the body to balance its own responses in the way it has evolved. However, cytokines may be ideal for isotype switching or selective enhancing at response initiation, e.g., for IgA with traces of TGF-β and IL-5,[199-201] preferably adsorbed on low-alum Algammulin. Study of switching rather than enhancing cytokines may be especially useful for vaccines.

9. HOW DO THE ADJUVANTS COMPARE?

Any useful comparison of adjuvants must be made concurrently with the same experimental protocol (antigen, animal species and mouse strain, dose regime and assay method), and relating the comparison studies available is in turn hampered by the very different protocols used. Doses often seem arbitrary especially for alum (ranging from 20 μg to several mg per mouse) and the alum itself is usually undefined, while IFA and CFA are fairly constant at the high foreign material content of 50 to 100 mg. Most tests use various inbred mouse strains while outbred strains are probably more relevant for vaccine development. Some tests use 'near self' antigens (e.g., human serum albumin in mice) whereas most commercial antigens will not have this degree of self homology. It is especially significant to note how much the responses vary with antigen and it is clear that each new immunogen should have careful optimization of adjuvant in the target species. The cytokine networks have not yet been unraveled for any immune stimulant.

Despite the difficulty in comparing adjuvants, some generalizations seem valid. Optimal formulation of all these commercial immune stimulants except alum (γ–IN with alum as Algammulin, MPL and lipid-conjugated MDP with detergent and oil droplets, saponins masked in ISCOMs or purified) can produce responses in mice equal to those of CFA that probably saturate the murine immune system. Figure 3 summarizes the types of response obtained. Rather surprisingly and in spite of apparently different modes of action, the final outcomes do not differ greatly. All amplify the 'unmodified' response, but in addition Algammulin, MDP, MPL and ISCOMs enhance protective Th1 Ig responses and Th1 CMI. Algammulin can also

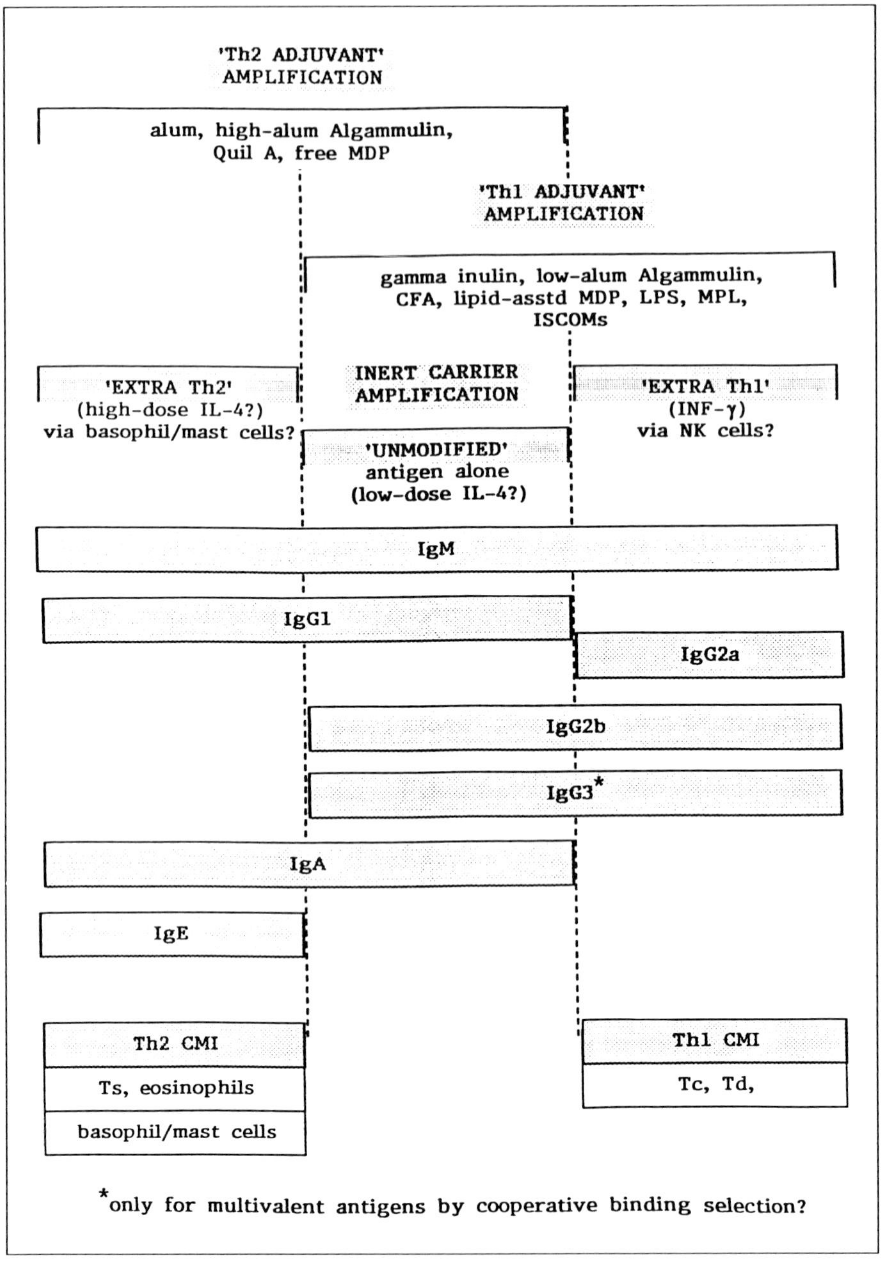

Fig. 3. Summary of the selective induction of different immune responses in the mouse by vaccine adjuvants.

be adjusted either to favor Th2 responses or to limit the IgE product of alum-adjuvanted vaccines as its enhancement of IgE can be fine-tuned up or down by adjusting the alum content. Th2 CMI enhancers are not reported but are worth looking for. Quil A and crude saponin are mainly inert enhancers but some isolated saponins have a humoral Th1 character; CMI enhancement is not yet reported for saponins. Algammulin was the most promising adjuvant for IgA in the comparisons available, and

Algammulin, MPL and possibly alum satisfy the requirements of causing interaction with identified, specific leukocyte receptors. Some questions are unanswered regarding possible self-tolerance suppression by strong, pure Th1 adjuvants, of possible nonspecific effects for MPL, saponins and oil droplets and toxicity for MDP analogues. Nevertheless, expecting that results from small rodents will apply broadly to humans, some useful choices are emerging that should satisfy a range of future vaccine needs.

10. CONCLUSIONS

We have addressed the question of the way in which vaccine adjuvants induce different immune responses in terms of the T cell subsets designated Th1 and Th2, with the suggestion that Th2 subsets may also comprise two functional pathways ('high-dose IL-4' and 'low-dose IL-4'). This has produced a fairly coherent picture of adjuvant action that allows some generalizations. Nevertheless it must be acknowledged that the basic concepts are derived largely from in vitro cloning studies and probably represent an oversimplification of a complex in vivo situation. It is to be expected that future work will modify and hopefully clarify some of this complexity.

REFERENCES

1. Cox JC, Coulter AR. Advances in adjuvant technology and application. In: Yong WK, ed. Animal Parasite Control utilizing Biotechnology. Boca Raton: CRC Press, 1992:49-112.
2. Gupta RK, Relyveld EH, Lindblad EB et al. Adjuvants - a balance between toxicity and adjuvanticity. Vaccine 1993; 11:293-306.
3. Gregoriadis G, Allison AC, Poste G, eds. Immunological Adjuvants and Vaccines. NATO ASI Series A: Life Sciences, Vol 179. New York: Plenum Press 1989.
4. Warren HS, Vogel FR, Chedid LA. Current status of immunological adjuvants. Ann Rev Immunol 1986; 4:369-88.
5. Nervig RM, Gough PM, Kaeberle ML et al, eds. Advances in Carriers and Adjuvants for Veterinary Biologics. Ames: Iowa State University Press 1986.
6. Adam A. Synthetic adjuvants. Modern Concepts in Immunology Vol 1. New York: John Wiley 1985.
7. Edelman R. Vaccine adjuvants. Rev Infect Dis 1980; 2:370-83.
8. Waksman BH. Adjuvants and immune regulation by lymphoid cells. Springer Semin Immunopathol 1979; 2:5-33.
9. Myers KR, Gustafson GL. Adjuvants for human vaccine usage: a rational design. In: Cryz SJ Jr, ed. Vaccines and Immunotherapy. New York: Pergamon Press 1991:404-11.
10. Holt LB. Quantitative studies in diphtheria prophylaxis: the primary response. Brit J Exp Pathol 1949; 30:289-97.
11. Freund J. The effect of paraffin oil and mycobacteria on antibody formation and sensitization. A review. Am J Clin Pathol 1951; 21:645-56.
12. Mitchison NA. Induction of immunological paralysis in two zones of dosage. Proc Roy Soc London Ser B 1964; 161:275-92.
13. Gray D, Skarvall H. B cell memory is short-lived in the absence of antigen. Nature, (London) 1988; 336:70-2.

14. Klaus GGB, Humphrey JH. A re-evaluation of the role of C3 in B-cell activation. Immunol Today 1986; 7:163-5.
14a. Redfield RR, Innis BL, Scott RM et al. Clinical evaluation of low-dose intradermally administered hepatitis B virus vaccine. A cost reduction strategy. J Amer Med Assoc 1985; 254:3203-6.
15. Van Nest GA, Steimer KS, Halgwood NL et al. Advanced adjuvant formulation for use with recombinant subunit vaccines. In: Brown F, Chanock R, Ginsberg HS et al, eds. Vaccines 92. Modern Approaches to New Vaccines Including Prevention of AIDS. Cold Spring Harbor: Cold Spring Harbor Laboratory Press, 1992:57-62.
16. Möller G. One non-specific signal triggers B lymphocytes. Transplant Rev 1975; 23:126-37.
17. Lanzavecchia A. Receptor-mediated antigen uptake and its effect on antigen presentation to class II-restricted T lymphocytes. Ann Rev Immunol 1990; 8:773-93.
18. Noelle RJ, Snow EC. T helper cell-dependent B cell activation. FASEB J 1991; 5:2770-6.
18a. Hodgkin PD, Kehry MR. B cell activation by T cells - the "TICCL" model. The Immunologist 1993; 1:5-8.
19. Rothman P, Lutzker S, Cook W et al. Mitogen plus interleukin 4 induction of Ce transcripts in B lymphoid cells. 1988; J exp Med 168:2385-89.
20. Colditz IG, Kerlin RL, Watson DL. Migration of neutrophils and their role in elaboration of host defense. In: Husband AJ, ed. Migration and Homing of Lymphoid Cells Vol 1 Boca Raton: CRC Press, 1988: 135-65.
21. Stryor L, Bourne HR. G proteins, a family of signal transducers. Ann Rev Cell Biol 1986; 2:391-419.
22. Gilman AG. G proteins, transducers of receptor-generated signals. Ann Rev Biochem 1987; 56:615-49.
23. Hamilton TA, Adams DO. Molecular mechanisms of signal transduction in macrophages. Immunol Today 1987; 8:151-8.
24. Müller-Eberhard HJ. The human complement protein C3: its unusual functional and structural versatility in host defense and inflammation. In: Weigle WO, ed. Advances in Immunopathology. Miami: Symp Specialists Inc, 1981:141-60.
25. Ross GD, Medof ME. Membrane complement receptors specific for bound fragments of C3. Adv Immunol 1985; 37:217-67.
26. Cooper PD. Solid phase activators of the alternative pathway of complement. In: Sim RB, ed. Activators and Inhibitors of Complement. Dordrecht: Kluwer Academic Publishers, 1993:69-106.
27. Mosmann TR, Coffman RL. Th1 and Th2 cells: different patterns of lymphokine secretion lead to different functional properties. Ann Rev Immunol 1989; 7:145-73.
28. Firestein GS, Roeder WD, Laxer JA et al. A new murine CD4+ T cell subset with an unrestricted cytokine profile. J Immunol 1989; 143:518-25.
29. Callard RE, Turner MW. Cytokines and Ig switching: evolutionary divergence between mice and humans. Immunol Today 1990; 11:200-203.
30. Scott P. Interferon-γ modulates the early development of Th1 and Th2 responses in a murine model of cutaneous leishmaniasis. J Immunol 1991; 147:3149-55.

31. Romagnani S. Induction of Th1 and Th2 responses: a key role for the 'natural' immune response? Immunol Today 1992; 13:379-81.
32. Finkelman FD, Holmes J, Katona IM et al. Lymphokine control of in vivo immunoglobulin secretion. Ann Rev Immunol 1990; 8:303-33.
33. Kelso A, Metcalf D. T lymphocyte-derived colony stimulating factors. Adv Immunol 1990; 48:69-105.
34. Bloom BR, Salgame P, Diamond B. Revisiting and revising suppressor T cells. Immunol Today 1992; 13:131-6.
35. Snapper CM, Finkelman FD, Paul WE. Differential regulation of IgG1 and IgE synthesis by interleukin 4. J Exp Med 1988; 167:183-96.
36. Paliard X, de Waal Malefijt R, Yssel H et al. Simultaneous production of IL-2, IL-4 and IFN-γ by activated human CD4+ and CD8+ T cell clones. J Immunol 1988; 141:849-55.
37. Romagnani S. Human Th1 and Th2 subsets: doubt no more. Immunol Today 1991; 12:256-7.
38. Urban JF, Madden KB, Svetic A et al. The importance of Th2 cytokines in protective immunity to nematodes. Immunol Rev 1992; 127:206-20.
39. Hocart MJ, Mackenzie JS, Stewart GA. The IgG subclass responses induced by wild-type, cold-adapted and purified haemagglutinin from influenza A/Queensland 16/72 in CBA/CaH mice. J Gen Virol 1988; 69:1873-82.
40. Hocart MJ, Mackenzie JS, Stewart GA. The IgG subclass response to influenza haemagglutinin in the mouse: effect of route of inoculation. J Gen Virol 1989; 70:809-18.
41. Hocart MJ, Mackenzie JS, Stewart GA. The immunoglobulin G subclass responses of mice to influenza A virus: the effect of mouse strain, and the neutralizing abilities of individual protein A-purified subclass antibodies. J Gen Virol 1989; 70:2439-48.
42. Balkovic ES, Florack JA, Six HR. Immunoglobulin G subclass antibody responses of mice to influenza virus antigens given in different forms. Antiviral Research 1987; 8:151-60.
43. Coutelier J-P, Van der Logt JTM, Heesen FWA et al. IgG_{2a} restriction of murine antibodies elicited by viral infections. J Exp Med 1987; 165:64-9.
44. Matthews TJ, Collins JJ, Rocoson GJ et al. Immunologic control of the ascites form of murine adenocarcinoma 755. IV Characterization of the protective antibody in hyperimmune serum. J Immunol 1981; 2332-36.
45. Herlyn D, Koprowski H. IgG_{2a} monoclonal antibodies inhibit human tumor growth through interaction with effector cells. Proc Nat Acad Sci US 1982; 79:4761-5.
46. Steplewski Z, Spira G, Blasczyc M et al. Isolation and characterization of anti- monosialoganglioside monoclonal antibody 19-9 class switch variants. Proc Nat Acad Sci US 1985; 82:3653-7.
47. Kaminski MS, Kitamura K, Maloney DG et al. Importance of antibody isotype in monoclonal anti-idiotype therapy of a murine B cell lymphoma. A study of hybridoma class switch variants. J Immunol 1986; 136:1123-30.
48. Wechsler DS, Konghavn PAL. Heat-labile IgG_{2a} antibodies effect cure of *Trypanosoma musculi* infection in C57BL/6 mice. J Immunol 1986; 137:2968-72.
49. Leatherbarrow RJ, Dwek RA. Binding of complement subcomponent C1q to mouse IgG_1, IgG_{2a}, IgG_{2b}: a novel C1q binding assay. Molec Immunol 1984; 21:321-7.

50. Nitta T, Saito-Taki T, Susuki T et al. Phospholipase A2 activity of Fcc2b receptors of thioglycollate-elicited murine peritoneal macrophages. J Leukocyte Biol 1984; 36:493-504.
51. Ralph P, Nakoinz I, Diamond B et al. All classes of murine IgG antibody mediate macrophage phagocytosis and lysis of erythrocytes. J Immunol 1980; 125:1885-8.
52. Ey PL, Russel-Jones GJ, Jenkin CR. Isotypes of mouse IgG$_{-1}$. Evidence for 'non- complement-fixing' IgG$_1$ antibodies and characterization of their capacity to interfere with IgG2 sensitization of target red blood cells for lysis by complement. Mol Immunol 1979; 17:699-710.
53. Greenspan NS, Cooper, LJN. Intermolecular cooperativity: a clue to why mice have IgG3? Immunol Today 1992; 13:164-8.
54. Riesen WF, Skvaril F, Braun DG. Natural infection of man with group A streptococci. Levels; restriction in class, subclass and type; and clonal appearance of polysaccharide group-specific antibodies. Scand J Immuno1976; 5:383-90.
55. Zauderer M, Askonas BA. Several proliferative phases precede maturation of IgG- secreting cells in mitogen-stimulated cultures. Nature (London) 1976; 260:611-3.
56. Horowitz S, Smolarski M, Arnon R. Protection against *Schistoma mansoni* achieved by immunization with sonicated parasite. Eur J Immunol 1982; 12:327-32.
57. Kenney JS, Hughes BW, Masada MP et al. Influence of adjuvants on the quantity, affinity, isotype and epitope specificity of murine antibodies. J Immunol Meth 1989; 121:157-66.
58. King PD, Katz DR. Mechanism of dendritic cell function. Immunol Today 1990; 11:206-11.
59. Schumaker VN, Calcott MA, Spiegelberg HL et al. Ultracentrifuge studies of the binding of IgG of different subclasses to the C1q subunit of the first component of complement. Biochemistry 1987; 16:5175-81.
60. Unkeless JC, Scigliano E, Freedman VH. Structure and function of human and murine receptors for IgG. Ann Rev Immunol 1988; 6:251-81.
61. Huber H, Douglas SD, Nusbacher J et al. IgG subclass specificity of human monocyte receptor sites. Nature (London) 1971; 229:419-20.
62. Van der Giessen M, Groenerboer-Kempers O. The subclasses of human IgG antibodies against tetanus toxoid. Clin Exp Immunol 1976; 25:117-21.
63. Ochs HD, Wedgwood RJ. IgG subclass deficiencies. Ann Rev Med 1987; 38:325-40.
63a. Matuhashi R, Ikegami H. Elevation of levels of IgE antibody to tetanus toxin in individuals vaccinated with diphtheria-pertussis-tetanus vaccine. J Infect Dis 1982; 146:290.
64. Salgame PR, Abrams JS, Clayberger C et al. Differing lymphokine profiles of functional subsets of human CD4 and CD8 T cell clones. Science 1991; 254:279-82.
65. Karagouni EE, Hadjipetrou-Kourounakis L. Regulation of isotype immunoglobulin production by adjuvants in vivo. Scand J Immunol 1990; 31:745-54.
66. Cooper PD, Steele EJ. The adjuvanticity of gamma inulin. Immunol Cell Biol 1988; 66:345-52.
67. Kensil CR, Patel U, Lennick M et al. Separation and characterization of saponins with adjuvant activity from *Quillaja saponaria* Molina cortex. J Immunol 1991; 146:431-7.

68. Stuart-Harris CH. Adjuvant influenza vaccines. Bull WHO 1969; 41:617-21.
69. White RG. The adjuvant effect of microbial products on the immune response. Ann Rev Microbiol 1976; 30:579-600.
70. Bomford R. The comparative selectivity of adjuvants for humoral and cell-mediated immunity. II Effect on delayed-type hypersensitivity in the mouse and guinea pig, and cell-mediated immunity to tumour antigens in the mouse of Freund's incomplete and complete adjuvants, Alhydrogel, *Corynebacterium parvum*, *Bordetella pertussis*, muramyl dipeptide and saponin. Clin Exp Immunol 1980; 39:435-41.
71. Dalsgaard K. Adjuvants. Vet Immunol Immunopathol 1987; 17:145-52.
72. Roberts AJ, de Avila DM, Gerber et al. Active immunization of beef heifers against luteinizing hormone. I Evaluation of protein carriers and adjuvants on antigenicity of LH. J Animal Sci 1990; 68:3742-6.
73. Johnston BA, Eisen H, Fry D. An evaluation of several adjuvant emulsion regimens for the production of polyclonal antisera in rabbits. Lab Animal Sci 1991; 41:15-21.
74. Gregoriadis G. Immunological adjuvants: a role for liposomes. Immunol Today 1990; 11:89-97.
75. Alving CR. Natural antibodies against phospholipid and liposomes in humans. Biochem Soc Trans 1984; 12:342-44.
76. Alving CR. Antibodies to liposomes, phospholipids and phosphate esters. Chem Phys Lipids 1984; 40:304-14.
77. Garcon N, Gregoriadis G, Taylor M et al. Mannose-mediated targeted immunoadjuvant action of liposomes. Immunol 1988; 64:743-5.
78. Shek PN, Sabiston BH. Immune responses mediated by liposome-associated protein antigens. I Potentiation of the plaque-forming cell response. Immunol 1981; 45:349-56.
79. Davis D, Davies A, Gregoriadis G. Liposomes as adjuvants with immunopurified tetanus toxoid: the immune response. Immunol Lett 1987; 14:341-8.
80. Relyveld EH. Preparation and use of calcium phosphate adsorbed vaccines. Develop Biol Stand 1986; 65:131-6.
81. Relyveld EH, Ickovic M-R, Henocq E et al. Calcium phosphate adjuvanted allergens. Annals Allergy 1985; 54:521-9.
82. Vassilev TL. Aluminium phosphate but not calcium phosphate stimulates the specific IgE response in guinea pigs to tetanus toxoid. Allergy 1978; 33:155-9.
83. Götze O, Müller-Eberhard HJ. The C3 activation system: an alternative pathway of complement activation. J Exp Med 1971; 134:90s-108s.
84. Müller-Eberhard HJ, Schreiber RD. Molecular biology and chemistry of the alternative pathway of complement. Adv Immunol 1980; 29:1-55.
85. Erdei A, Füst G, Gergely J. The role of C3 in the immune response. Immunol Today 1991; 12:332-7.
86. Rosen H, Law SKA. The leukocyte cell surface receptors for the iC3b product of complement. Curr Topics Microbiol Immunol 1990; 153:99-122.
87. Fearon DT, Ahearn JM. Complement receptor type 1 (C3b/C4b receptor: CD35) and complement receptor type 2 (C3d/Epstein-Barr virus receptor: CD21). Curr Topics Microbiol Immunol 1990; 153:83-98.
88. Lambris JD, Becherer JD, Servis C et al. Use of synthetic peptides in exploring and modifying complement reactivities. In: Sim RB, ed. Activators and Inhibitors of Complement. Dordrecht: Kluwer Academic Publishers, 1993:201-32.

89. Cooper PD, Carter M. Anticomplementary action of polymorphic 'solubility forms' of particulate inulin. Molec Immunol 1986; 23:895-901.
90. Cooper PD, Steele EJ. Algammulin: a new vaccine adjuvant comprising gamma inulin particles containing alum. Vaccine 1991; 9:351-7.
91. Cooper PD, Carter M. The anti-melanoma activity of inulin in mice. Molec Immunol 1986; 23:903-8.
92. Cooper PD, Steele EJ, McComb C et al. Gamma inulin and Algammulin: two new vaccine adjuvants. In: Ginsberg HS, Brown F, Chanock R et al, eds. Vaccines 93. Modern Approaches to New Vaccines Including Prevention of AIDS. Cold Spring Harbor: Cold Spring Harbor Laboratory Press, 1993:25-30.
93. Kyme HJ, Cooper PD, Deol HS et al. In vitro assessment of a new alum-polysaccharide adjuvant (Algammulin) with a defined recombinant antigen against a sheep parasite. Aust Soc Immunol Abstr, Melbourne 1990:72.
94. Dinarello CA. Interleukins, tumour necrosis factors (cachectin) and interferons as endogenous pyrogens and mediators of fever. In: Pick E, ed. Lymphokines. Vol 14. New York: Academic Press, 1987:1-31.
95. Green S, Dobrjansky A, Chiasson MA et al. *C parvum* as the priming agent in the production of tumour necrosis factor in the mouse. J Nat Cancer Inst 1977; 59:1519-22.
96. Lachmann PJ. Complement. In: Sela M, ed. The Antigens. Vol 5. New York: Academic Press, 1979:283-303.
97. Melchers F, Erdei A, Schultz T et al. Growth control of activated, synchronized murine B cells by the C3d fragment of human complement. Nature (London) 1985; 317:264-7.
98. Thyphronitis G, Kinoshita T, Inoue K et al. Modulation of mouse complement receptors 1 and 2 suppresses antibody responses in vivo. J Immunol 1991; 147:224-30.
99. Erdei A, Spaeth E, Alsenz J et al. Role of C3b receptors in the enhancement of interleukin-2-dependent T cell proliferation. Mol Immunol 1984; 21:1215-21.
100. Bartok I, Erdei A, Mousaki A et al. Interaction between C3 and IL-2; inhibition of C3b binding to CR1 by IL-2. Immunol Letters 1989; 21:131-7.
101. Arvieux J, Yssel H, Colomb MG. Antigen-bound C3b and C4b enhance antigen- presenting cell function in activation of human T-cell clones. Immunol 1988; 65:229-36.
102. Erdei A, Batjay Zs, Fabry Zs et al. Appearance of acceptor-bound C3b on HLA-DR positive macrophages and on stimulated U937 cells; inhibition of Fcc-receptors by the covalently fixed C3 fragments. Mol Immunol 1988; 25:295-303.
103. Maison CM, Villiers CL, Colomb MG. Secretion, cleavage and binding of complement component C3 by the human monocyte cell line U937. Biochem J 1989; 261:407-13.
104. Czop JK. Phagocytosis of particulate activators of the alternative complement pathway: effects of fibronectin. Adv Immunol 1986; 38:361-98.
105. Herbert WJ. Mineral oil adjuvants and the immunization of laboratory animals. In: Weir DM, ed. Handbook of Experimental Immunology. 3rd ed. Oxford: Blackwell, 1978:A3.1-15.
106. Nail SL, White JL, Hem SL. Structure of aluminum hydroxide gel 1. Initial precipitate. 2. Aging mechanism. J Pharm Sci 1976; 65:1188-95.
107. Stewart-Tull DES. Recommendations for the assessment of adjuvants

(immunopotentiators). In: Gregoriadis G, Allison AC, Poste G, eds. Immunological Adjuvants and Vaccines. Nato ASI Series A: Life Sciences Vol 179. New York: Plenum Press, 1989:213-26.
108. Jensen OM, Koch C. On the effect of $Al(OH)_3$ as an immunological adjuvant. APMIS 1988; 257-64.
109. Bomford R. Relative adjuvant efficacy of $Al(OH)_3$ and saponin is related to the immunogenicity of the antigen. Int Archs Allergy Appl Immunol 1984; 75:280-1.
110. Cooper PD, McComb C, Steele EJ. The adjuvanticity of Algammulin, a new vaccine adjuvant. Vaccine 1991; 9:408-15.
111. Hamaoka T, Katz DH, Benacerraf B. Hapten-specific IgE antibody responses in mice. II Cooperative interactions between adoptively transferred T and B lymphocytes in the development of IgE response. J Exp Med 1973; 138:538-56.
112. Mancino D, Ovary Z. Adjuvant effects of amorphous silica and of aluminum hydroxide on IgE and IgG1 antibody production in different inbred mouse strains. Int Arch Allergy Appl Immunol 1980; 61:253-8.
112a. Ramanathan VD, Badenoch-Jones P, Turk JL. Complement activation by aluminium and zirconium compounds. Immunol 1979; 37:881-8.
113. Mannhalter JW, Neychev HO, Zlabinger GJ et al. Modulation of the human immune response by the non-toxic and non-pyrogenic adjuvant aluminium hydroxide: effect on antigen uptake and antigen presentation. Clin Exp Immunol 1985; 61:143-51.
114. Walls RS. Eosinophil response to alum adjuvants: involvement of T cells in non-antigen dependent mechanisms. Proc Soc Exp Biol Med NY 1977; 156:431-5.
115. Sakata KM, Tashiro K, Hirashima M et al. Selective regulation of chemotactic lymphokine production. 1. Selective potentiation of eosinophil chemotactic lymphokine production in alum hydroxy gel- and *Bordetella pertussis* vaccine-treated guinea pigs. J Immunol 1985; 135:3463-7.
116. Kishimoto T, Ishizaka K. Regulation of antibody response in vitro. VI Carrier-specific helper cells for IgG and IgE antibody response. J Immunol 1973; 111:720-32.
117. Grun JL, Maurer PH. Different T helper cell subsets elicited in mice utilizing two different adjuvant vehicles: the role of endogenous interleukin 1 in proliferative responses. Cell Immunol 1989; 121:134-45.
118. Wodnar-Filipowicz A, Heusser CH, Moroni C. Production of the haemopoietic growth factors GM-CSF and interleukin-3 by mast cells in response to IgE receptor- mediated activation. Nature (London) 1989; 339:150-2.
119. Plaut M, Pierce JH, Watson CJ et al. Mast cell lines produce lymphokines in response to cross-linkage of FcεRI or to calcium ionophores. Nature (London) 1989; 339:64-7.
120. Holmes KL, Palfree RG, Hammerling U et al. Alleles of the Ly-17 alloantigen define polymorphisms of the murine IgG Fc receptor. Proc Nat Acad Sci US 1985; 82:7706-10.
121. Hibbs ML, Hogarth PM, McKenzie IF. The mouse Ly-17 locus identifies a polymorphism of the Fc receptor. Immunogenetics 1985; 22:335-48.
122. Mark WH, Kimura S, Hammerling U. Biochemical characterization of murine lymphoid alloantigen Ly-m20.2, a cell surface marker controlled by a gene linked to the Mls locus. J Immunol 1985; 135:2635-41.

123. Nagel JE, White C, Ming SL et al. IgE synthesis in man. II Comparison of tetanus and diphtheria IgE antibody in allergic and nonallergic children. J Allergy Clin Immunol 1979; 63:308-14.
124. Jones GL, Spencer L, Lord R et al. Peptide vaccines derived from a malarial surface antigen: effects of dose and adjuvants on immunogenicity. Immunol Letters 1990; 24:253-60.
125. Saul A, Lord R, Jones GL et al. Protective immunization with invariant peptides of the *Plasmodium falciparum* antigen MSA2. J Immunol 1992; 148:208-11.
126. Cooper PD, Turner R, McGovern J. Algammulin (gamma inulin/alum hybrid adjuvant) has greater adjuvanticity than alum for hepatitis B surface antigen in mice. Immunol Letters 1990; 27:131-4.
127. Palmer DG, Cooper PD, Carnegie PR et al. A new polysaccharide adjuvant (Algammulin) useful for the improvement of cell-mediated immune responses in sheep. Aust Soc Parasitol Abstr 1990; Fremantle WA.
128. Freund J. The mode of action of immunological adjuvants. Adv Tuberc Res 1956; 7:130-48.
129. Bomford R. The comparative selectivity of adjuvants for humoral and cell-mediated immunity. I Effect on the antibody response to bovine serum albumin and sheep red blood cells of Freund's incomplete and complete adjuvants, Alhydrogel, *Corynebacterium parvum, Bordetella pertussis,* muramyl dipeptide and saponin. Clin Exp Immunol 1980; 39:426-34.
130. Revoltella R, Ovary Z. Reaginic antibody production in different mouse strains. Immunology 1969; 17:45-54.
131. Berman PW, Gregory T, Crase D et al. Protection from genital herpes simplex virus type 2 infection by vaccination with cloned type 1 glycoprotein D. Science 1985; 227:1490-2.
132. Pearson CM. Development of arthritis, periarthritis and periostitis in rats given adjuvant. Proc Soc Exp Biol Med NY 1956; 91:95-101.
133. Allison AC. Autoimmune diseases: concepts of pathogenesis and control. In: Talal N, ed. Autoimmunity: Genetic, Immunologic, Virologic and Clinical Aspects. New York: Academic Press, 1977:92-139.
134. Ellouz F, Adam A, Ciorbaru R et al. Minimal structural requirements for adjuvant activity of bacterial peptidoglycan derivatives. Biochem Biophys Res Commun 1974; 59:1317-25.
135. Audibert F, Przewlocki G, Leclerc CD et al. Enhancement by murabutide of the immune response to natural and synthetic hepatitis B surface antigens. Infect Immun 1984; 45:261-6.
136. Lefrancier P, Demier M, Jamet X et al. Apyrogenic, adjuvant-active N-acetylmuramyldipeptides. J Med Chem 1982; 25:90-3.
137. Bahr GM, Chedid LA, Behbehani K. Induction, in vivo and in vitro, of macrophage membrane interleukin-1 by adjuvant-active synthetic muramyl peptides. Cell Immunol 1987; 107:443-54.
138. Allison AC, Byars NE. An adjuvant formulation that selectively elicits the formation of antibodies of protective isotypes and of cell-mediated immunity. J Immunol Meth 1986; 95:157-68.
139. Audibert F, Chedid L, Lefrancier P et al. Distinctive adjuvanticity of synthetic analogs of mycobacterial water-soluble components. Cell Immunol 1976; 21:243-9.
140. Kishimoto T, Hirai Y, Nakanishi K et al. Regulation of antibody response in

different immunoglobulin classes. VI Selective suppression of IgE response by administration of antigen-conjugated muramyl peptides. J Immunol 1979; 123:2709-15.
141. Leclerc C, Audibert F, Chedid L. Influence of a synthetic adjuvant (MDP) on qualitative and quantitative changes of serum globulins. Immunol 1978; 35:963-70.
142. Ohkuni H, Norose Y, Ohta M et al. Adjuvant activities in production of reaginic antibody by bacterial cell wall peptidoglycan or synthetic N-acetylmuramyl dipeptides in mice. Infect Immun 1979; 24:313-8.
142a. Butler JE, Richerson HB, Swanson PA et al. The influence of muramyl peptide on the secretory immune response. Ann NY Acad Sci 1983; 409:669-87.
142b. Leclerc C, Bourgeois E, Chedid L. Demonstration of muramyl dipeptide (MDP)-induced T-suppressor cells responsible for MDP immunosuppressive activity. Eur J Immunol 1982; 12:249-52.
142c. Ferguson TA, Krieger NJ, Pesce A. Enhancement of antigen specific suppression by muramyl dipeptide. Infect Immun 1983; 39:800-6.
143. Parant MA, Audibert FM, Chedid LA et al. Immunostimulant activities of a lipophilic muramyl dipeptide derivative and of desmuramyl peptidolipid analogs. Infect Immun 1980; 27:826-31.
144. Staruch MJ, Wood DD. The adjuvanticity of interleukin 1 in vivo. J Immunol 1983; 130:2191-4.
145. Kurt-Jones EA, Beller DI, Mizel SB et al. Identification of membrane-associated interleukin 1 in macrophages. Proc Nat Acad Sci US 1985; 82:1204-8.
146. Damais C, Parant M, Chedid L et al. In vitro spleen cell responsiveness to various analogs of MDP (N-acetylmuramyl-L-alanyl-D-isoglutamine), a synthetic immunoadjuvant, in MDP high-responder mice. Cell Immunol 1978; 35:173-9.
147. Watson J, Whitlock C. Effect of a synthetic adjuvant on the induction of primary immune responses in T-cell depleted spleen cultures. J Immunol 1978; 121:383-9.
148. Odean MJ, Frane CM, Van derVieren M et al. Involvement of gamma interferon in antibody enhancement by adjuvants. Infect Immun 1990; 58:427-32.
149. Oppenheim JJ, Kovacs EJ, Matsushima K et al. There is more than one interleukin 1. Immunol Today 1986; 7:45-56.
150. Zidek Z, Masek K, Jiricka Z. Arthritogenic activity of a synthetic immunoadjuvant, muramyl dipeptide. Infect Immun 1982; 35:674-9.
151. Parant M. Biologic properties of a new synthetic adjuvant, muramyl dipeptide (MDP). Springer Semin Immunopathol 1979; 2:101-18.
152. Waters R, Terrell T, Jones GH. Uveitis induction in the rabbit by muramyl dipeptides. Infect Immun 1986; 51:816-25.
153. Allison AC, Byars NE, Waters RV. Immunologic adjuvants: efficacy and safety considerations. In: Nervig RM, Gough PM, Kaeberle ML et al, eds. Advances in Carriers and Adjuvants for Veterinary Biologics. Ames: Iowa State University Press 1986: 91-103.
154. Reichert CM, Carelli C, Jolivet M et al. Synthesis of conjugates containing N- acetylmuramyl-L-alanyl-D-isoglutaminyl (MDP). Their use as hapten-carrier systems. Mol Immunol 1980; 17:357-63.
155. Raetz, CRH. Biochemistry of endotoxins. Ann Rev Biochem 1990; 59:129-70.
156. Taylor PW. Non-immunoglobulin activators of the complement system. In: Sim RB, ed. Activators and Inhibitors of Complement. Dordrecht: Kluwer Academic Publishers, 1993:37-68.

157. Bergstedt-Lindqvist S, Sideras P, Macdonald HR et al. Regulation of Ig class secretion by soluble products of certain T cell lines. Immunol Rev 1984; 78:25-50.
158. Martinez-Alonso C, Coutinho A, Augustin A. Immunoglobulin C-gene expression. I The commitment to IgG subclass of secretory cells is determined by the quality of the nonspecific stimuli. Eur J Immunol 1980; 10:698-702.
159. Snapper CM, Paul WE. Interferon-γ and B cell stimulatory factor-1 reciprocally regulate Ig isotype production. Science 1987; 236:944-7.
160. Ohta M, Nakashima I, Kato N. Adjuvant action of bacterial lipopolysaccharide in induction of delayed-type hypersensitivity to protein antigens. II Relationships of intensity of the action to that of other immunological activities. Immunobiol 1982; 163:460-9.
161. Lynn WA, Golenbock DT. Lipopolysaccharide antagonists. Immunol Today 1992; 13:271-276.
162. Adams DO, Hamilton TA. The cell biology of macrophage activation. Ann Rev Immunol 1984; 2:283-318.
163. Fidler IJ. Intracellular activation of tumoricidal properties in mouse macrophages and human monocytes by recombinant mouse or human gamma interferon encapsulated in liposomes. Ann Inst Past/Immunol 1986; 137C:212-5.
164. Meltzer MS, Hoover DL, Gilbreath MJ et al. Experimental variables for induction of activated cytotoxic macrophages. Ann Inst Past/Immunol 1986; 137C:206-11.
165. Schreiber RD, Celada A. Molecular characterization of interferon-c as a macrophage- activating factor. Lymphokines 1983; 11:87-118.
166. Revel M, Chebat S. Interferon-activated genes. Trends Biochem Sci 1986; 11:166-70.
167. Gery I, Kruger J, Spiesel SZ. Stimulation of B lymphocytes by endotoxin. Reactions of thymus-deprived mice and karyotypic analysis of dividing cells in mice bearing T6T6 thymus grafts. J Immunol 1972; 108:1088-91.
168. Qureshi N, Takayama K, Ribi E. Purification and structural determination of nontoxic lipid A obtained from the lipopolysaccharide of *Salmonella typhimurium.* J Biol Chem 1982; 257:11808-15.
169. Ribi E. Structure-function relationship of bacterial adjuvants. In: Nervig RM, Gough PM, Kaeberle ML et al, eds. Advances in Carriers and Adjuvants for Veterinary Biologics. Ames: Iowa State University Press 1986: 35-49.
170. Tomai, MA, Solem LE, Johnson AG et al. The adjuvant properties of a nontoxic monophosphoryl lipid A in hyporesponsive and aging mice. J Biol Resp Modif 1987; 6:99-107.
171. Baker PJ, Hiernaux JR, Fauntleroy MB et al. Inactivation of suppressor T cell activity by non-toxic monophosphoryl lipid A. Infect Immun 1988; 56:1076-83.
172. Takayama K, Qureshi E, Ribi E et al. Separation and characterization of toxic and non- toxic forms of lipid A. Rev Inf Dis 1984; 6:439-43.
173. Vosika GJ, Barr C, Gilbertson D. Phase I study of intravenous modified lipid A. Cancer Immunol Immunother 1984; 18:107-12.
174. Mitchell MS, Kan-Mitchell J, Kempf RA et al. Active specific immunotherapy for melanoma: phase I trial of allogeneic lysates and a novel adjuvant. Cancer Res 1988; 48:5883-93.
174a. Miller JJ 3rd, Olds LC. Antibodies to lipid A in pauciarticular juvenile arthritis: clinical studies. J Rheumatol 1992; 19:959-63.

175. Dalsgaard K. Saponin adjuvants. III Isolation of a substance from Quillaja saponaria Molina with adjuvant activity in foot-and-mouth disease vaccines. Arch Gesamte Virusforsch 1974; 44:243-54.
176. Morein B, Sundqvist B, Höglund S et al. ISCOM, a novel structure for antigenic presentation of membrane proteins from enveloped viruses. Nature (London) 1984; 308:457-60.
177. Morein B, Lövgren K, Höglund S. Immunostimulating complex. In: Gregoriadis G, Allison AC, Poste G, eds. Immunological Adjuvants and Vaccines. NATO ASI Series A: Life Sciences, Vol 179. New York: Plenum Press 1989: 153-61.
178. Chavali SR, Francis T, Campbell JB. An in vitro study of immunomodulatory effects of some saponins. Int J Immunopharmacol 1987; 9:675-83.
179. Flebbe LM, Braley-Mullen H. Immunopotentiating effects of the adjuvants SGP and Quil A. I Antibody responses to T-dependent and T-independent antigens. Cell Immunol 1986; 99:119-27.
180. Flebbe LM, Braley-Mullen H. Immunopotentiating effects of the adjuvants SGP and Quil A. II Identification of responding cell populations. Cell Immunol 1986; 99:128-39.
181. Lövgren K. The serum antibody response distributed in subclasses and isotypes after intranasal and subcutaneous immunization with influenza virus immunostimulating complexes. Scand J Immunol 1988; 27:241-5.
182. Jones PD, Tha Hla R, Morein B et al. Cellular immune responses in the murine lung to local immunization with influenza A virus glycoproteins in micelles and immunostimulatory complexes (iscoms). Scand J Immunol 1988: 27:645-52.
183. Fossum C, Bergstrom M, Lovgren K et al. Effect of iscoms and their adjuvant moiety (matrix) on the initial proliferation and IL-2 responses: comparison of spleen cells from mice inoculated with iscoms and/or matrix. Cell Immunol 1990; 129:414-25.
184. Overnes G, Nesse LL, Waldeland H et al. Immune response after immunization with an experimental *Toxoplasma gondii* ISCOM vaccine. Vaccine 1991; 9:25-8.
185. Takehashi H, Takeshita T, Morein B et al. Induction of CD8+ cytotoxic T cells by immunization with purified HIV-1 envelope protein in ISCOMs. Nature (London) 1990; 344:873-5.
186. Morein B, Lövgren K, Höglund S et al. The ISCOM: an immunostimulating complex. Immunol Today 1987; 8:333-8.
187. Tung HS, Ju S-T, Sato S et al. Production of large amounts of antibodies in individual mice. J Immunol 1976; 116:676-81.
188. Specter S, Friedman H, Chedid L. Dissociation between the adjuvant vs mitogenic activity of a synthetic muramyl dipeptide for murine splenocytes. Proc Soc Exp Biol Med NY 1977; 155:349-93.
189. Leclerc C, Lowy I, Chedid L. Influence of MDP and of some analogous synthetic glycopeptides on the in vitro mouse spleen cell viability and immune response to sheep erythrocytes. Cell Immunol 1978; 38:286-93.
190. Wraith DC, Vessey AE, Askonas BA. Purified influenza virus nucleoprotein protects mice from lethal infection. J Gen Virol 1987; 68:433-40.
191. Good MF. A malaria vaccine strategy based on the induction of cellular immunity. Immunol Today 1992; 13:126-30.

192. Perlmutter RM, Hansburg D, Briles DE et al. Subclass restriction of murine anti- carbohydrate antibodies. J Immunol 1978; 121:566-72.
193. Snapper CM, McIntyre TM, Mandler R et al. Induction of IgG3 secretion by interferon- gamma: a model for T cell-independent class switching in response to T cell-independent type 2 antigens. J Exp Med 1992; 175:1367-71.
194. Shapiro ED, Ward JI. The epidemiology and prevention of disease caused by *Haemophilus influenzae* type b. Epidemiol Rev 1991; 13:113-42.
195. Reed SG, Pihl DL, Conlon PJ et al. IL-1 as adjuvant. Role of T cells in the augmentation of specific antibody production by recombinant human IL-1α. J Immunol 1989; 142:3129-33.
196. Ramshaw IA, Andrew ME, Phillips SM et al. Recovery of immunodeficient mice from a vaccinia virus/IL-2 recombinant infection. Nature (London) 1987; 329:545-6.
197. Playfair JH, DeSouza JB. Recombinant gamma interferon is a potent adjuvant for a malaria vaccine in mice. Clin Exp Immunol 1987; 67:5-10.
198. Finkelman FD, Katona IM, Mosmann TR et al. Interferon-γ regulates the isotypes of Ig secreted during in vivo humoral immune responses. J Immunol 1988; 140:1022-7.
199. Coffman RL, Schrader B, Carty J et al. A mouse T cell product that preferentially enhances IgA production. I Biologic characterization. J Immunol 1987; 139:3685-90.
200. Bond MW, Schrader B, Mosmann TR et al. A mouse T cell product that preferentially enhances IgA production. II Physicochemical characterization. J Immunol 1987; 139:3691-6.
201. Coffman RL, Lebman DA, Schrader B. Transforming growth factor-β specifically enhances IgA production by lipopolysaccharide-stimulated murine B lymphocytes. J Exp Med 1989; 170:1039-44.

CHAPTER 10

Rational Designs for Attenuated Live Virus Vaccines

R. Mark L. Buller

The use of attenuated live viruses as vaccines to protect against disease has spanned many centuries. As early as the 10th century A.D., it was recognized that inoculations (variolation) with scab material from an individual who had a milder form of smallpox could offer limited protection from the severe form of the disease. This practice gave way to the Jennerian approach, in which an animal strain of virus (cowpox virus) was used to immunize humans against a severe disease (smallpox) caused by a closely related human virus (variola virus).[1] When cross-protecting animal viruses were not available as a vaccine option, the disease-causing viruses were sequentially blind-passaged through animals, tissue explants or tissue culture followed by testing of the virus strain for the loss of virulence prior to efficacy testing in human populations. The viral vaccines currently in use for polio and chicken pox were developed in this manner.

With the advent of molecular genetics, the design of viral vaccines took on a more rational approach with the development of reassortment vaccines to achieve the necessary balance between immunogenicity and attenuation. Reassortment vaccines take advantage of the segmented genome of certain RNA viruses which allows the construction of a virus vaccine by substituting gene(s) for the immunoprotective antigens of the human pathogen for homologous genes in a closely related virus species which is naturally attenuated for replication in humans (i.e., human rotavirus VP7 in a rhesus rotavirus reassortment).[2]

For a great many of the other pathogenic viruses, current live virus vaccine strategies have focused on defining and attenuating or inactivating

Strategies in Vaccine Design, edited by Gordon L. Ada, D.Sc.

the genes or portions of genes which are responsible for virus virulence (without interfering with important antigenic epitopes). Virus attenuation through the introduction into the genome of single or multiple mutations in the form of deletions theoretically rules out reversion to the virulent phenotype which has been observed with the classically attenuated live vaccines such as the Sabin oral polio vaccine.[3] Recently the first gene-deleted vaccine (for immunization against pseudorabies virus) was licensed for use.[4] In the first part of this selected review, we will examine the attempts to balance immunogenicity with attenuation through the specific deletion of virus genes and, in the second part, briefly examine the recent advances in molecular genetics which have permitted the introduction of attenuating mutations into positive-strand and (to a lesser extent) negative-strand RNA viruses.

GENE-DELETED VIRUS VACCINE DESIGN

Poxviruses

Variola virus, the causative agent of smallpox, was eliminated from human populations through a worldwide immunization program employing a live, closely related poxvirus, vaccinia virus. Immunization with vaccinia virus (VV; for review see Moss[5]) was not without its own health risks, with the severity and frequency of VV-associated complications dependent in part on the VV strain utilized for immunizations.[1, 6]

With the eradication of smallpox, the need to improve the safety of the VV vaccine lacked a rational basis until the early 1980s, when two studies proposed the development of VV as an expression vector which could be employed as a live recombinant virus vaccine for the prevention of other infectious diseases.[7, 8] Because of the broad host range of VV, VV-based vaccines could be applicable to the management of both human and veterinary diseases.

Although low cost, heat stability and ease of administration would be important attributes of a VV vaccine vector, concerns were again raised as to the potential for VV-related complications which reached 1254 cases per million primary immunizations with the New York City Board of Health (NYCBH) strain of VV.[9] Even though the NYCBH VV strain was one of the safest virus strains employed in the smallpox eradication program,[1, 6] its frequency of complications had been viewed in the light of a 20% mortality rate for infections with variola major. It would be desirable, however, to further reduce the potential for VV-related complications prior to the reintroduction of VV-based recombinant vaccines for human immunizations. In addition, proposals for the use of VV-based vaccines in domesticated animals or for the control of rabies in the wild stimulated discussion on the potential spread of the VV vaccine strain into non-target animal species, including man (see review by Binns and Smith[10]). These concerns initiated new research on the genetic basis of poxvirus host range and virulence.

The construction of a viable VV deletion mutant vP811 (top of Table 1), in which 55 open reading frames (ORFs) were deleted, suggested that at least 25% of the virus-encoded ORFs were not essential for replication in tissue culture and were probably involved in various aspects of virus replication and spread in the animal.[11,12] This large number of nonessential

Table 1. Selected vaccinia virus open-reading frames not essential for growth in tissue culture

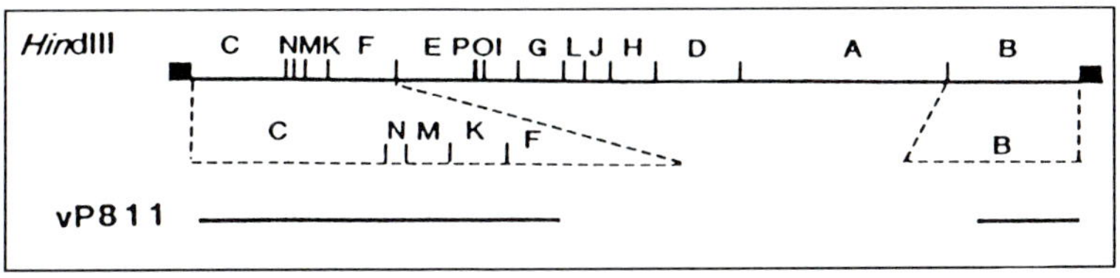

ORF[b]	Gene Bank Homology	Function	Important for Virus Replication *in Vivo*
C22L[c]	Tumor necrosis factor receptor	Binds TNF-α	Yes[122]
C13L-C10L[d]	Ankyrin repeat	Tissue culture hr	Not known[123, 124]
C11R	EGF	Growth factor	Yes[20, 21]
C12L	Serine protease inhibitor	Not known	Not known[125]
C7L[e]	Not known	Tissue culture hr	Not known[11]
C3L[e]	C4B binding protein	Blocks complement action	Yes[126, 127]
NIL[e]	Not known	Not known	Yes[128]
K1L[e]	Ankyrin repeat	Tissue culture hr	Not known[16]
K2L	Serine protease inhibitor	Blocks cell fusion	No[129, 130]
K3L	elF-2-α	Blocks interferon action	Not known[131]
F2L	Retroviral protease	Not known	Not known[132]
I4L	Ribonucleotide reductase	Nucleic acid metabolism	Yes[22, 133]
F13L	None	Extracellular virus	Yes[134]
E3L	dsRNA binding domain	Blocks interferon action	Not known[135]
D8L	Carbonic anhydrase	Cell surface binding	Yes[136, 137]
J2R[e]	Thymidine kinase	Nucleic acid metabolism	Yes[138]
A34R	C-type animal lectins	Extracellular virus	Not known[139, 154]
A42R	Profilin	Not known	Not known[140]
A44L	3β-hydroxy-5-ene steroid dehydrogenase	3β-hydroxy steroid dehydrogenase	Yes[141]
A45R	Superoxide dismutase	Not known	Not known[132]
A48R	Thymidylate kinase	Nucleic acid metabolism	Yes
A50R	DNA ligase	Nucleic acid metabolism	Yes[143]
A53R	Tumor necrosis factor receptor	Not known	Not known[144]
A56R[e]	Ig super family	Extracellular virus	Yes[132, 145]
B5R	Complement control protein	Extracellular virus	Yes[146, 147]
B8R	IFN-γ receptor	Binds IFN-γ	Not known [148]
B13R[d,e]	Serine protease inhibitor	Inhibits IL-1 and AA metabolism	Yes[17, 149]
B16R	Strong to IL-1 type 2 receptor	Binds IL-1	Yes[18, 19, 150]
B19R	Weak to IL-1 type 2 receptor	Not known	Not known[150]

[a] Horizontal line delineates the approximate boundaries of the deletion in vP811.[11]

[b] ORF designations are from VV strain Copenhagen,[132] although data are included for homologous genes in other vaccinia virus strains and poxviruses.

[c] This ORF is fragmented in VV strain Copenhagen but intact in cowpox virus (Pickup, personal communication) and myxoma virus[122]

[d] ORF designation from WR strain.

[e] ORFs deleted in NYVAC strain of VV as well as A25L/26L, C6L, C5L, C4L, C2L, C1L I4L, N2, M1 and M2.

genes provides numerous potential targets for virus attenuation, which may provide the opportunity to "fine-tune" the in vivo properties of the virus. Inactivation of a virus gene does not always result in attenuation of the virus at the expense of immunogenicity of the foreign antigen. For example, human papillomavirus L1 polypeptide was more immunogenic in a VV recombinant lacking ORF B13R than in its presence[13] which (by analogy to the cowpox virus/chick embryo model) may be due to the massive influx of inflammatory cells into the virus-induced lesion.[14, 15]

Table 1 is a selected list of ORFs of the Copenhagen strain of VV which have been shown, or are thought, to be required for virus replication and spread in vivo. These ORFs can be roughly divided into four groups with functions responsible for virus host range (K1L is required for virus replication in RK-13 cells[16]), production of extracellular virus (F13L), inhibition of host defense mechanisms at different levels (B13R inhibits IL-1β convertase[17] and B15R binds soluble IL-1[18, 19]), and stimulation of host cell metabolism (the product of ORF C11R, vaccinia growth factor [VGF] has properties similar to epidermal growth factor[20, 21]). Some of these ORFs have been examined in the mouse LD_{50} assays for their relative importance to vaccinia virus virulence. As shown in Table 2, there are wide fluctuations in LD_{50} values depending on the ORF inactivated, which lends credence to the notion that the attenuation level of VV can be fine-tuned. It is also clear that the level of attenuation gained by the inactivation of an ORF is

Table 2. Relative virulence of selected vaccinia virus mutants by the intracranial route in the mouse[a]

Vaccinia virus strain[b]	*Gene inactivated*	LD_{50} of mutant virus *relative to wild-type[c]*	*Reference No.[a]*
WR	TK	40,000	138
	VGF	20,000	20
	ORF N1L	13,000	128
	HA	3,500	145
	IL-1r homolog	355	18
	VCBP	57	151
	ORF C20L	7.5-50	145
	3β-hydroxy-steroid dehydrogenase	5-27	152
	RR	17	133
NYCBH	TK	50	22
	RR	794	22
	HA	7,943	22
Wyeth	TK	28	138
	VGF	1.3	22

[a] Serial dilutions of virus were inoculated by the intracranial route into BALB/c mice. The values were normalized to a WT value of 1.

[b] The Wyeth and WR strains of VV were derived from the NYCBH strain, see Fenner.[1]

[c] Value was calculated as LD_{50} mutant ÷ LD_{50} WT.

dependent on the VV strain (Table 2; compare LD_{50} values of strain WR TK^- [40,000] and Wyeth TK^- [28]; WR RR^- [17], and NYCBH RR^- [794]). Furthermore, the inactivation of a VV gene like RR can have a dramatic effect in the i.c. mouse model, but can cause little reduction of VV replicaton in the mouse skin.[22]

The knowledge gained in the molecular characterization of VV virulence genes has been employed in the construction of a VV vector (NYVAC) designed for human vaccine applications.[23] NYVAC differs from the parental Copenhagen strain by the precise deletion of 18 ORFs (see Table 1) which resulted in poor to no growth in six tested human-derived cell lines (MRC-5, WISH, Detroit 532, HEL 299, JT-1 and HNK). The NYVAC strain of VV was shown to be more highly attenuated than the Wyeth vaccine strain by the following criteria: 1) induration or ulceration at the site of inoculated rabbit skin, 2) clearance of infectious virus from infected rabbit skin, and 3) LD_{50} determinations for intraperitoneal injections of immunodeficient mice and intradermal and intracranial injections of rabbits and mice, respectively. These data support the notion that the NYVAC strain in humans will probably be more attenuated than the NYCBH strain. Even with this attenuated phenotype, NYVAC-based recombinant viruses retained the ability to induce in animal models strong immune responses to certain foreign antigens which were protective on challenge with rabies (NYVAC-RG)[23] or Japanese encephalitis virus (NYVAC-JEV).[24] Taken together, these data suggested that extensive replication of the VV vaccine was not important in conferring immunity to challenge, especially if multiple immunizations were involved. This hypothesis is supported by studies with fowlpox or canarypox vectors, which do not replicate in mammalian cells yet induce protective immunity to challenge with feline leukemia virus in cats (ALVAC-FL)[25] or rabies in dogs or cats (vFP-3[26], vCP16[27]). For an informative review, see Tartaglia et al.[28] Both replication-competent and -incompetent recombinant poxvirus vectors are now being tested in human clinical trials to ascertain safety and immunogenicity.[29-31]

Although the results to date with the highly attenuated NYVAC and avipoxvirus vectors in the small animal models are encouraging, immunogenicity and protection studies with a large number of antigens will be needed in non-human primates including chimpanzees to determine the general applicability of these vectors. We are always reminded of the promising studies with VV strain WR recombinants expressing respiratory syncytial virus F or G proteins which protected mice,[32] cotton rats,[33,34] and monkeys,[35] but not chimpanzees[36] (and presumably not man) from severe disease on challenge with respiratory syncytial virus. Similarly, a thymidine kinase insertion recombinant of the WR strain of VV expressing the Epstein-Barr virus gp340 glycoprotein protected the cottontop tamarins against Epstein-Barr virus-induced malignant lymphoma, whereas a similar construct based on the more attenuated Wyeth strain of VV did not.[37]

Herpesviruses

Herpesvirus infections constitute an extremely prevalent health risk for humans and economically important livestock. Infections are characterized by a primary disease of varying severity based on the age and animal species and is followed, in most cases, by virus latency.[38,39] This disease course emphasizes the need to develop prophylactic herpesvirus vaccines which limit virus replication to the site of initial infection and below the level of virus replication required to establish latency. Live gene-deleted herpesvirus vaccines have been developed for herpes simplex (HSV) and pseudorabies viruses, which are attenuated yet immunogenic, and incorporate genetic markers to assist differentiation between field virus infections and vaccine immunization (see review by Kit[4,40]). The experience with the pseudorabies vaccine design should facilitate human HSV vaccine research.

Pseudorabies virus

Pseudorabies virus (PRV) or Aujeszky's disease is caused by swine herpesvirus-1 which (in unvaccinated populations) induces abortions and stillbirths in pregnant sows, neurological disorders and mortality in piglets and respiratory ailments in adult pigs. Pigs that survive an acute infection often are latently infected and capable of reactivation and transmission to other pigs.[4, 40, 41]

Although conventional modified live PRV vaccines have been in use for a number of years, they have failed both in experimental tests[42, 43] and in the field[44] to prevent infection and the establishment of latency by virulent PSV. In addition, some of these vaccine strains were insufficiently attenuated for pregnant and newborn pigs. The current strategy for the control of PRV does not rely on the development of a vaccine that induces sterilizing immunity, but rather on the construction of safer vaccines which are genetically marked to facilitate the differentiation of uninfected immunized pigs from those infected with PRV field isolates. This would allow a systematic and intensive immunization campaign, followed by the serologic screening of pigs for evidence of infection and the culling of infected pigs. The construction of the gene-deleted marker PRV vaccines was dependent on a compilation of studies describing the major virulence genes of the virus and the viral antigens important in the induction of PRV immunity (see reviews by van Oirschot,[41] Kit[4,40]).

Modified live-virus marker vaccines licensed in the U.S. have reduced PRV virulence by deletion of TK, gI, gIII, and/or gp63 and have used the loss of gI, gX, or gIII as a diagnostic marker for detection of field virus infection of immunized populations.

Herpes simplex virus

HSVs infect the mucosal membranes and multiply in epithelia cells including sensory cells. Infection of the sensory nerve ending within these cells results in transport to the sensory nerve nucleus where the virus can remain latent for the life of the cell. Upon reactivation of the virus from the latent state, it migrates back to the sensory cell, replicates and is transmitted into the environment, all in the presence of virus-neutralizing antibody.[38,39]

The optimal design of a HSV live attenuated vaccine should focus at the inactivation of genes or DNA sequences which severely restrict the acute-phase replication of the virus and block the establishment and maintenance of—and reactivation from—latency, yet express virus antigens required for induction of protective immunity against both HSV-1 and HSV-2 infection (see review by Whitley and Meignier[45]). As with vaccinia virus, some of the virus genes important for virus-induced disease are nonessential for replication in tissue culture (at least 18 out of a total of 74 genes for HSV-1).[38] Some of these nonessential genes were deleted in the construction of two prototype HSV vaccines (R7017 and R7020[46]).

The R7017 strain was constructed from the F strain of HSV-1 by the deletion of 700 bp from within the coding sequence of the TK gene (which is important for neurovirulence)[47] and a second, larger, 14.5 kbp deletion spanning a region from the immediate early α27 gene in the long repeat element, across the internal inverted repeats to the immediate early α4 gene in the short element, which had the additional effect of preventing isomerization of the genome during virus replication. Glycoprotein (g) genes D, G, I and part of E lost to this 14.5 kbp deletion were reintroduced from HSV-2, giving this virus strain a unique pattern of type I- and II-specific antigens which would broaden the spectrum of the immune response and permit the serologic detection of infections of HSV-2, but not HSV-1, in R7017 vaccinees. Strain R7020 differed from strain R7017 by having the TK gene reinserted into the large deletion, making this virus susceptible to antiviral chemotherapy with acyclovir.[46]

The virulence of both R7017 and R7020 strains was greatly diminished as compared to WT virus in the various animal models, including intraocular inoculations of the mouse, rabbit and owl monkey; intravaginal inoculations of the guinea pig and owl monkey; and intracerebral inoculations of the mouse.[46,48] Interestingly, there were few detectable differences in attenuation between the TK^+ R7020 and the TK^-R7017 strains, although R7020 virus appeared to establish latent infections slightly more frequently than R7017 (tk^-) virus but less so than WT virus.[46] In addition, the attenuated phenotype of both R7017 and R7020 strains was genetically stable after multiple passages in mouse brains.[46] Although less immunogenic than WT virus, immunizations of mice[46] and owl monkeys[48] with R7017 and R7020 strains protected against severe disease on challenge, but did not block the establishment of latency by WT virus. Since both R7017 and R7020 strains were similarly attenuated and immunogenic, the tk^+ R7020 virus will probably be the preferred strain for clinical trials. Although the results of the R7017 and R7020 strains in animal models give reason for optimism, the failure of PRV vaccines in the natural host to prevent the establishment of latency by virulent field isolates may foreshadow the clinical experience with the R7017 and R7020 strains. It may be that the design of a human HSV vaccine for sterilizing immunity is not attainable, and a more modest performance goal may have to be established.

Adenoviruses

Of the 47 serotypes of human adenovirus (Ad), approximately one-third are associated with human disease while the rest are responsible for subclinical infections. In both cases, the virus is thought to persist for extended lengths of time in the host. Although Ads are associated with diseases of the respiratory tract, the eye, gastrointestinal tract and the urinary bladder, vaccines have only been developed against Ad types 4 and 7 and are only for use by the military.[49,50] Oral administration of unattenuated Ad4 and Ad7 enteric-coated capsules over an approximate 20-year period and in millions of military recruits established the safety, immunogenicity and efficacy of these vaccines. These vaccines were never licensed for use in the general population due to concerns about potential oncogenicity and pathogenicity in infants and immunocompromised individuals.[51] The admirable safety record of the Ad types 4 and 7 vaccines, the potential advantage of the oral route of administration over the parenteral routes for the induction of mucosal immunity, and the detailed understanding of the molecular genetics of the prototypic Ad viruses have suggested that Ad, like VV, be considered as a vector for immunization in the human population. The methodology for constructing Ad recombinant vectors[51-53] and the foreign immunogens expressed by them[52] have been recently reviewed. As with VV, Ad recombinant vectors can be constructed to be replication-competent or -incompetent in vivo depending on the sites selected for insertion of foreign DNA.

Compared to VV, the size of DNA fragments and the number of insertion sites in the Ad genome are severely restricted. Whereas VV vectors can received as much as 25 kbp of DNA,[54] Ad can accept 2 kbp[55] or a maximum of approximately 7 kbp with compensating deletions from early transcription regions of the genome. The E1, E3 and the junction of E4 and the inverted terminal repeat regions of the Ad genome have been utilized most often for insertions of foreign DNA. The E1 region is composed of the E1A and E1B transcription units. The former encodes five proteins; two of the major proteins (243 and 289 aa) appear involved in the immortalization of primary cells in cooperation with the E1B region, the transactivation of cellular promoters and the transrepression of both viral and cellular promoters.[56] The latter also encodes multiple proteins[57] with a 19 kDa and 55 kDa protein important for neoplastic transformation in cooperation with E1A. In addition (or perhaps related) to its role in transformation, the 19 kDa protein appears to suppress apoptosis[58] and the cytolysis of human cells induced by TNF.[58,59] Disruption of the E1 region by insertion or substitution of foreign DNA generates an Ad recombinant which undergoes abortive infection unless it is grown in human 293 cells expressing the Ad E1 region in *trans*;[60] nevertheless with $E1^-$ Ad vectors, the expression of foreign genes in vitro is not restricted to cells complementing the E1 defect but, on the contrary, can be obtained at high levels in various tissue culture lines.[61-63] These replication-defective Ad recombinant vectors have also been shown to induce neutralizing antibodies to the expressed protein and to protect with varying efficiencies against virus challenge in various animal models (Ad5/gp50 pseudorabies virus, rabbits and mice;[61] Ad5/HBs hepatitis B virus, chimpanzees;[63] and Ad5/gp340/220 Epstein-Barr virus, cottontop tamarin[62]). Replication-defective Ad vectors should reduce concerns about the safety of live Ad vaccines for possible use in humans.

Vaccine design strategies which require a replication-competent virus have most often made use of the E3 region for insertion of foreign DNA. The E3 region also is nonessential for replication in the lungs of hamsters[64] or cotton rats[65] but is maintained in natural isolates of Ad, indicating these genes are important in natural infections of humans.[66,67] This supports an in vivo role for this region in the natural host and infers that inactivation of E3 genes may affect virus virulence. For a detailed description of the functions of the E3 region refer to Wold and Gooding.[68] There are nine predicted Ad-2/5 E3 proteins, six of which have been identified in infected cells, and a further four for which functions have been assigned: the gp19K binds to certain class I antigens,[69] preventing their transport to the cell surface[70,71] and lysis of Ad-infected cells by Ad-specific cytotoxic T lymphocytes (CTL);[72] the 14.7K protein prevents tumor necrosis factor (TNF)-induced lysis of 14 of 15 mouse cell lines infected with Ad;[73-75] the 10.4 and 14.5K proteins exist as a complex[76] and also prevent TNF cytolysis of 11 of 15 Ad-infected mouse cell lines,[75] and downregulate the epidermal growth factor receptor in Ad-infected cells.[76,77] It is interesting that at least 4 of the 25 to 30 early Ad proteins function in blocking TNF cytolysis of Ad-infected cells.

As compared to the E1 region, the main advantage in expression of foreign genes from within the E3 is the likelihood of obtaining greater antigenic mass and, hopefully, increased immunogenicity and protection from pathogen challenge in vivo, whereas the major disadvantage may lie in too little attenuation. The expression level of a number of genes from within E1 or E3 appears to be comparable in tested cell lines.[64,78] Although both constructions appear immunogenic as indicated by the detection of specific neutralizing antibody in various animal models, in certain cases the $E3^-$ replication-competent Ad recombinant viruses seem to offer better protection to pathogen challenge (Ad5/gB HSV-1, mice[79] and Ad5/G vesicular stomatitis virus, mice[80]). A further consideration is the fact that the conditional replication of E1-substituted Ad recombinants in 293 cells precludes its propagation in cell lines such as WI38, which have been approved for production of virus vaccines; however, the main question in evaluating the E1- and E3-derived recombinant vectors is that of safety: Does inactivation of E3 functions decrease the risk of adenovirus-related side effects to an acceptable level for general use as a human vaccine vector?

To date, the studied functions of the E3 region appear targeted at the inflammatory and/or the immune responses to infection. The gp19K protein protects virus-infected cells from destruction by Ad-specific CTL, whereas the 14.7 and 10.4/14.5K proteins prevent cytolysis induced by TNF produced either nonspecifically by natural killer cells and/or macrophages or through immune recognition by $CD4^+$ T lymphocytes. Together, these virus functions may have principal roles in the establishment of persistent infections. Preliminary results from studies in small animals provide some support for a role of E3 functions in the regulation of the host response to infection, if not in the maintenance of viral persistence. Ginsberg and coworkers,[65] using the Ad5/cotton rat model, found the lymphocyte and macrophage/monocyte inflammatory response into the cotton rat's lung was exacerbated with Ad mutants lacking gp19K as compared to WT. Also, an E3 mutant expressing the gp19K but lacking at least the 10.4 and 14.7 proteins (and sensitive to TNF lysis in vitro) did not produce a significantly greater inflammatory infiltration in the cotton rat's lungs than did WT virus, although there were greater numbers and pockets of polymorphonuclear leukocytes. At this time, the molecular basis for these observations is not clear. The data do support the notion that live $E3^-$ Ad vaccine vectors may have altered pathogenicity in humans; however, it is not clear if this will be an increase in virulence or attenuation. It should be remembered that the unattenuated Ad vaccines used for military recruits presumably had an intact E3 region.

The third major insertion site is located at the right-hand end of the Ad genome, located between the start site for E4 transcription and the right-hand inverted terminal repeat element.[81,82] A number of genes have been recombined into this site and expressed to high levels (Ad7/gp160 HIV-1, in vitro;[83] Ad4,7/HBs, hepatitis B virus, dogs[82]). This insertion site usually has a compensating deletion in E3, and the Ad recombinants replicate unconditionally in tissue culture.

Lentiviruses

Currently, there are over 11 HIV-1 vaccine trials in seronegative individuals;[84] however, the lack of an animal model which faithfully mimics AIDS and the scarcity and exorbitant cost of the current alternative, chimpanzees, have contributed to the slow pace in vaccine design. Only purified subunit protein vaccines or live recombinant virus vectors expressing gp160 or other HIV-1 proteins are in trials, in spite of the record that live attenuated vaccines induce the longest-lasting immunity. Although live attenuated HIV-1 vaccines are not in consideration for clinical trials, studies with a strain of simian lentivirus (SIV) isolated from macaque monkeys have suggested that a live attenuated HIV-1 vaccine is at least a theoretical possibility (see review by Desrosiers[85]); however, it must be remembered that SIV differs from HIV-1 in several respects and, in particular, the V3 region of HIV-1 does not appear to have a functional homolog in SIV.

Infection of rhesus monkeys with SIV_{mac} results in an AIDS-like illness.[86] The availability of a pathogenic molecular clone of SIV_{mac}[87] and its complete nucleotide sequence[88] allowed the introduction of mutations into genes nonessential for replication in tissue culture, but possibly important for virus pathogenesis in the studied animal model. SIV_{mac} and HIV-1 have in common at least two gene functions (see Table 3; vpr/vpx and nef) nonessential for replication in tissue culture. Single or multiple deletions have been made in nonessential genes of the SIV_{mac} genome and the NRE region of the LTR which may be important for transcriptional control in vivo yet is dispensable for virus replication in tissue culture. These mutants are currently being evaluated in the rhesus monkey model to determine the optimal genetic manipulation(s) to obtain a live attenuated SIV_{mac} which is safe yet protects against a mucosal or intravenous challenge with relevant doses of cell-free or cell-associated virus.[85] Encouraging is the observation that six rhesus monkeys infected with a SIV_{mac} *nef*$^-$ have remained disease-free for three years, although a persistent low grade infection was detected. Eleven out of 12 control monkeys that received WT virus have died.[85,89] Two and a quarter years after immunization with SIV_{mac} *nef*$^-$, monkeys were challenged with live pathogenic cloned or uncloned SIV_{mac} WT. The monkeys survived challenge and displayed no evidence of disease nor could WT virus be isolated from cells 40 weeks post-challenge. Two of the four immunized

Table 3. Nonessential SIV and HIV Genes

Gene	SIV_{mac}	HIV-1	In vivo role[b]	Proposed function[c]
vpr/vpx[a]	+	+	?	Supports replication in macrophages?
nef	+	+	Yes	Regulation of gene expression?
vpu	–	+	?	Export of virions from cell
vif	+	+	?	Needed early during infection; essential?

[a] vpx may be a duplicated vpr gene;[153] thus, it can be speculated that vpr and vpx are interchangeable.

[b] SIV_{mac} model.

[c] See Desrosiers[85] for additional information and references.

and challenged monkeys were challenged a second time with a larger dose of 1000 rhesus monkey infectious doses of uncloned SIV_{mac} with little or no effect.[89] Although there are many road blocks to the utilization of a live attenuated lentivirus vaccine, these results give an experimental model where theoretical concerns can be tested.

GENE-MODIFIED VIRUS VACCINE DESIGN

POSITIVE-STRAND RNA VIRUSES

Development of full-length cDNA clones of the genomes of positive-strand RNA viruses was the first step in developing a rational vaccine strategy (polio,[90] Sindbis virus,[91,92] Dengue virus,[93] Venezuelan equine encephalitis virus[94]). cDNAs allowed the comparison of the nucleotide sequences of virulent virus strains with their attenuated counterparts (hepatitis A virus,[95] poliovirus[96]). Sequence differences were tested for importance in virus attenuation by the construction, first of chimeric viruses (Sindbis virus,[97] hepatitis A virus,[98] poliovirus,[3,99,100] Dengue virus[101,102]) and second by the introduction of specific mutations into the full-length cDNA clones (poliovirus,[3] Venezuelan equine encephalitis virus,[94] Sindbis virus[92,103]). In many cases, the attenuating mutations were found to reside in the envelope or capsid proteins (poliovirus;[3] Sindbis virus, E1,[97,104] E2;[105,106] Venezuelan equine encephalitis virus, E2[94]) which are important in determining tissue and cell tropism, and other mutations, as in the case of poliovirus[99,107,108] and Sindbis virus,[103,109,110] mapped to regulatory regions in the nontranslated portions of the genome.

This approach to vaccine construction seems promising, as a series of Venezuelan equine encephalitis virus mutants in the E2 gene have been constructed and shown to be both immunogenic and protective against challenge with virulent virus in the mouse and hamster models.[94] A number of groups are involved in the construction and evaluation of new poliovirus vaccine strains which will not revert to neurovirulence (see review by Racaniello[3]).

Based on its safety record and immunogenicity via the oral route of administration, poliovirus (like VV and Ad) is being studied as an expression vehicle for foreign sequences, especially those important for immunity to mucosal route pathogens. For example, the antigenic site N-Ag1 of P1/Sabin was replaced with an epitope of the transmembrane protein gp41 of HIV-1[111] or a portion of the L1 protein of human papillomavirus 16.[112] Similarly, Sindbis virus has been shown to be an efficient, broad host range vector for gene expression in animal cells.[113] Finally, experiments with Dengue chimeric viruses containing sequences from Dengue virus and the distantly related tick-borne encephalitis virus suggest the possibility of employing Dengue virus as a vector for the expression of closely related mosquito-borne viruses such as Japanese encephalitis virus, which continues to be a major public health problem in the Far East.[102]

NEGATIVE-STRAND RNA VIRUSES

Because the viral genome of RNA negative-strand viruses is not infectious alone or as a cDNA, the fine analysis of markers of virus attenuation and the ability to specifically mutate the virus genome has been hindered.

Recently, Luytjes and his colleagues[114] developed an efficient method to introduce synthetic gene segments into infectious influenza virus. Using this approach, attenuated chimeric influenza A viruses have been constructed, in one case with replacement of the 5′ and 3′ noncoding region with the homologous area from influenza B virus[115] and in another by substituting a foreign epitope for a portion of the neuraminidase molecule.[116] Although the cold-adapted live influenza virus vaccines hold promise for use in the general population,[117,118] field reversion of the vaccine virus to a virulent form is a concern which now can be addressed through the introduction of additional attenuating mutations.[119] Similar studies are being carried out in the respiratory syncytial virus,[120] Sendai virus[121] and other systems.

CONCLUSIONS

Molecular genetic approaches permit the deletion of whole genes or specific sequences to achieve a balance between virus attenuation and immunogenicity in both RNA and DNA viruses with encouraging results.

In certain cases, protective immunity has been obtained with replication-defective Ad and poxvirus recombinant vectors in small animal and lower primate models.

Deletion of sequences is an advantage over substitution mutations (which often characterized classically attenuated virus strains) in being stable without reversion to the virulent genotype.

In addition to attenuation of virus virulence, this approach allows 1) the genetic marking of the virus vaccine strain for detecting field virus infections of immunized populations; 2) the maintenance of critical antigenic epitopes in the protein targeted for modification; and 3) the addition of mutations which will improve the manufacturing or stability of the virus vaccine.

ACKNOWLEDGMENTS

I thank Dr. Gunasegaran Karupiah for critically reading this manuscript and Mr. Cornelio Duarte for archival research and NIAID intramural program support.

REFERENCES

1. Fenner F, Henderson I, Arita L et al. Smallpox and its eradication. Geneva: World Health Organization 1988:245-76.
2. Flores J, Kapikian AZ. Rotavirus vaccines. In: Davies JE, ed. Vaccines: New Approaches to Immunological Problems. Boston: Butterworth-Heinemann, 1992:255-88.
3. Racaniello VR. Poliovirus vaccines. In: Davis JE, ed. Vaccines: New Approaches to Immunological Problems. Boston: Butterworth-Heinemann, 1992:205-22.
4. Kit S. Genetically engineered vaccines for control of Aujeszky's disease (pseudorabies). Vaccine 1990;5:420-24.
5. Moss B. Vaccinia virus. In: Fields BN, Knipe DM et al., eds. Virology. 2nd ed. New York: Raven Press, Ltd, 1990:2079-111.

6. Buller RML, Palumbo GJ. Safety and attenuation of vaccinia virus. In: Smith GL, Binns M, eds. Recombinant Poxviruses. Boca Raton: CRC Press, 1992:235-67.
7. Panicali D, Paoletti E. Construction of poxviruses as cloning vectors: insertion of the thymidine kinase gene from herpes simplex virus into the DNA of infectious vaccinia virus. Proc Natl Acad Sci USA 1982;79:4927-31.
8. Mackett M, Smith GL, Moss B. Vaccinia virus: a selectable eukaryotic cloning and expression vector. Proc Natl Acad Sci USA 1982;79:7415-19.
9. Lane JM, Ruben FL, Neff JM et al. Complications of smallpox vaccination, 1968: results of ten statewide surveys. J Infect Dis 1970;122:303-09.
10. Binns MM, Smith GL (eds). Recombinant Poxviruses. Boca Raton: CRC Press, 1992:1-343.
11. Perkus ME, Goebel SJ, Davis SW et al. Deletion of 55 open reading frames from the termini of vaccinia virus. Virology 1991;180:406-10.
12. Buller RML, Palumbo GJ. Poxvirus pathogenesis. Microbiol Revs 1991;55:80-122.
13. Zhou J, Crawford L, McLean L et al. Increased antibody responses to human papillomavirus type 16 L1 protein expressed by recombinant vaccinia virus lacking serine protease inhibitor genes. J Gen Virol 1990;71:2185-90.
14. Palumbo GJ, Pickup DJ, Fredrickson TN et al. Inhibition of an inflammatory response is mediated by a 38 kDa protein of cowpox virus. Virology 1989;172:262-73.
15. Fredrickson TN, Sechler JMG, Palumbo GJ et al. Acute inflammatory response to cowpox virus infection of the chorioallantoic membrane of the chick embryo. Virology 1992;187:693-704.
16. Gillard S, Spehner D, Drillien R et al. Localization and sequence of a vaccinia virus gene required for multiplication in human cells. Proc Natl Acad Sci USA 1986;83:5573-77.
17. Ray CA, Black RA, Koronheim SR et al. Viral inhibition of inflammation: cowpox virus encodes an inhibitor of the interleukin-1β converting enzyme. Cell 1992;69:597-604.
18. Spriggs MK, Hruby DE, Maliszewski CR et al. Vaccinia and cowpox viruses encode a novel, secreted interleukin-1 binding protein. Cell 1992;71:145-52.
19. Alcami A, Smith GL. A soluble receptor for interleukin-1β encoded by vaccinia virus: a novel mechanism of virus modulation of the host responses to infection. Cell 1992;71:153-60.
20. Buller RML, Chakrabarti S, Cooper JA et al. Deletion of the vaccinia virus growth factor gene reduces virus virulence. J Virol 1988;62:866-74.
21. Buller RML, Chakrabarti S, Moss B et al. Cell proliferative response to vaccinia virus is mediated by VGF. Virology 1988;164:182-92.
22. Lee MS, Roos JM, McGuigan LC et al. Molecular attenuation of vaccinia virus: mutant generation and animal characterization. J Virol 1992;66:2617-30.
23. Tartaglia J, Perkus ME, Taylor J et al. NYVAC: a highly attenuated strain of vaccinia virus. Virology 1992;188:217-32.
24. Konishi E, Pincus S, Paoletti E et al. A highly attenuated host range-restricted vaccinia virus strain, NYVAC, encoding the prM, E, and NS1 genes of Japanese encephalitis virus prevents JEV viremia in swine. Virology 1992;190:454-58.
25. Tartaglia J, Jarrett O, Neil JC et al. Protection of cats against feline leukemia virus by vaccination with a canarypox virus recombinant, ALVAC-FL. J Virol 1993:67:2370-75.

26. Taylor J, Weinberg R, Languet B et al. Recombinant fowlpox virus inducing protective immunity in non-avian species. Vaccine 1988;6:466-72.
27. Taylor J, Trimarchi C, Weinberg R et al. Efficacy studies on a canarypox-rabies recombinant virus. Vaccine 1991;9:190-93.
28. Tartaglia J, Cox WI, Taylor J et al. Live vectors as vaccines: highly attenuated poxvirus vectors. AIDS Res Human Retrovir 1992:8:1445-47.
29. Cooney EL, Collier AC, Greenberg PD et al. Safety of and immunological response to a recombinant vaccinia virus vaccine expressing HIV envelope glycoprotein. Lancet 1991;337:565-72.
30. Cadoz M, Strady A, Meignier B et al. Immunisation with canarypox virus expressing rabies glycoprotein. Lancet 1992;339:1429-32.
31. Graham BS, Matthews TJ, Belshe RB et al. Augmentation of human immunodeficiency virus type 1 neutralizing antibody by priming with gp160 recombinant vaccinia and boosting with rgp160 in vaccinia-naive adults. J Infect Dis 1993;167:533-37.
32. Wertz GW, Stott EJ, Young KK-Y et al. Expression of the fusion protein of human respiratory syncytial virus from recombinant vaccinia virus vectors and protection of vaccinated mice. J Virol 1987;61:293-98.
33. Elango N, Prince GA, Murphy BR et al. Resistance to human respiratory syncytial virus (RSV) infection induced by immunization of cotton rats with a recombinant vaccinia virus expressing the RSV G glycoprotein. Proc Natl Acad Sci USA 1986;83:1906-11.
34. Olmstead RA, Elango N, Prince GA et al. Expression of the F glycoprotein of respiratory syncytial virus by a recombinant vaccinia virus: comparison of the individual contributions of the F and G glycoproteins to host immunity. Proc Natl Acad Sci USA 1986;83:7462-67.
35. Olmstead RA, Buller RML, Collins PL et al. Evaluation in non-human primates of the safety, immunogenicity and efficacy of recombinant vaccinia viruses expressing the F or G glycoprotein of respiratory syncytial virus. Vaccine 1988:6:519-24.
36. Collins PL, Purcell RH, London WT et al. Evaluation in chimpanzees of vaccinia virus recombinants that express the surface glycoproteins of human respiratory syncytial virus. Vaccine 1990;8:164-69.
37. Morgan AJ, Mackett M, Finerty S et al. Recombinant vaccinia virus expressing Epstein-Barr virus glycoprotein gp340 protects cottontop tamarins against EB virus-induced malignant lymphomas. J Med Virol 1988;25:189-95.
38. Roizman B, Sears AE. Herpes simplex viruses and their replication. In: Fields BN, Knipe DM et al, eds. Virology. 2nd ed. New York: Raven Press, Ltd, 1990:1795-841.
39. Whitley RJ. Herpes simplex viruses. In: Fields BN, Knipe DM et al, eds. Virology. 2nd ed. New York: Raven Press, Ltd, 1990:1843-87.
40. Kit S, Kit M. Genetically engineered herpesvirus vaccines. Prog Med Virol 1991;38:128-66.
41. van Oirschot JT, Gielkens ALJ, Moormann RJM et al. Marker vaccines, virus protein-specific antibody assays and the control of Aujeszky's disease. Vet Microbiol 1990;23:85-101.
42. Vannier P. Experimental infection of fattening pigs with pseudorabies (Aujeszky's disease) virus: efficacy of attenuated live- and inactivated-virus vaccines in pigs with or without passive immunity. Am J Vet Res 1985;46:1498-502.

43. Schoenbaum MA, Beran GW, Murphy DP. Pseudorabies virus latency and reactivation in vaccinated swine. Am J Vet Res 1990;51:334-38.
44. Cowen P, Li S, Guy JS et al. Reactivation of latent pseudorabies virus infection in vaccinated commercial sows. Am J Vet Res 1990;51:354-58.
45. Whitley RJ, Meignier B. Herpes simplex viruses. In: Davis JE, ed. Vaccines: New Approaches to Immunological Problems. Boston: Butterworth-Heinemann, 1992:223-54.
46. Meignier B, Longnecker R, Roizman B. In vivo behavior of genetically engineered herpes simplex viruses R7017 and R7020: construction and evaluation in rodents. J Infect Dis 1988;158:602-14.
47. Field HJ, Wildy P. The pathogenicity of thymidine kinase-deficient mutants of herpes simplex virus in mice. J Hyg 1978;81:267-77.
48. Meignier B, Martin B, Whitley RJ et al. In vivo behavior of genetically engineered herpes simplex viruses R7017 and R7020. II. Studies in immunocompetent and immunosuppressed owl monkeys (*Aotus trivirgatus*). J Infect Dis 1990;162:313-21.
49. Horwitz MS. Adenoviruses. In: Fields BN, Knipe DM et al, eds. Virology. 2nd ed. New York: Raven Press, Ltd, 1990:1723-40.
50. Horwitz MS. Adenoviridae and their replication. In: Fields BN, Knipe DM et al, eds. Virology. 2nd ed. New York: Raven Press, Ltd, 1990:1679-721.
51. Graham FL, Prevec L. Adenovirus-based expression vectors and recombinant vaccines. In: Davis JE, ed. Vaccines: New Approaches to Immunological Problems. Boston: Butterworth-Heinemann, 1992:363-90.
52. Berkner KL. Expression of heterologous sequences in adenoviral vectors. Curr Top Microbiol Immunol 1992;159:39-66.
53. Graham FL, Prevec L. Manipulation of adenovirus vectors. In: Murray EJ, ed. Methods in Molecular Biology. Gene Transfer and Expression Protocols, Vol. 7. Clifton: Humana Press, 1991:109-29.
54. Smith GL, Moss B. Infectious poxvirus vectors have capacity for at least 25,000 base pairs of foreign DNA. Gene 1983;25:21-28.
55. Jones N, Shenk T. Isolation of deletion and substitution mutants of adenovirus type 5. Cell 1978;13:181-88.
56. Moran E, Mathews MB. Multiple functional domains in the adenovirus E1A gene. Cell 1987;48:177-78.
57. Lewis JB, Anderson CW. Identification of adenovirus type 2 early region 1B proteins that share the same N terminus as do the 495R and 155R proteins. J Virol 1987;61:3879-88.
58. White E, Sabbatini P, Debbas M et al. The 19-kilodalton adenovirus E1B transforming protein inhibits programmed cell death and prevents cytolysis by tumor necrosis factor α. Mol Cell Biol 1992;12:2570-80.
59. Gooding LR, Aquino L, Duerksen-Hughes PJ et al. The E1B 19000-molecular-weight protein of group C adenoviruses prevents tumor necrosis factor cytolysis of human cells but not of mouse cells. J Virol 1991;65:3083-94.
60. Graham FL, Smiley J, Russell WC et al. Characteristics of a human cell line transformed by DNA from human adenovirus 5. J Gen Virol 1977;36:59-72.
61. Eliot M, Gilardi-Hebenstreit P, Toma B et al. Construction of a defective adenovirus expressing the pseudorabies virus glycoprotein gp50 and its use as a live vaccine. J Gen Virol 1990;71:2425-31.
62. Ragot T, Finerty S, Watkins PE et al. Replication-defective recombinant adenovirus expressing the Epstein-Barr virus (EBV) envelope glycoprotein

gp340/220 induces protective immunity against EBV-induced lymphomas in the cottontop tamarin. J Gen Virol 1993;74:501-7.
63. Levrero M, Barban V, Manteca S et al. Defective and nondefective adenovirus vectors for expressing foreign genes in vitro and in vivo. Gene 1991;101:195-202.
64. Morin JE, Lubeck MD, Barton JE et al. Recombinant adenovirus induced antibody response to hepatitis B virus surface antigen in hamsters. Proc Natl Acad Sci USA 1987;84:4626-30.
65. Ginsberg HS, Lundholm-Beauchamp U, Horswood RL et al. Role of early region 3 (E3) in pathogenesis of adenovirus disease. Proc Natl Acad Sci USA 1989;86:3823-27.
66. Adrian T, Best B, Hierholzer JC et al. Molecular epidemiology and restriction site mapping of adenovirus type 3 genome types. J Clin Microbiol 1989;27:1329-34.
67. Adrian T, Becker M, Hierholzer JC et al. Molecular epidemiology and restriction site mapping of adenovirus type 7 genome types. Arch Virol 1989;106:73-84.
68. Wold WSM, Gooding LR. Region E3 of Adenovirus: A cassette of genes involved in host immunosurveillance and virus-cell interactions. Virol 1991;184:1-8.
69. Kvist S, Ostberg L, Persson H et al. Molecular association between transplantation antigens and cell surface antigen in adenovirus-transformed cell line. Proc Natl Acad Sci USA 1978;75:5674-78.
70. Andersson M, Pääbo S, Nilsson T et al. Impaired intracellular transport of class I MHC antigens as a possible means for adenoviruses to evade immune surveillance. Cell 1985;43:215-22.
71. Burgert H-G, Kvist S. An adenovirus type 2 glycoprotein blocks cell surface expression of human histocompatibility class I antigens. Cell 1985;41:987-97.
72. Rawle FC, Tollefson AE, Wold WSM et al. Mouse anti-adenovirus cytotoxic T lymphocytes. Inhibition of lysis by E3 gp19K but not E3 14.7K. J Immunol 1989;143:2031-37.
73. Gooding LR, Elmore LW, Tollefson AE et al. A 14,700 MW protein from the E3 region of adenovirus inhibits cytolysis by tumor necrosis factor. Cell 1988;53:341-46.
74. Gooding LR, Sofola IO, Tollefson AE et al. The adenovirus E3-14.7K protein is a general inhibitor of tumor necrosis factor-mediated cytolysis. J Immunol 1990;145:3080-86.
75. Gooding LR, Ranheim TS, Tollefson AE et al. The 10,400- and 14,500-dalton proteins encoded by region E3 of adenovirus function together to protect many but not all mouse cell lines against lysis by tumor necrosis factor. J Virol 1991;65:4114-23.
76. Tollefson AE, Stewart AR, Yei S et al. The 10,400- and 14,500-dalton proteins encoded by region E3 of adenovirus form a complex and function together to down-regulate the epidermal growth factor receptor. J Virol 1991;65:3095-105.
77. Carlin CR, Tollefson AE, Brady HA et al. Epidermal growth factor receptor is down-regulated by a 10,400 MW protein encoded by the E3 region of adenovirus. Cell 1989;57:135-44.
78. Ballay A, Levrero M, Buendia M-A et al. In vitro and in vivo synthesis of the hepatitis B surface antigen and of the receptor for polymerized human serum albumin from recombinant human adenovirus. EMBO J 1985;4:3861-65.

79. McDermott MR, Graham FL, Hanke T et al. Protection of mice against lethal challenge with herpes simplex virus by vaccination with an adenovirus vector expressing HSV glycoprotein B. Virology 1989;169:244-47.
80. Prevec L, Schneider M, Rosenthal KL et al. Use of human adenovirus-based vectors for antigen expression in animals. J Gen Virol 1989;70:429-34.
81. Saito I, Oya Y, Yamamoto K et al. Construction of nondefective adenovirus type 5 bearing a 2.8 kilobase hepatitis B virus DNA near the right end of its genome. J Virol 1985;54:711-19.
82. Mason BB, Davis AR, Bhat BM et al. Adenovirus vaccine vectors expressing hepatitis B surface antigen: importance of regulatory elements in the adenovirus major late intron. Virology 1990;177:452-61.
83. Chanda PK, Natuk RJ, Mason BB et al. High level expression of the envelope glycoproteins of the human immunodeficiency virus type 1 in presence of rev gene using helper-independent adenovirus type 7 recombinants. Virology 1990;175:535-47.
84. Barrett PN, Dorner F. Vaccines in AIDS: present state of knowledge. Int Arch Allergy Immunol 1993;100:93-8.
85. Desrosiers RC. HIV with multiple gene deletions as a live attenuated vaccine for AIDS. AIDS Res Human Retrovir 1992;8:411-21.
86. Desrosiers RC. The simian immunodeficiency viruses. Annu Rev Immunol 1990;8:557-78.
87. Kestler H Kodama T, Ringler D et al. Induction of AIDS in rhesus monkeys by molecularly cloned simian immunodeficiency virus. Science 1990;248:1109-12.
88. Regier DA, Desrosiers RC. The complete nucleotide sequence of a pathogenic molecular clone of simian immunodeficiency virus. AIDS Res Hum Retrovir 1990;6:1221-32.
89. Daniel MD, Kirchhoff F, Czajak SC et al. Protective effects of a live attenuated SIV vaccine with a deletion in the *nef* gene. Science 1992;258:1938-41.
90. Racaniello VR, Baltimore D. Cloned poliovirus complementary DNA is infectious in mammalian cells. Science 1981;214:916-19.
91. Strauss EG, Strauss JH. Mutants of alphaviruses: genetics and physiology. In: Schlesinger RW, ed. The Togaviruses: Biology, Structure, Replication. New York: Academic Press, 1984:393-426.
92. Rice CM, Levis R, Strauss JH et al. Production of infectious RNA transcripts from Sindbis virus cDNA clones: mapping of lethal mutations, rescue of a temperature-sensitive marker, and in vitro mutagenesis to generate defined mutants. J Virol 1987;61:3809-19.
93. Lai C-J, Zhao B, Hori H et al. Infectious RNA transcribed from stably cloned full-length cDNA of Dengue type 4 virus. Proc Natl Acad Sci USA 1991;88:5139-43.
94. Davis NL, Powell N, Greenwald GF et al. Attenuating mutations in the E2 glycoprotein gene of Venezuelan equine encephalitis virus: construction of single and multiple mutants in a full-length cDNA clone. Virology 1991;183:20-31.
95. Cohen JI, Rosenblum B, Ticehurst JR et al. Complete nucleotide sequence of an attenuated hepatitis A virus: comparison with wild-type virus. Proc Natl Acad Sci USA 1987;84:2497-501.
96. Toyoda H, Kohara M, Kataoka Y et al. Complete nucleotide sequence of all three poliovirus serotype genomes: implication for genetic relationship, gene function and antigenic determinants. J Mol Biol 1985;174:561-85.

97. Polo JM, Davis NL, Rice CM et al. Molecular analysis of Sindbis virus pathogenesis in neonatal mice by using virus recombinants constructed in vitro. J Virol 1988;62:2124-33.
98. Cohen JI, Rosenblum B, Feinstone SM et al. Attenuation and cell culture adaptation of hepatitis A virus (HAV): a genetic analysis with HAV cDNA. J Virol 1989;63:5364-70.
99. Omata T, Kohara M, Kuge S et al. Genetic analysis of the attenuation phenotype of poliovirus type 1. J Virol 1986;58:348-58.
100. Westrop GD, Evans DMA, Minor PD et al. Investigation of the molecular basis of attenuation in the Savin type 3 vaccine using novel recombinant polioviruses constructed from infectious cDNA. In: Rowlands DJ, Mayo MA, Mahy BWJ, eds. Molecular Biology of Positive Strand RNA Viruses. London: Academic Press, 1987:53-60.
101. Bray M, Lai C-J. Construction of intertypic chimeric Dengue viruses by substitution. Proc Natl Acad Sci USA 1991;88:10342-46.
102. Pletnev AG, Bray M, Huggins J et al. Construction and characterization of chimeric tick-borne encephalitis/Dengue type 4 viruses. Proc Natl Acad Sci USA 1992;89:10532-36.
103. Kuhn RJ, Griffin DE, Zhang H et al. Attenuation of Sindbis virus neurovirulence by using defined mutations in nontranslated regions of the genome RNA. J Virol 1992;66:7121-27.
104. Polo JM, Johnston RE. Attenuating mutations in glycoproteins E1 and E2 of Sindbis virus produce a highly attenuated strain when combined in vitro. J Virol 1990;64:4438-44.
105. Davis NL, Fuller FJ, Dougherty WG et al. A single nucleotide change in the E2 glycoprotein gene of Sindbis virus affects penetration rate in cell culture and virulence in neonatal mice. Proc Natl Acad Sci USA 1986;83:6771-75.
106. Schoepp RJ, Johnston RE. Directed mutagenesis of a Sindbis virus pathogenesis site. Virology 1993;193:149-59.
107. Evans DMA, Dunn G, Minor PD et al. Increased neurovirulence associated with a single nucleotide change in a noncoding region of the Sabin type 3 poliovaccine genome. Nature 1985;314:548-50.
108. Iizuka N, Kohara M, Hagino-Yamagishi K et al. Construction of less neurovirulent polioviruses by introducing deletions into the 5′ noncoding sequence of the genome. J Virol 1989;63:5354-63.
109. Niesters HGM, Strauss JH. Defined mutations in the 5′ nontranslated sequence of Sindbis virus RNA. J Virol 1990;64:4162-68.
110. Niesters HGM, Strauss JH. Mutagenesis of the conserved 51 nucleotide region of Sindbis virus. J Virol 1990;64:1639-47.
111. Evans DJ, McKeating J, Meridith JM et al. An engineered poliovirus chimera elicits broadly reactive HIV-1 neutralizing antibodies. Nature 1989;339:385-88.
112. Almond JW, Burke KL. Poliovirus as a vector for the presentation of foreign antigens. Semin Virol 1990;1:11-20.
113. Xiong C, Levis R, Shen P et al. Sindbis virus: an efficient, broad host range vector for gene expression in animal cells. Science 1989;243:1188-91.
114. Luytjes W, Krystal M, Enami M et al. Amplification, expression, and packaging of a foreign gene by influenza virus. Cell 1989;59:1107-13.
115. Muster T, Subbarao EK, Enami M et al. An influenza A virus containing influenza B virus 5′ and 3′ noncoding regions on the neuraminidase gene is attenuated in mice. Proc Natl Acad Sci USA 1991;88:5177-81.

116. Castrucci MR, Bilsel P, Kawaoka Y. Attenuation of influenza A virus by insertion of a foreign epitope into the neuraminidase. J Virol 1992;66:4647-53.
117. Steinhoff MC, Halsey NA, Fries LF et al. The A/Mallard/6750/78 avian-human, but not the A/Ann Arbor/6/60 cold-adapted, influenza A/Kawasaki/86 (H1N1) reassortant virus vaccine retains partial virulence for infants and children. J Infect Dis 1990;163:1023-28.
118. Steinhoff MC, Halsey HA, Wilson MH et al. Comparison of live attenuated cold-adapted and avian-human influenza A/Bethesda/85 (H3N2) reassortant virus vaccines in infants and children. J Infect Dis 1990;162:394-401.
119. Cox NJ, Kitame F, Kendal AP et al. Identification of sequence changes in the cold-adapted, live attenuated influenza vaccine strain, A/Ann Arbor/6/60 (H2N2). Virology 1988;167:554-67.
120. Collins PL, Mink MA, Stec DS. Rescue of synthetic analogs of respiratory syncytial virus genomic RNA and effect of truncations and mutations on the expression of a foreign reporter gene. Proc Natl Acad Sci USA 1991;88:9663-67.
121. Park KH, Hunag T, Correia FF et al. Rescue of a foreign gene by Sendai virus. Proc Natl Acad Sci USA 1991;88:5537-41.
122. Upton C, Macen JL, Schreiber M et al. Myxoma virus expresses a secreted protein with homology to the tumor necrosis factor receptor gene family that contributes to viral virulence. Virology 1991;184:370-82.
123. Spehner D, Gillard S, Drillien R et al. A cowpox virus gene required for multiplication in Chinese hamster ovary cells. J Virol 1988;62:1297-1304.
124. Chen W, Drillien R, Spehner D et al. Restricted replication of ectromelia virus in cell culture correlates with mutations in virus-encoded host range gene. Virology 1992;187:433-42.
125. Kotwal GJ, Moss B. Vaccinia virus encodes two proteins that are structurally related to members of the plasma serine protease inhibitor superfamily. J Virol 1989;63:600-06.
126. Kotwal GJ, Moss B. Vaccinia virus encodes a secretory polypeptide structurally related to complement control proteins. Nature 1988;335:176-81.
127. Isaacs SV, Kotwal GJ, Moss B et al. Vaccinia virus complement control protein prevents antibody-dependent complement-enhanced neutralization of infectivity and contributes to virulence. Proc Natl Acad Sci USA 1992;89:628-32.
128. Kotwal GJ, Hügin AW, Moss B. Mapping and insertional mutagenesis of a vaccinia virus gene encoding a 13,800 Da secreted protein. Virology 1989;171:579-87.
129. Law KM, Smith GL. A vaccinia serine protease inhibitor which prevents virus-induced cell fusion. J Gen Virol 1992;73:549-57.
130. Turner PC, Moyer RW. An orthopoxvirus serpinlike gene controls the ability of infected cells to fuse. J Virol 1992;66:2076-85.
131. Beattie E, Tartaglia J, Paoletti E. Vaccinia virus-encoded eIF-2α homolog abrogates the antiviral effect of interferon. Virology 1991;183:419-22.
132. Goebel SJ, Johnson GP, Perkus ME et al. The complete DNA sequence of vaccinia virus. Virology 1990;179:247-66.
133. Child SJ, Palumbo GJ, Buller RML et al. Insertional inactivation of the large subunit of ribonucleotide reductase encoded by vaccinia virus is associated with reduced virulence in vivo. Virology 1990;174:625-29.
134. Blasco R, Moss B. Extracellular vaccinia virus formation and cell-to-cell virus transmission are prevented by deletion of the gene encoding the 37,000-dalton outer envelope protein. J Virol 1991;65:5910-20.

135. Chang H-W, Watson JC, Jacobs BL. The E3L gene of vaccinia virus encodes an inhibitor of the interferon-induced, double-stranded, RNA-dependent protein kinase. Proc Natl Acad Sci USA 1992;89:4825-29.
136. Niles EG, Seto J. Vaccinia virus gene D8 encodes a virion transmembrane protein. J Virol 1988;62:3772-78.
137. Rodriguez J-R, Rodriguez D, Esteban M. Insertional inactivation of the vaccinia virus 32-kilodalton gene is associated with attenuation in mice and reduction of viral gene expression in polarized epithelial cells. J Virol 1992;66:183-89.
138. Buller RML, Smith GL, Cremer K et al. Decreased virulence of recombinant vaccinia virus expression vectors is associated with a thymidine kinase-negative phenotype. Nature 1985;317:813-15.
139. Duncan SA, Smith GL. Identification and characterization of an extracellular envelope glycoprotein affecting vaccinia virus egress. J Virol 1992;66:1610-21.
140. Blasco R, Cole NB, Moss B. Sequence analysis, expression, and deletion of a vaccinia virus gene encoding a homolog of profilin, a eukaryotic actin-binding protein. J Virol 1991;65:4598-608.
141. Moore JB, Smith GL. Steroid hormone synthesis by a vaccinia enzyme: a new type of virus virulence factor. EMBO J 1992;11:1973-80.
142. Hughes SJ, Johnston LH, de Carlos A et al. Vaccinia virus encodes an active thymidylate kinase that complements a cdc8 mutant of *Saccharomyces cerevisiae.* J Biol Chem 1991;266:20103-09.
143. Kerr SM, Johnston LH, Odell M et al. Vaccinia DNA ligase complements *Saccharomyces cerevisiae* cdc9, localizes in cytoplasmic factories and affects virulence and virus sensitivity to DNA damaging agents. EMBO J 1991;10:4343-50.
144. Howard ST, Chan YS, Smith GL. Vaccinia virus homologues of the Shope fibroma virus inverted terminal repeat proteins and a discontinuous ORF related to the tumor necrosis factor receptor family. Virology 1991;180:633-47.
145. Flexner C, Hügin A, Moss B. Prevention of vaccinia virus infection in immunodeficient mice by vector-directed IL-2 expression. Nature 1987;330:259-301.
146. Engelstad M, Howard ST, Smith GL. A constitutively expressed vaccinia gene encodes a 42-kDa glycoprotein related to complement control factors that forms part of the extracellular virus envelope. Virology 1992;188:801-10.
147. Wolffe EJ, Isaacs SN, Moss B. Deletion of the vaccinia virus B5R gene encoding a 42 kiloxdalton membrane glycoprotein inhibits extracellular virus envelope formation and dissemination. J Virol 1993;67:4732-41.
148. Upton C, Mossman K, McFadden G. Encoding of a homolog of the IFN-γ receptor by myxoma virus. Science 1992;258:1369-72.
149. Palumbo GJ, Glasgow WC, Buller RML. Poxvirus-induced alteration of arachidonate metabolism. Proc Natl Acad Sci USA 1993;90:2020-24.
150. Smith GL, Chan YS, Howard ST. Nucleotide sequence of 42 kbp of vaccinia virus strain WR from near the right inverted terminal repeat. J Gen Virol 1991;72:1349-76.
151. Hugin A, Issacs S, Kotwal G et al. personal communication.
152. Buller RML, Blasco R, Moss B. personal communication.
153. Tristem M, Marshall C, Karpas A et al. Origin of *vpx* in lentiviruses. Nature 1990;347:341-42.
154. Blasco R, Sisler J, Mass B. Dissociation of progeny vaccinia virus from the cell membrane is regulated by a viral envelope glycoprotein. J Virol 67:3319-25

CHAPTER 11

The Modulation of Immune Responses by Cytokines Encoded in Recombinant Vaccine Vectors

Alistair J. Ramsay
Janet C. Ruby
Ian A. Ramshaw

INTRODUCTION

Virus vector vaccines

Conventional vaccines, consisting of attenuated strains of pathogens or inactivated preparations, have certain disadvantages including high production costs, low immunogenicity, instability, and in some cases, a requirement for adjuvants. Furthermore, alternative vaccines based upon purified immunogens or synthetic peptides frequently elicit poor protective immune responses. A major factor in the efficacy of infectious virus vaccines is their ability to replicate and persist in the host for several days, allowing prolonged and enhanced production of desired antigens in host cells. If this standard is to be achieved using genetically engineered products, research effort must be made in the areas of cell-mediated and humoral immunogenicity and other host responses, as well as in the context of vaccine safety.

Vaccinia and other poxvirus vectors now being developed have the capacity to carry enough heterologous DNA to encode single or multiple genes for immunogenic proteins and allow faithful transcription and translation from inserted genes and appropriate post-translational processing and

Strategies in Vaccine Design, edited by Gordon L. Ada, D.Sc..

transport. Vaccinia also stimulates good cell-mediated and humoral immunity, is highly stable, easily administered intradermally and has been successful as a vaccine in the eradication of smallpox. Indeed, recombinant vaccinia viruses (rVV) have been used in animals, and in some cases in limited human studies, as vectors to deliver many vaccine antigens of biological importance.[1] Experience obtained during the smallpox campaign, however, revealed that the frequency of complications associated with various VV strains was high, though the LC16 or NYCBH strains, which have had extensive human and animal testing, may represent reasonable choices as vaccine vehicles in humans. Nevertheless, a major concern about the use of VV as a vaccine vector for humans is one of safety. Other poxviruses with restricted host ranges (avipoxviruses) are also being tested as vaccine vectors and appear to be safe, as determined in laboratory animals[2] and humans.[3] Adenovirus and herpes virus have also been described as potential vaccine vectors, however by far the most widely studied is vaccinia.

THE IMPORTANCE OF CYTOKINES IN THE IMMUNE RESPONSE

The generation of an effective immune response requires the interaction of several cell types and the subsequent release of cytokines by the activated cells. Cytokines are a group of signaling molecules which not only determine the magnitude but also the type of immune response mounted against an antigen. Indeed, it now appears that the immunity induced by an infectious agent is determined, in part, by the pattern of cytokines secreted by immune cells, in particular different subsets of T cells.[4] One subset (Th1) secretes the cytokines interleukin-2 (IL-2) tumor necrosis factor-α (TNF-α) and interferon-γ (IFN-γ) and promotes cell-mediated immunity, while an-

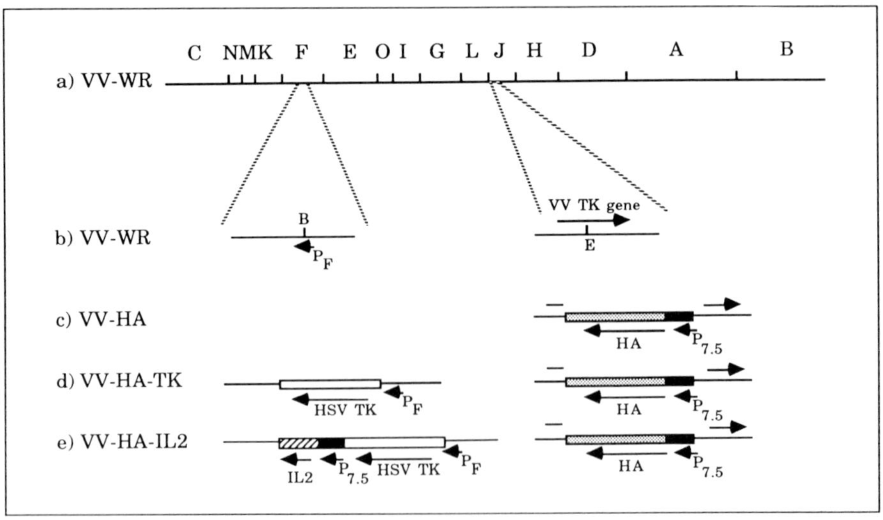

Fig. 1. Genomic configuration of VV-HA-IL-2. A Hind III map of vaccinia virus, strain VV-WR, is shown with insertion points at the EcoRI (E) and BamHI (B) sites in the J and F fragments, respectively. Arrows indicate orientations of the vaccinia virus thymidine kinase (TK) gene, vaccinia promoters P_F and $P_{7.5}$, the influenza virus HA gene, the herpes simplex virus (HSV) TK gene (as a selectable marker) and the murine IL-2 coding sequences. Constructs encoding HA and cytokine genes IL-5 or IL-6 are also referred to in the text.

other population (Th2) secretes IL-4, IL-5, IL-6 and IL-10 and preferentially induces antibody responses.[5] Cytokines also influence the development of these different T cell subpopulations. For example, IL-4 produced by the Th2 subset promotes Th2 development but inhibits the growth of Th1 populations, while Th1-derived IFN-γ suppresses the Th2 response. The extensive range of potential immune responses to an infectious agent is therefore tightly regulated by the cytokines produced by immune cells. Given these findings, it is not surprising that attempts have been made to modify the immune response by the administration of recombinant cytokines. This work has been hampered, however, by the short half-life of these factors in vivo and by difficulties in targeting recombinant material to sites of immune reactivity, with very high, and consequently non-physiological concentrations required for observable effects. In order to address some of

Table 1. Comparison of the known functions of cytokines with their effects when expressed by recombinant vaccinia viruses.

Cytokine	Major Known Functions	Effects on immunity when expressed by rVV
Th1 type factors		
IL-2	T cell growth factor, activates B cells, monocytes and NK cells	Attenuates growth of virus, stimulates natural killer cells to produce IFN-γ
TNF-α	Anti-viral activity in vitro, activates cytotoxic T cells	Limits growth of rVV allowing T cell-deficient mice to resolve infection
IFN-γ	Upregulates MHC molecules on antigen-presenting cells	Limits growth of rVV allowing T cell-deficient mice to resolve infection
Th2 type factors		
IL-4	Regulates antibody responses, especially IgE	Increases pathogenicity of rVV
IL-5	Regulates antibody production	Stimulates antigen-specific mucosal IgA responses
IL-6	Involved in the maturation of B cells to ASC	Stimulates antigen-specific systemic IgG1 and mucosal IgA responses, recruits T helper cells
Other factors		
IL-1α	Activates T cells	Enhances memory antibody responses
IL-1β	Activates T cells	?
IL-7	Early activator of T and B cells	Stimulates T cell and nonspecific antiviral immunity
TGF-β	Suppresses T and B cell function in vitro, activates T cell memory	?

these problems, we have constructed recombinant poxvirus vectors encoding cytokine genes (Fig. 1). Thus, during replication in vivo, the virus produces the encoded factor which is secreted from infected cells, i.e. the extent and sites of virus replication determine the level and sites of production of the cytokine. In this way, we hoped to approximate the physiological state more closely than other methods of cytokine delivery. Using this system, we have begun to study the immunoregulatory and antiviral properties of a number of cytokines. Our findings suggest that expression of selected cytokines may allow manipulation of the microenvironment to favor development of appropriate protective immune responses and, where required, suitable attenuation of the vector (summarized in Table 1).

CYTOKINES WHICH ALTER VIRUS PATHOGENICITY

CO-EXPRESSION OF IL-2 ATTENUATES VACCINIA VIRUS

Our studies began with the observation, by ourselves and others that insertion of the gene for IL-2 into the VV genome resulted in a highly attenuated rVV.[6,7] IL-2 has immunostimulatory influence on natural killer (NK) cells, large granular lymphocytes and B cells. Immunodeficient (athymic nude) mice are able to resolve infection with VV encoding IL-2 (VV-IL-2), but develop progressive vaccinal disease and die when given control virus (Fig. 2). In normal mice, the extensive virus growth and resultant tissue destruction which occurs, especially in ovaries, following VV infection, is absent in animals given VV-IL-2.[8] This dramatic reduction in the pathogenicity of the rVV is dependent on IL-2 expression and not simply the insertion of a foreign gene.

These are important findings relating to the safety of virus vector vaccines for human use. A major obstacle in this regard, particularly in the case of VV, has been the danger of serious side effects if virus is inadvertently given to immunodeficient individuals, in the face of a substantial current rate of HIV infection and other conditions affecting immunocompetence. Indeed, at least one individual with subclinical HIV infection has developed

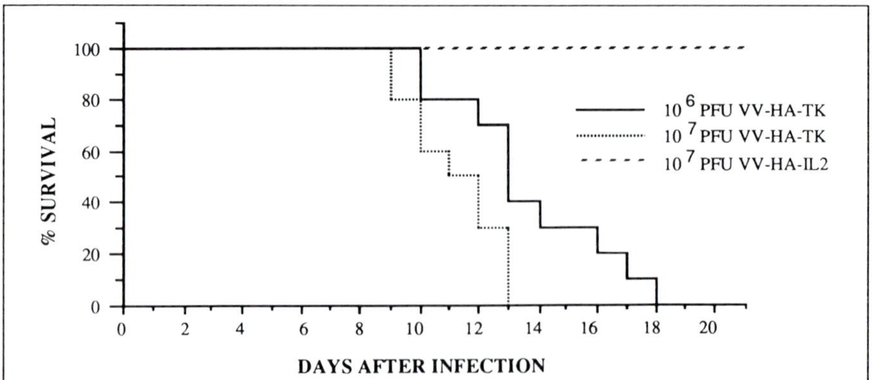

Fig. 2. Survival of athymic, nude mice infected with vaccinia virus encoding IL-2. Groups of five female nude mice were given intravenous inocula of 10^7 plaque-forming units (PFU) of VV-HA-IL-2 or 10^6 or 10^7 PFU of the control virus VV-HA-TK. The figure shows that mice survive infection with a 10-fold higher dose of VV-HA-IL-2 compared to the control virus, of which 10^6 PFU was lethal.

disseminated vaccinal disease after routine vaccination.[9] It has also been found that antiviral serum IgG antibody responses in primates vaccinated with VV-IL-2 are of similar magnitude to control responses, despite attenuation and decreased replication of the IL-2 virus.[10,11] Furthermore, when we infect immunodeficient mice with a double construct encoding both IL-2 and the hemagglutinin (HA) gene of influenza virus (strain A/PR/8/34), they are subsequently resistant to challenge with wild-type influenza virus of the same strain.[12] These mice, of course, fail to survive immunization with control rVV expressing HA but no IL-2. Thus, the use of this strategy, i.e., co-expression of IL-2 along with protective foreign antigen, allows protective immunization of severely immunocompromised individuals with an otherwise potentially lethal antigen.

We have since conducted a detailed analysis of mechanisms involved in IL-2-mediated recovery of immunodeficient mice from virus infection. In brief, it appears that vector-expressed IL-2 attracts NK cells to the site of infection and stimulates their production of interferon-γ (IFN-γ).[8,13] Indeed, our data suggest that recovery from VV-IL-2 infection is critically dependent on this host-derived factor, as monoclonal antibodies to IFN-γ, given prior to infection with VV-IL-2, completely inhibit the protective effect of the IL-2.[13]

Antiviral activity of Th1 cytokines

It is well-established that IFN-γ and tumor necrosis factor-α (TNF-α) are potently antiviral molecules and exhibit a wide range of actions which are likely to contribute to clearance of virus infection. For example, IFN-γ enhances NK cell cytotoxicity,[14] activates macrophages[15] and upregulates expression of class I MHC molecules on target cells, thereby increasing the efficiency of target cell recognition.[16] Tumor necrosis factor-α exhibits antiviral activity in vitro against several RNA and DNA viruses. Synergy with IFN-γ and IFN-β dramatically enhances the antiviral effects of TNF-α, which include inhibition of virus replication,[17] the induction of an antiviral state and the lysis of virus infected cells.[18]

We have found that rVV engineered to express murine IFN-γ[19] or TNF-α,[20] like VV-IL-2, also exhibit markedly reduced pathogenicity. Although the expression of these factors did not affect growth of rVV in tissue culture, a potent antiviral activity led to their rapid clearance in vivo. In contrast to the mechanisms involved in IL-2 virus clearance, however, neither factor appears to enhance the NK cell response, or any other cellular or antibody-mediated response, beyond those induced by the control virus. Indeed, sublethal irradiation of euthymic mice prior to infection had little effect on the growth of either the IFN-γ or TNF-α viruses, but abrogated the capacity of these mice to control infection with the IL-2 virus. The reduced pathogenicity of these viruses cannot, therefore, be attributed to the induction of an enhanced antiviral host response and it may well be that these factors directly suppress the growth of the rVV in vivo. Likely antiviral actions of these factors encoded in rVV are outlined in Figure 3.

We now have evidence that IL-7, originally described as a growth factor for both T and B cells but not regarded as a Th1 factor, also attenuates the growth of rVV in immunodeficient animals, albeit not as effectively as IL-2, IFN-γ or TNF-α (unpublished data). In normal mice, rVV-expressing IL-7 is cleared

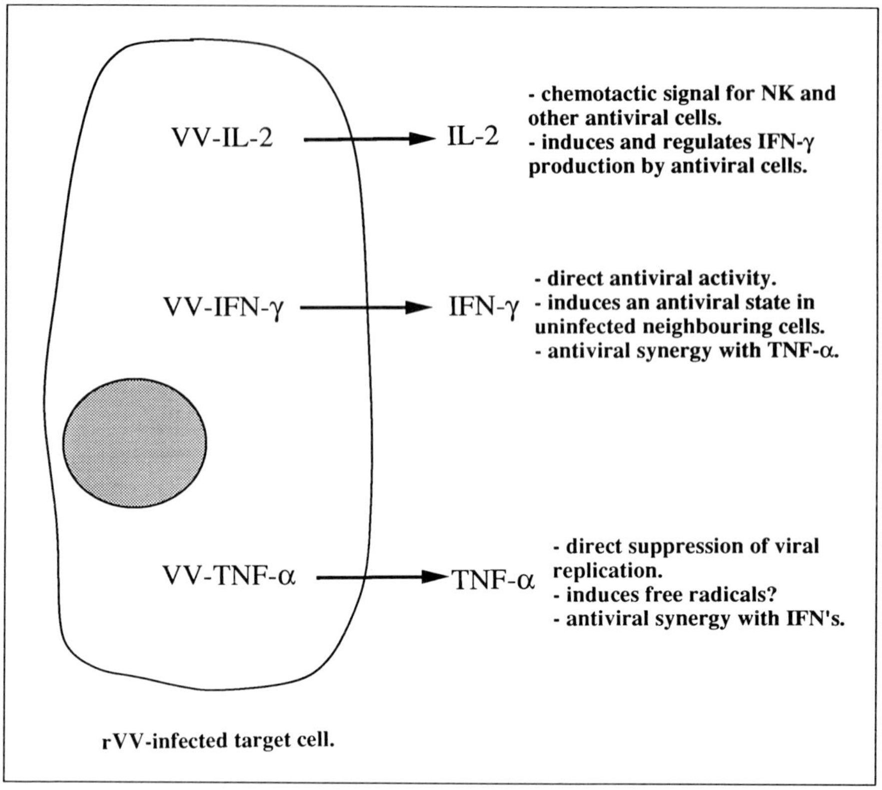

Fig. 3. Antiviral actions of virus-encoded Th1-type cytokines secreted from cells infected with recombinant vaccinia viruses.

faster than control virus and stimulates enhanced specific and nonspecific antiviral cellular immune functions. Thus, we have described a number of cytokines which, when encoded in rVV, dramatically attenuate virus virulence. These constructs nevertheless retain immunogenicity and have been used to boost responses in both primates and mice in the face of pre-existing immunity.[10,21]

It is important to stress here that the cytokines produced by these constructs act in a highly localized manner. There are many published observations of severe pathology caused by TNF, nevertheless we found that mice given virus encoding this factor remained healthy throughout the experimental period. In addition, the vector-directed expression of antiviral cytokines in mice given simultaneous inocula of cytokine-encoding virus and control virus did not dramatically alter the growth of the latter.

The Physiological Response to Virus Infection

Our rationale for encoding IFN-γ or TNF-α in rVV was based on their demonstrated antiviral activity in vitro and we considered that their expression in vivo could have a direct effect on virus growth. The results appear to represent strong evidence that virus-encoded TNF-α and IFN-γ are acting in a directly antiviral manner in vivo. It was quite clear that in the absence of antiviral effector T cells, animals were able to resolve an otherwise lethal infection provided a source of either IL-2, IFN-γ or TNF-α was present at foci of virus replication. These data suggest that cytokines play an important role as antiviral effector molecules in the T cell response to virus infection.

It has been shown previously that $CD8^+$ T cells are a dominant factor in recovery from poxvirus infection in mice.[22] It has also been known for some time that antiviral T cells secrete IFN-γ in an antigen-specific manner. Indeed we have shown that at the height of the cellular response to VV infection, $CD8^+$ T cells are the major producers of this factor.[23] When treated with neutralizing antibody against IFN-γ during the course of infection with wild-type VV, mice succumb to an otherwise nonlethal inoculum, highlighting the importance of IFN-γ in recovery.[24] Such treatment did not affect the generation of the $CD8^+$ T cells. Furthermore, the ability of $CD8^+$ T cell isolates to transfer specific antiviral reactivity to infected recipient mice was critically dependent on IFN-γ. Thus, treatment of recipients with anti-IFN-γ antibodies completely blocked the ability of the transferred cells to control virus growth. This antibody did not affect the proliferation, migratory patterns or the in vitro cytolytic capacity of the transferred cells, neither did upregulation of class I major histocompatibility complex molecules by IFN-γ appear to be an important factor in this model. These findings have important implications in our understanding of how individuals resolve virus infections. Based on their activity in vitro, it has been assumed that cytolytic activity is the major effector mechanism of T cells in vivo. Our findings indicate that the principal function of antiviral T cells may be to focus cytokines, such as IFN-γ and TNF-α, at sites of viral replication thereby limiting the spread of virus.[25] The activity of these factors, perhaps in synergy would not only control virus growth, but would also induce an antiviral state in neighboring uninfected cells.

CYTOKINES WITH IMMUNOREGULATORY ACTIVITY

The Th1 cytokine profile of IL-2, IFN-γ and TNF-α is also typical of many antigen-specific $CD8^+$ T cell clones.[26] Functions mediated by these cells are largely concerned with cytotoxic activity and it is likely that a Th1-like immune response is the most appropriate in defense against viruses and other intracellular pathogens.[4] In contrast, Th2-type cells provide help for antibody production by B cells. The Th2 cytokines, including IL-4, IL-5 and IL-6, stimulate B cell growth and differentiation in vitro, while immune responses characterized by the production of these factors in vivo correlate with high levels of antibody synthesis.[4] Interleukin-4 also inhibits the synthesis of IFN-γ by Th1 cells,[27] and may, in this way, counteract the antiviral activity of both $CD4^+$ and $CD8^+$ virus-specific T cells.

There are no reports of the control of virus infection by Th2-type factors. Indeed, IL-4 increases virus pathogenicity when encoded in rVV (unpublished data). Interleukin-5 and IL-6 have no obvious effect on virus replication but display a remarkable capacity to modulate antibody responses to heterologous vaccine antigen co-expressed by the rVV vector.[28,29] These examples of immune deviation and the selective induction of particular types of immune responses by vector-encoded cytokines, of obvious relevance to vaccine design, are detailed below.

A Th2 factor which inhibits antiviral immunity

Recombinant VV which express IL-4 exhibit sustained growth in normal mice for many days after control virus is cleared (unpublished data). Based on its in vitro immunoregulatory actions which are outlined above, IL-4 might be expected to inhibit the activity of Th1 cells and, therefore, the normal development of the antiviral cellular immune response. Our preliminary findings suggest that this may indeed be the case in vivo, as cell-mediated immune responses against rVV expressing IL-4 are markedly depressed. Others have recently shown that IL-4 has the capacity in vitro to change the phenotype of T cell subpopulations normally associated with antiviral immune responses to one normally involved with helper activity for antibody responses, i.e., a Th2 phenotype, and suggest that the overexpression of this factor may underlie, at least in part, the decline in effective antiviral immunity observed during diseases associated with immunodeficiency, such as AIDS.[30] Designers of vaccines should clearly take account of the deleterious effects that the inappropriate induction of particular patterns of cytokine synthesis may have on the optimal development of immune responses following immunization.

Th2 factors selectively enhance mucosal antibody responses

Immunodeficient mice, which are able to survive challenge with rVV expressing IL-2, IFN-γ or TNF-α, as described earlier, succumb to infection with rVV encoding either of the Th2-type factors, IL-5 or IL-6 as rapidly as with control virus. In normal mice, viruses encoding these factors exhibit growth kinetics similar to those of the control virus, whereas VV-HA-IL-2 is recovered at greatly reduced titers and is cleared rapidly. Despite having no apparent direct antiviral activity, however, vector-expressed IL-5 and IL-6 clearly modulate antiviral antibody responses, in particular those at mucosae.

Mucosal surfaces represent by far the most common route of infection by pathogens causing both mucosal and systemic disease; however, events controlling the development of local, protective antibody responses are poorly understood. The mucosal immune response is characterized by the production of antibodies of the IgA isotype by plasma cells lying beneath the epithelial basement membrane and present in secretory glandular tissue.[31] Efforts to design effective "mucosal vaccines", given greater prominence by the current HIV epidemic, have been hampered by an incomplete understanding of factors controlling the development of mucosal immunity, although it is now clear that T cell-derived cytokines play a major role. In particular, IL-5 and IL-6, have been shown to increase IgA reactivity of activated mucosal B cells in vitro, either alone, in synergy or in combination with other factors.[32,33] In addition, mucosal tissues contain large numbers of cells capable of producing IL-5 and IL-6. It is thought likely, therefore, that T cell-derived cytokines normally direct the development of IgA B cells arriving in the submucosa following their exposure to antigen in the organized mucosal lymphoid tissues.

To study the influence of these factors on the development of mucosal IgA reactivity in vivo, we co-expressed the IL-5 or IL-6 genes in rVV along with the HA gene of influenza virus, i.e., a heterologous vaccine antigen (construction as in Fig. 1). These constructs were given to mice intranasally and the development of immunocytes secreting antibodies specific for co-expressed HA in their lungs was monitored.[28,29] As shown in Table 2, significantly greater numbers of anti-HA IgA antibody-secreting cells (ASC) were found in the lungs of mice given

Table 2. Anti-HA IgA responses in lungs of mice immunized with rVV

Days after immunization[a]	Anti-HA IgA ASC/10^6 cells[b]		Reciprocal IgA antibody titer[c]		
	VV-HA-TK	VV-HA-IL5	VV-HA-TK	VV-HA-IL5	VV- HA-IL6
3	<50	<50	ND	ND	ND
7	80	100	ND	ND	ND
10	100	233	ND	ND	ND
14	180	766	<5	5	5
21	160	400	<5	5	20
28	<50	100	5	20	20
42	<50	<50	ND	ND	ND
unimmunized	<50	<50	<5	<5	<5

[a] Mice were immunized intranasally with 10^7 PFU of rVV under light ether anesthesia.

[b] Lung cells were isolated by collagenase digestion and assayed for antibody-secreting cells (ASC) by ELISPOT when indicated. Values represent mean counts from triplicate wells in two separate assays. Cells were pooled from five mice within each group and SEM were <15% in each case.

[c] Lung lavage fluids were assayed by ELISA. Figures are mean titers for groups of five mice.

VV-HA-IL-5 than in those given the control virus VV-HA-TK (which expresses HA but no IL-5 or IL-6). The elevated response was first detected on day 10 after infection and peaked on day 14, at four-fold greater than control levels. This had declined by day 21, although anti-HA IgA ASC were found at significantly higher levels at this stage than in mice given control virus and was still present on day 28, by which time responses in the control group had fallen below detectable levels. It was unlikely that different patterns of growth and persistence of VV-HA-TK and VV-HA-IL-5 influenced these responses, as the kinetics of replication of both viruses were similar. Moreover, the ability of monoclonal antibodies specific for IL-5 to abolish the elevated response confirms that this factor was responsible for upregulating anti-HA IgA levels.[28] We also measured anti-HA IgA antibody levels in lung lavage fluids, finding significant increases in IgA titers in mice given rVV expressing IL-5 by 28 days post-infection, and IL-6 at both 21 and 28 days (Table 2).

Our data suggest that rVV-encoded IL-5 and IL-6, produced at foci of infection, are acting either directly, or in concert with host-derived factors, to enhance the differentiation of newly-arrived virus-specific IgA plasma cell precursors into antibody-secreting cells and support an important role for these factors in the physiological development of mucosal IgA responses. In terms of improvement of vector vaccines, IL-5 and IL-6, when expressed locally, are clearly able to selectively enhance specific mucosal IgA reactivity to co-expressed heterologous vaccine antigen. Thus, one of the major problems associated with the potential use of infectious vector vaccines, their low immunogenicity, may be overcome by the selective co-expression of cytokines. This finding may be of particular importance for the enhancement of mucosal immune responses which are often difficult to induce and are notoriously short-lived. In this context, we are currently looking at the ability of these constructs to prime for enhanced protective mucosal IgA responses to challenge with wild-type influenza virus. Our approach may also be useful for stimulating mucosal immunity to a wide range of vector-encoded antigens, including HIV glycoprotein. In this respect, further experiments are underway using a range of other established vectors engineered to encode cytokine genes, including avipoxvirus (see below), adenovirus and Salmonella, which may be more suitable for mucosal immunization, particularly by the oral route.

Th2 Factors Modulate Systemic Antibody Responses

The isotype and subclass of an antibody response is an important determinant of its protective efficacy. Virus infections of mice typically elicit serum antibody responses dominated by the IgG2a subclass.[34] The Th1-type factor, IFN-γ, enhances the production of IgG2a by murine B cells both in vitro[35] and in vivo[36] and may be responsible for the predominance of IgG2a as it is normally produced in response to virus infection. Other cytokines may promote the synthesis of different IgG subclasses, e.g., IL-4, acts as a switch factor for IgG1 production in vitro.[35] Mice given systemic inocula of rVV encoding IFN-γ mount antiviral antibody responses which are of similar magnitude to those elicited by control virus and largely IgG2a, the subclass in serum normally associated with protection from infection with influenza virus.[34] In contrast, rVV encoding IL-6 induce a response to co-expressed HA antigen which is predominantly of the IgG1 subclass.[21] The time course of the response occurred in parallel to that of the growth of the virus in infected tissues, after a lag of some 4-5 days. The manner by which vector-encoded IL-6 promotes IgG1 reactivity remains to be clarified. The ability to influence antibody subclass selection, thereby skewing antiviral reactivity away from the subclass normally induced by virus infection, is a previously undescribed activity of this factor. It is reminiscent, however, of the above mentioned activity of IL-4, and represents a further example of the ability of Th2-type cytokines to selectively induce particular and characteristic types of immune reactivity when present as a component of vector vaccines. In summary, strong specific antibody responses were selectively induced to heterologous vaccine antigen by co-expressed cytokines, as was the case in the studies on rVV-induced mucosal immunity, findings of importance for vector vaccine strategies.

Avipoxviruses, an Alternative Vector System

We have now extended these studies to include the avipoxviruses (APV), the replication of which is restricted to avian species.[2,3] Avipoxviruses undergo an abortive infection in mammals. Recombinant APV can, nevertheless, express foreign gene products in mammalian cells, including those encoding heterologous proteins, when these are driven by an early promoter. This process results in the induction of immune responses in the absence of sustained productive vector replication. Thus, a strong safety barrier exists against vaccine-induced complications and cross-contamination, even in immunosuppressed individuals. An important component of our work involves the development of rAPV encoding cytokine genes. Preliminary findings suggest that the co-expression of cytokine genes with heterologous vaccine antigen in rAPV constructs enhances antibody responses to the latter and may also lead to the selective induction of particular immune responses, much as described above for rVV vectors. Apart from their outstanding safety advantages, an important feature of rAPV vectors would appear to be their capacity for sustained presentation of encoded gene products to the immune system, in the face of negligible host responses to the vectors themselves.

CONCLUSIONS

Live recombinant vaccines have great potential for human vaccination, especially for use in developing countries. Before they can be considered for widespread introduction, however, questions of safety, especially in immunodeficient individuals, and efficacy need to be addressed. The engineering of vectors which encode cytokine genes may help overcome many of the problems associated with this form of vaccine delivery. The expression of cytokine genes may prevent complications associated with the inadvertent vaccination of immunodeficient individuals by attenuating the vaccine vector. Of particular importance, indications are that with the appropriate choice of cytokines it will also be possible to design a vaccine that selectively enhances desirable primary immune responses and primes for appropriate responses upon exposure to infectious antigen. Furthermore, although the classic use of a vaccine is to prevent an initial infection, it is feasible that these constructs may be used to ameliorate the progression of disease. For example, vaccines co-expressing cytokine genes and HIV genes could be used in HIV-seropositive individuals, not only to render the vaccine safe, but with the possibility that vector-encoded cytokines would overcome immunological defects caused by HIV infection and deviate immune reactivity into a form appropriate to controlling disease. This approach is also currently finding much favor as a potential means of tumor therapy and vaccination, through the immunostimulatory actions of cytokines encoded in virus vectors or transfected tumor cells.

REFERENCES

1. Moss B. Vaccinia virus: A tool for research and vaccine development. Science 1992; 252:1662-1667.
2. Taylor J, Weinberg R, Languet B et al. Recombinant fowlpox virus inducing protective immunity in non-avian species. Vaccine 1988; 6:497-503.
3. Cadoz M, Strady A, Meignier B et al. Immunisation with canarypox virus expressing rabies glycoprotein. Lancet 1992; 339:1429-1432.
4. Mosmann TR, Schumacher JH, Street NF et al. Diversity of cytokine synthesis and function of mouse CD4+ T cells. Immunol Rev 1991; 123:209-229.
5. Scott P, Kaufman S. The role of T cell subsets and cytokines in the regulation of infection. Immunol Today 1991; 12:346-348.
6. Ramshaw IA, Andrew ME, Phillips SM et al. Recovery of immunodeficient mice from a vaccinia virus/IL-2 recombinant infection. Nature 1987; 329:545-546.
7. Flexner C, Hugin A, Moss, B. Prevention of vaccinia virus infection in immunodeficient mice by vector-directed IL-2 expression. Nature 1987; 330:259-261.
8. Karupiah G, Coupar BEH, Andrew ME et al. Elevated natural killer cell responses in mice infected with recombinant vaccinia virus encoding murine IL-2. J Immunol 1990; 144:290-298.

9. Redfield RR, Wright DC, James WD et al. Disseminated vaccinia in a military recruit with human immunodeficiency virus (HIV) disease. New Eng J Med 1987; 316:673-676.
10. Ruby J, Brinkman C, Jones S et al. Response of monkeys to vaccination with recombinant vaccinia virus which coexpress HIV gp160 and human interleukin-2. Immunol Cell Biol 1990; 68:113-117.
11. Flexner C, Moss B, London T et al. Attenuation and immunogenicity in primates of vaccinia virus recombinants expressing human interleukin-2. Vaccine 1990; 8:17-21.
12. Karupiah G, Ramsay AJ, Ramshaw IA et al. Recombinant vaccine vector-induced protection of athymic, nude mice from influenza A virus infection. Analysis of protective mechanisms. Scand J Immunol 1992; 36:99-105.
13. Karupiah G, Blanden RV, Ramshaw IA. Interferon-γ is involved in the recovery of athymic nude mice from recombinant vaccinia/interleukin 2 infection. J Exp Med 1990; 172:1495-1503.
14. Perussia B, Santoli D, Trinchieri G. Interferon modulation of natural killer cell activity. Ann NY Acad Sci 1980; 350:55-66.
15. Schultz RM, Kleinschmidt WJ. Functional identity between murine gamma interferon and macrophage activating factor. Nature 1983; 305:239-240.
16. Bukowski JF, Welsh RM. Interferon enhances the susceptibility of virus-infected fibroblasts to cytotoxic T cells. J Exp Med 1985; 161:257-262.
17. Feduchi E, Carrasco L. Mechanism of inhibition of HSV-1 replication by tumour necrosis factor and interferon-γ. Virology 1991; 180:822-825.
18. Wong GHW, Goeddel DV. Tumour necrosis factors α and β inhibit virus replication and synergize with interferons. Nature 1986; 323:819-822.
19. Kohonen-Corish M, King N, Woodhams C et al. Immunodeficient mice recover from infection with vaccinia virus expressing interferon-γ. Eur J Immunol 1990; 20:157-161.
20. Sambhi SK, Kohonen-Corish M, Ramshaw IA. Local production of tumour necrosis factor encoded by recombinant vaccinia virus is effective in controlling viral replication in vivo. Proc Natl Acad Sci USA 1991; 88:4025-4029.
21. Ramshaw I, Ruby J, Ramsay A et al. Expression of cytokines by recombinant vaccinia viruses: A model for studying cytokines in virus infections in vivo. Immunol Rev 1992; 127:157-182.
22. Blanden RV. T cell responses to viral and bacterial infection. Transplant Rev 1974; 19:56-88.
23. Ruby J, Sedger L, Ramshaw I. Cytokine production in virus infected mice: a single cell analysis. Viral Immunol 1993; 6:125-134.
24. Ruby J, Ramshaw I. The antiviral activity of immune $CD8^+$ T cells is dependent on interferon-γ. Lymphokine Cytokine Res.1991; 10:353-358.
25. Ramsay AJ, Ruby J, Ramshaw IA. A case for cytokines as effector molecules in the resolution of virus infection. Immunol Today 1993; 14:155-157.
26. FongTAT, Mosmann TR. Alloreactive murine CD8+ T cell clones secrete the TH1 pattern of cytokines. J Immunol 1990; 144:1744-1752.
27. Fiorentino DF, Bond MW, Mosmann TR. Two types of mouse T helper cell. IV. TH2 clones secrete a factor that inhibits cytokine production by TH1 clones. J Exp Med 1989; 170:2081-2095.
28. Ramsay AJ, Kohonen-Corish M. Interleukin-5 expressed by a recombinant virus vector enhances specific mucosal IgA responses in vivo. Eur J Immunol 1993; 23:3141-3145.

29. Ramsay AJ. Vector-encoded IL-5 and IL-6 enhance specific mucosal IgA reactivity in vivo. In: Jackson, S et al eds. Recent Advances in Mucosal Immunology. New York: Plenum Press, In press.
30. Erard F, Wild MT, Garcia-Sanz JA et al. Switch of CD8 T cells to noncytolytic CD8-CD4- cells that make TH2 cytokines and help B cells. Science 1993; 260: 1802-1805.
31. Mestecky J, McGhee JR. Immunoglobulin A (IgA): Molecular and cellular interactions involved in IgA biosynthesis and immune response. Adv Immunol 1987; 40:153-245.
32. Harriman GR. Kunimoto DY, Elliot JF et al. The role of IL-5 in IgA B cell differentiation. J.Immunol 1988; 140:3033-3039.
33. Beagley KW, Eldridge JH, Lee F et al. Interleukins and IgA synthesis. Human and murine interleukin 6 induce high rate IgA secretion in IgA-committed cells. J Exp Med 1989; 169:2133-2148.
34. Hocart MJ, MackenzieJS, Stewart GA. The IgG subclass responses to influenza virus haemagglutinin in the mouse: Effect of route of inoculation. J Gen Virol 1989; 70:809-818.
35. Snapper CM, Paul WE. Interferon-γ and B cell stimulatory factor-1 reciprocally regulate Ig isotype production. Science 1987; 236:944-947.
36. Finkelman FD, Holmes J, Katona IM et al. Lymphokine control of in vivo immunoglobulin isotype selection. Ann Rev Immunol 1990; 8:303-333.

CHAPTER 12

Vaccines to Prevent Sexually Transmitted Diseases: The Challenge of Generating Protective Immunity at Genital Mucosal Surfaces

Christopher J. Miller
Nancy J. Alexander
Michael B. McChesney

INTRODUCTION

Vaccination against microbial agents is the most cost effective approach to reducing morbidity and mortality in a population. In developing countries with a minimum of medical infrastructure, vaccines may offer the only practical strategy to reduce the impact of infectious disease. Two recent developments have combined to spur effort in the development of vaccines to prevent sexually transmitted diseases (STDs). The obviously immense social and economic costs of the HIV pandemic and the recognition of the serious and potentially devastating consequences of the more traditional STD pathogens have convinced the medical research community to devote increasing resources to the prevention of STDs. The challenges and opportunities involved in attempting to develop anti-STD vaccines have been presented in recent reviews[1,2] and we will not repeat the insightful observations contained in these contributions. Instead, we will use these reviews as a foundation on which to highlight potential strategies to produce effective anti-STD immune responses at genital mucosal surfaces. Because women and their offspring are disproportionately affected by the sequelae of STD infection, initial attempts to generate STD vaccines should be directed toward protecting women from STDs. Of course, a vaccine which prevents STDs

Strategies in Vaccine Design, edited by Gordon L. Ada, D.Sc.

in women will decrease the incidence of STD in heterosexual males as well. For these reasons this chapter will concentrate on the subject of anti-STD immunity in the female genital tract.

MUCOSAL IMMUNITY: OVERVIEW

Abundant information is available on generating immune responses at the mucosal surface of the gastrointestinal (GI) tract.[3-6] Efforts to produce protective immunity in the GI tract have been greatly aided by a detailed understanding of the intestinal mucosal immune system. Our understanding of the genital mucosal immune system is nascent and it is likely that successful STD vaccines will require more knowledge about the mechanisms involved in generating an immune response in these tissues.[7] Our current understanding of the mucosal immune system in genital tract has been the subject of a recent reviews.[8,9] The nature of the local immune system in the female tract is summarized below.

Gut-associated and bronchial-associated lymphoid tissues (GALT and BALT) constitute the largest accumulation of lymphoid tissue in the body. Plasma cells in these regions release secretory IgA which is the most important immunoglobulin in conferring resistance to virus infection at mucosal surfaces. In the intestinal tract, the mucosal immune response is achieved through the uptake of antigen by M cells in the columnar epithelium. M cells pass the antigen to antigen-presenting cells (APC) in the lamina propria. The APCs process and present the antigen to antigen-specific B and T cell precursors in Peyer's patches and draining lymph nodes. Mature B and T cells enter the efferent lymph, pass through the thoracic duct, enter the circulating blood and reach distant mucosal sites where they pass through the endothelium of post-capillary venules. The migration of mature B and T cells from the blood into the mucosal tissues is thought to be mediated by the specific binding of adhesion molecules on the cytoplasmic membranes of lymphocytes and endothelial cells.[10-12] Thus, B and T lymphocytes which are stimulated following exposure at a mucosal surface are 'predestined' to seek out other mucosal sites. This specific migration of lymphocytes is the basis for the common mucosal immune system.[7] The concept of a common mucosal immune system[6,13-15] implies that immune responses may occur at mucosal surfaces which are distinct from the site of mucosal immunization. The extent that this concept extends to the genital tract is ill defined. However several recent studies have demonstrated vaginal secretory Ig following immunization at distant mucosal sites. In mice intranasal and intragastric immunization with streptococcal antigen conjugated to cholera toxin subunit B (CT-B) resulted in specific IgA responses in saliva, tracheal wash, gut wash and vaginal wash.[16] In rhesus macaques, the detection of specific antibody in vaginal secretions following oral immunization with yeast retrotransposon Ty virus-like particles carrying SIV-p27 and conjugated to CT-B was variable, but when orally immunized animals were boosted vaginally, specific IgA responses were detected in the vaginal secretions of all animals.[17] Guinea pigs immunized enterically with *C. psittaci* are protected from challenge at both the conjunctival and vaginal mucosa.[18] Thus there is an indication that, at least with some antigens, the genital tract is part of a common mucosal immune system.

Function of S-IgA

S-IgA antibodies are likely to play an important role in mucosal immunity, because they are present at the sites of initial contact of pathogens with host cells. Virus-neutralizing antibodies at mucosal surfaces are important in preventing local infection and disease.[19] The view that has emerged is that S-IgA/viral binding in the mucus layer can prevent virus attachment to epithelial cells and thus block their subsequent penetration. However, this idea may be too simplistic. In some cases the mechanism of neutralization is a transcriptional block of virus replication in the infected epithelial cell. For influenza virus the mechanism for this transcriptional block may involve a conformational change in HA following antibody binding, which results in transmission of a signal to the transcriptase complex inside the virus.[20] The epithelial cells infected by virus in the upper respiratory tract are involved with IgA transport, and are therefore the site of antigen-IgA neutralization that results in blocked viral nucleotide transcription. Intracellular neutralization was recently reported with in vitro infection of Sendai virus.[21] IgA was capable of blocking Sendai virus replication by binding to viral proteins within epithelial cells. Thus by eliciting an IgA response, three mechanisms of virus elimination may be induced: prevention of virus attachment by formation of immune complexes in the mucous layer, transport of immune complexes from the lamina propria across the epithelium into the secretions and interruption of virus replication within the target cell.[22]

THE MUCOSAL IMMUNE SYSTEM OF THE FEMALE REPRODUCTIVE TRACT

The mucosa of the vagina consists of a non-keratinized, stratified squamous epithelium and an underlying vascular submucosa. The ectocervix has a similar architecture, while the endocervix consists of a simple columnar epithelium covering a vascular submucosa. The mechanism of antigen uptake and processing in the female reproductive tract has only recently been elucidated. M cells have not been described in the vagina or cervix; but Langerhans cells and macrophages are present in the vaginal mucosa. In mice, antigen absorption in the vagina occurs via $CD4^+$ Langerhans cells.[23] Langerhans cell are MHC class II, $CD4^+$ dendritic cells located within squamous epithelia throughout the body. Langerhans cells are common in the skin where they can bind antigen, migrate to the draining lymph node and there transform into interdigitating dendritic cells in the T cell-rich paracortex.[24-27]

The lower female reproductive tract has the ability to initiate an immune response. Vaginal antibodies are induced as a result of natural or experimental infection of the lower reproductive tract with a variety of pathogens. Women with genital herpes simplex virus infection have secretory IgA in their vaginal secretion.[28] Following intravaginal immunization with inactivated polio vaccine, women produce specific secretory IgA in vaginal secretions.[29] Intravaginal immunization with *Candida albicans* also induces high titers of specific secretory IgA in vaginal secretions.[30] The lower female reproductive tract can mount an immune response to protein antigens.[31, 32] However, the response to these non-replicating antigens is short-lived and weak. Often, large doses of antigen and adjuvants are required to generate significant responses to vaginal immunization.[33] This relative inability of the mucosal immune system in the female genital tract to respond to non-replicating antigens may be important in preventing women from developing anti-sperm immune responses that could prevent fertilization. In fact, the presence of anti-sperm antibodies in women is associated with infertility.[34]

The immune system in the genital tract of the female rhesus macaque consists of a resident population of monocyte/macrophages, T and B cells in the submucosa of the vagina and cervix.[35] These cells are specifically localized in the superficial submucosa, just beneath the vaginal epithelium. A similar population of lymphocytes and macrophages has been described in the submucosa of the human cervix where they have been called mucosal-associated lymphoreticular tissue (MALT).[36] Langerhans cells are abundant in the vaginal and ectocervical mucosa of women[36-40] and rhesus macaques,[35] and dendritic processes extend to the lumen of the vagina. A large number of $CD8^+$ T lymphocytes are located within the epithelium and superficial submucosa of the vagina in rhesus macaques.[35] The function of these cells is unknown but studies are underway to determine if they are cytotoxic T lymphocytes (CTLs).

It is likely that in the vagina, both Langerhans cells and macrophages are capable of acting as APCs and initiating an immune response. One hypothesis to explain the generation of a primary immune response in the female genital tract is that antigen contacts APCs (Langerhans cell in the epithelium or macrophage in the submucosa), which then migrate to draining lymph nodes. Once in the lymph nodes, the APCs stimulate B and T lymphocytes, including memory subpopulations, which enter the blood stream via the efferent lymph and thoracic duct. The T and B lymphocytes (including memory cells) migrate to the genital tract. Upon exposure to the antigen, these cells participate in a secondary immune response.

In rats, the presence of IgG and IgA antibodies in uterine secretions is hormonally regulated. IgG and IgA levels are maximum at pro-estrus, but IgG drops markedly at estrus.[41] Human cervical mucus from normal women sampled throughout the menstrual cycle contained albumin/IgG ratios which approximate those in serum, suggesting that the IgG is derived from the blood circulation.[42] IgA levels in cervical mucus have been assessed and ~85-90% is locally produced S-IgA (reviewed in ref. 43). The effect of estrogen on local IgA synthesis in women is unclear. One study reported that more IgA is present at midcycle when compared with IgG,[44] while another study stated that the levels of IgG and IgA were consistently lower at midcycle.[45] These observations emphasize the importance of hormonal regulation of local antibody production in genital secretions. The finding of reduced IgA (but not IgG) in vaginal secretions of hysterectomised mice[46] is indirect evidence that IgA is locally produced in the upper reproductive tract. In hysterectomized women, IgG levels in cervical mucus are reduced 50% while IgA levels were less than 10% of normal.[44]

Recent studies have shed light on the cellular origin of Ig isotypes present in reproductive tract secretions of women. The lamina propria of the endo- and ectocervix contain the highest numbers of plasma cells, with significant numbers also present in the fallopian tube and in the vagina.[43,47] The major Ig isotype of the plasma cells present in these tissues is IgA, with smaller numbers of IgM^+ and IgG^+ plasma cells. Further, most of the IgA^+ plasma cells contain J chain, and this clearly suggests that the IgA produced in these regions is largely polymeric.[43,47,48] Interestingly, an approximately equal distribution of IgA_1 and IgA_2

plasma cells were noted, a pattern similar to that of the lower regions of the GI tract. Women with a variety of sexually transmitted diseases have increased numbers of plasma cells (especially IgA plasma cells) in the submucosa of the endocervix.[49] Finally, the columnar epithelial cells of the genital tract produce secretory component, which is required for transport of polymeric IgA into the reproductive tract secretions. These studies indicate that certain regions, e.g., the fallopian tubes, ecto- and endocervix and perhaps the vagina, exhibit characteristics of mucosal effector sites.

THE NATURAL HISTORY OF STDS AS IT RELATES TO VACCINE DEVELOPMENT

Of the successful vaccines currently used, most have been produced by empirical approaches. Although this approach has worked well against some systemic and mucosal infections, attempts to prevent STD disease or transmission, with the possible exception of hepatitis B virus, have been unsuccessful. Most STD pathogens have a common feature: they usually infect women by crossing or directly infecting the mucosal surfaces of the genital tract. This fact presents an opportunity to prevent or limit these infections by generating protective immune responses at these mucosal surfaces. However, some of these pathogens such as herpes simplex virus (HSV), human papilloma virus (HPV) and syphilis can also infect cutaneous surfaces of the external genitalia. These cutaneous surfaces are not protected by genital secretions and thus stimulating genital secretory immune responses would not be expected to prevent infection at these surfaces. In men, STDs commonly infect the cutaneous surfaces of the external genitalia or the dry mucosal surface of the foreskin and glans. HSV, HPV and syphilis rarely infect the male urethra and it is unlikely that a genital secretory immune response in the male reproductive tract will prevent infection with these agents. Infection with two STD pathogens, gonorrhea and chlamydia, is initiated at mucosal surfaces in both men and women and it seems likely that a genital secretory immune response could prevent infection with these agents.

The mechanism of HIV transmission is less clear. There is abundant evidence that HIV is transmitted across the genital mucosa of women (reviewed in ref. 8) however the site of transmission in men is not clear. Epidemiological studies suggests that the presence of an intact foreskin is one of the risk factors associated with HIV infection in men.[50,51] Studies in chronically SIV-infected rhesus macaques found virus infected cells in the stratified squamous mucosal epithelium of the foreskin.[52] This finding, together with the observation that SIV can be transmitted to male rhesus macaques by placing cell-free virus onto the foreskin and glans of the penis,[53] suggests that target cells for SIV are present in the epithelium of the foreskin and glans. Langerhans cells are the most abundant $CD4^+$ cell type present in this tissue, although lesser numbers of macrophages and T cells are also found in the foreskin.[52] Thus HIV may be transmitted to men across a relatively dry mucosal surface. If HIV is transmitted across the foreskin and glans epithelium, secretory IgA in genital tract secretions is likely to have little effect on transmission. However, the presence of anti-HIV IgA in the semen of an infected individual may bind free virus and make that individual less infectious.

The cutaneous regions of the external genitalia and the mucosal surfaces of the lower reproductive tract have overlapping lymphatic drainage and immune responses to both sites occur in the same regional lymph nodes. Thus cellular immune responses generated by an optimum immunization strategy are likely to be found in the cutaneous surfaces of the external genitalia, the genital mucosa and the draining lymph nodes. Because most of the agents that infect the cutaneous surfaces of the external genitalia are intracellular (HSV, HPV, HIV) or are normally controlled by cellular immunity (syphilis, see below), cellular immune responses in these sites may be sufficient to limit infection or prevent disease.

The organisms that cause STDs are divergent and the nature of the disease produced by these agents varies. STD pathogens consist of two types of organisms. One type causes primarily genital mucosal disease (gonorrhea, chlamydia) and the other type uses the genital tract as a route of entry to initiate disseminated infections (HIV, HSV, syphilis, hepatitis B). Localized infections with regional sequelae are produced by some of the agents. Uncomplicated gonococcal infection is limited to the mucous membranes of the genitourinary tract.[54] The neutrophilic exudate that is associated with gonococcal urethritis does not control the infection. To prevent infection with gonorrhea, vaccines should generate specific immunity in the genital secretions and tissues. HPV infects squamous epithelial cells that line the mucosal surfaces of the reproductive tract. In women, the most serious lesion associated with HPV infection is cervical carcinoma.[55-58] There is no evidence of systemic dissemination of HPV infection, thus any vaccine designed to prevent or limit HPV infection must generate an immune response at the mucosal surface of the genital tract. Chlamydia infects mucosal surfaces throughout the genital tract. The chronic inflammation of trachoma and chlamydial salpingitis develops after reinfection. Humans and monkeys systemically immunized with *C. trachomatis* developed more severe ocular disease upon infection.[59-64,54-60] Thus, anti-chlamydial vaccines must avoid producing immunopathology while preventing attachment and uptake of the organism into epithelial cells. For this agent, specific IgA immunity may be more desirable than cellular immunity.

Systemic and potentially fatal infection can result from infection with other STD agents. Herpes simplex virus type-2 (HSV-2) infects epithelial cells initially, but subsequently travels up sensory nerve axons to sensory and autonomic ganglia. This latent infection can be reactivated resulting in recurrent genital lesions and virus shedding (for a review of HSV-2 pathogenesis see ref. 65). Perhaps the most serious consequence of HSV-2 infection is the intrapartum transmission of HSV-2 to neonates. HSV-2 vaccines could be designed to prevent primary infection by generating genital mucosal immunity, to eliminate latent infection through systemic immunity or to prevent reactivation and shedding by inducing a combination of mucosal and systemic immunity. The acute and chronic lesions characteristic of syphilis consist of mononuclear cell infiltrates; in gummatous lesions the cellular infiltrate is typical of a delayed hypersensitivity (DH) response with macrophage and lymphocyte infiltrates surrounding areas of necrosis.[66] The majority of infiltrating cells in these lesions are $CD4^+$ T cells in primary lesions and $CD8^+$ T cells in secondary lesions.[67] To prevent infection with syphilis, a vaccine should generate specific immunity in the genital tract but, if the goal is to prevent only the serious consequences associated with systemic disease then a systemic immune response may be sufficient. Although the mechanism of HIV transmission remains undefined,[8] infection of $CD4^+$ cells in lymphoid tissue and blood is the ultimate consequence of HIV transmission. Because there is no conclusive evidence that HIV infection can be cleared by host immune responses, efforts to develop a prophylactic vaccine have been directed toward preventing infection rather than eliminating primary infection. Thus it may be necessary to prevent interaction of HIV with target cells in the genital tract. This could best be accomplished by generating anti-HIV immunity (including secretory IgA) in the genital tract. An additional challenge lies in preventing genital transmission of cell-associated HIV.[68]

IMMUNE RESPONSES TO STDS

STDs have infected humans for a very long time and reports of infection extend to the beginning of recorded history. Although there are genital mucosal immune responses to sexually transmitted pathogens, these responses rarely constitute protective immunity. Women with acute gonococcal infection have specific IgG and IgA responses in vaginal secretions.[69, 70] Cellular immune responses to gonococcal infection exist but the significance of these responses are unclear.[71] Despite these responses both men and women are commonly reinfected with gonorrhea and infection can persist for months in untreated individuals.[72] The presence of anti-chlamydial IgA in genital mucosal secretions is associated with a significant reduction in recovery of chlamydia from cervical secretions.[73] Chlamydia can grow in unstimulated macrophages, but are killed by interferon-gamma-activated macrophages (reviewed in ref. 74). Protective immunity does develop following chlamydial infection but the response wanes and reinfection is common.[75] Despite the fact that individuals treated for syphilis can be reinfected, immunity to *T. pallidum* does develop (reviewed in ref. 66). Attachment of *T. pallidum* to eukaryotic cells can be blocked by specific antibody (reviewed in ref. 66) which suggests that a vaccine-generated immune response may be able to prevent the initial infection of target cells in the genital tract. In the rabbit model of syphilis, development of systemic T cell responses correlates with the onset of cellular infiltration at the site of primary infection.[76] It has been proposed that a continuing T cell response is required to maintain *T. pallidum* infection latency.[66] It has also been postulated that those persons who fail to develop a strong DH response early in infection progress to subsequent stages. The preferential stimulation of the Th1 subset of CD4 T cells and the subsequent induction of strong DH responses may protect infected individuals from activation of latent infection (see below).

HPV infections are localized to the genital epithelium and cells of the immune system have little access to the HPV antigens. HPV-specific CTL responses can be induced in mice immunized with vaccinia expressing an HPV-16 antigen.[77] Serum antibodies to HSV-2 are detected in the first few weeks post-infection.[78,79] Antibodies to HSV are present in cervicovaginal secretions[80-83] and S-IgA levels are inversely correlated with the isolation of HSV-2 from the genital tract.[28] Prior infection and subsequent immunity to HSV-1 lowers the risk of acquiring genital infection with HSV-2.[84-87] The risk of recurrence of asymptomatic HSV-2 is directly correlated with serum levels of complement-independent neutralizing antibody.[88] There have been a few reports describing the genital secretory immune response to HIV.[89,90] In women, both IgA and IgG, directed at HIV-1 core and envelope antigens, can be detected in the vaginal secretions, but neutralizing activity has not been demonstrated. It was recently reported that anti-HIV IgG is the predominant component of the HIV-specific immunity in vaginal secretions.[91]

The ability of these organisms to escape the immune response is an indication of the extent to which these agents have adapted to their host. This adaptation allows STDs to persist and be transmitted in a population despite the presence of immunity. It seems likely that one strategy employed by these agents to achieve this adaptation is to display antigens that evoke a strong but ineffective immune response. This antigenic camouflage is used to hide from the immune system those components of the organisms that are required for survival and transmission. Thus one of the challenges to generating effective anti-STD immunity is to select critical antigens (binding epitopes, etc.) for incorporation into candidate vaccines.

VACCINE DESIGN

While vaccines are generally beneficial to the recipient, immune responses elicited by vaccination can result in paradoxical inflammatory responses and severe disease when the primed host encounters a pathogen, as occurred with formalin-inactivated measles virus, respiratory syncitial virus (RSV) and caprine arthritis-encephalitis virus vaccines. This aberrant vaccine-induced immunity has been attributed to immune responses that differ from normal immune responses to the pathogen: either due to the loss of protective epitopes or to the induction of "non-protective" immunity to denatured antigens in the vaccine. But the actual mechanisms are not known.[92] Recent studies in the RSV/cotton rat system demonstrate that animals immunized with formalin-inactivated virus or a glycoprotein subunit vaccine and challenged with RSV have more severe disease than naive animals.[93] The enhanced pathology in vaccinated animals may be due to an exaggeration of normal antiviral immune responses in the vaccinated animals.[94] Caution must be used when attempting to vaccinate against infections that can produce disease through immunopathogenic mechanisms. Several organisms that cause STDs (syphilis, chlamydia, HSV and possibly HIV) have an underlying immunopathogenic mechanism of disease, thus a vaccine has the potential to exacerbate the clinical course of these infections.

The challenge of developing effective anti-STD mucosal immune responses in the genital tract is paralleled by the effort to develop immunocontraceptive vaccines. The work in this field supports the notion that systemic immunization alone does not produce strong immunity in the reproductive tract. A recombinant vaccinia vector expressing the human sperm antigen LDH-C4 resulted in strong serum antibody responses but specific antibodies were not detected in the reproductive tract of female baboons.[65] Studies in both mice and monkeys indicate that vaginal and uterine immunization with immunogens results in weak genital immune responses, but combined systemic and mucosal immunization increases the vaginal S-IgA levels in monkeys immunized with a variety of antigens including SIV p27.[17,95] In mice, uterine antibody levels were highest when systemic immunization was followed by gastric and then intrauterine boosting.[95] These observations suggest that combining systemic and mucosal routes of immunization may be the best strategy to elicit strong genital immunity.

Recently (reviewed in ref. 96 and chapters by Schearer et al and Bretscher in this volume), it has been suggested that preferential stimulation of one subset of CD4⁺ T helper cells (Th1 cells) may be a desirable property of vaccines, including HIV vaccines. This hypothesis is based on several observations including mice exposed to a low dose of *Leishmania major* "lock" the immune system in a Th1 immune response with activation of DH responses that protect the animals from subsequent rechallenge.[97] Thus it may be desirable to preferentially stimulate Th1 T cells and subsequent cellular immune responses against intracellular STD pathogens. Although it is not clear that this type of response is desirable for all STD vaccines, a thorough study of the Th1/Th2 system in these infections is warranted. It is very likely that different adjuvants, vectors and routes of immunization will influence the specific Th subset that is stimulated. A detailed discussion of the role of Th cell subsets in the induction of mucosal immunity is included in recent reviews.[3,4,8,98]

MUCOSAL IMMUNIZATION AGAINST STDS

There is evidence that local antiviral immunity can be induced in the female genital tract. In the guinea pig model of vaginal herpes infection, glycoprotein vaccines produce a marked reduction in recurrence and shedding of HSV-2. This reduction is associated with the presence of specific antibody in secretions.[99] In addition, CTL may be important in preventing infection following mucosal exposure to viruses. In mice, intravaginal immunization with a live-attenuated HSV-2 induced protection from lethal intravaginal challenge with virulent HSV-2.[100] The protective immune response in the animals was associated with lymphoid hyperplasia in the genital lymph nodes and decreased replication of the virulent HSV-2 challenge virus in the genital tract.[101] These investigators demonstrated that the protective immunity could be passed from vaccinated mice to naive mice by adoptive transfer of T lymphocytes in the genital lymph nodes, but not from other lymphoid sites.[101,102] These T cells preferentially migrate into HSV-2 infected tissue.[102] This work demonstrates that, in the HSV-2/mouse model, protective genital mucosa immunity is due to migration of CTL from the genital lymph nodes into the genital mucosa. A number of human clinical trials of HSV vaccines have been undertaken with varying degrees of success (reviewed in ref. 103) and it seems likely that a vaccine capable of reducing genital secretion of HSV-2 will become available. It is less clear that a vaccine capable of preventing primary infection will be developed in the near future.

Therapeutic and prophylactic vaccines against bovine papillomavirus type-4 have been developed using recombinant proteins[104,105] and efforts to develop recombinant HPV vaccines are underway. Virus-like particles (VLPs) are formed when the L1 coat protein of HPV-11 is expressed in a recombinant baculovirus system.[106] These particles react with sera from individuals infected with HPV-11 and display conformational epitopes characteristic of native virions.[106] Experiments using similar HPV L1 VLPs produced in a different expression system demonstrate that these particles retain neutralizing conformational epitopes.[107] It may be possible to use these or similar antigens to generate protective genital secretory immunity against genital papillomavirus infection or to treat HPV-related cervical carcinoma.

Immunity to genital chlamydial infection can be generated by enteric immunization. Guinea pigs infected intestinally with *C. psittaci* are protected from challenge at both the conjunctival and vaginal mucosa.[18] Complete protection from challenge with *T. pallidum* following vaccination can occur but only after prolonged immunization schedules.[108] This protection against *T. pallidum* was not associated with "immobilizing" antibody.

The majority of the HIV vaccine studies to date have been limited to parenteral immunization schedules. In the animal model systems (HIV-1/chimpanzee, HIV-2/macaque, SIV/macaque) in which vaccine efficacy against challenge has been tested, protection has been obtained using inactivated whole virus, modified live virus and envelope-based vaccines (reviewed in ref. 109). Protection has been associated with anti-envelope antibody in some studies, but a correlation between protection and neutralizing antibody is far from clear. The same inactivated whole or modified live SIV vaccine formulations and immunization schedules that protect rhesus macaques against i.v. challenge do not protect against low dose vaginal mucosal challenge with cell-free SIV.[110] Thus, systemic immunity alone cannot prevent the genital transmission of SIV and novel immunization routes must be developed in an attempt to generate protective immunity against HIV in the genital tract of women. It was recently reported that macaques mucosally (orally and vaginally) immunized with SIV gag p27 hybridized to the yeast retrotransposon virus-like particle (Ty-VLP) and then boosted intramuscularly developed a strong genital mucosal immune response to the immunogen.[17] In most of the animals in this report the systemic boost significantly enhanced the genital immune response. In order to maximize the mucosal immune response to this antigen, the p27 Ty-VLP was covalently linked to CT-B and cholera vibrio were included in the capsules used for oral immunization. There was also specific sensitization of T cells in genital and mesenteric lymph nodes.[17] It was recently reported that rhesus macaques mucosally and systemically immunized with a microencapsulated whole-killed SIV preparation were protected from vaginal challenge with virulent SIV.[111]

ANTIGEN DELIVERY SYSTEMS

MUCOSAL ADJUVANTS: CHOLERA TOXIN AND CHOLERA TOXIN SUBUNIT B

Oral administration of most protein antigens does not induce mucosal immunity but rather, oral tolerance. The secretory immune response to most antigens can be markedly enhanced through the use of mucosal adjuvants. Cholera toxin (CT) has been shown to enhance the immunogenicity of even poor mucosal immunogens when mixed or conjugated together and given orally. CT is the most potent mucosal immunogen yet identified and its properties are exactly those one would desire for an effective mucosal vaccine (reviewed in ref. 112). CT is an effective oral adjuvant because it elicits strong secretory IgA and mucosal T cell responses (reviewed in ref. 112). It does not induce oral tolerance and even abrogates oral tolerance to orally administered antigens.[112,113] CT stimulates homing of antigen-specific B cells to distant mucosal sites such as the lung and salivary glands and it leads to long-lasting antigen-specific memory B and T cells in the lamina propria (reviewed in ref. 112). CT is composed of two components (one subunit of CT-A and five subunits of CT-B). Because CT can cause side effects in humans, recent efforts have used CT-B as an oral adjuvant (reviewed in ref. 112) and have met with mixed success. In one report, orally administered mixtures of KLH and CT-B were unable to stimulate mucosal immunity unless very small amounts of the holotoxin were added.[114] The use of CT-B/antigen conjugates has been reported to be effective in some cases but not in others (reviewed in ref. 112). The results of these studies make it clear that CT is a more effective mucosal adjuvant than CT-B but because CT-B has been used effectively in humans, without detectable side effects,[115-117] it is more acceptable for clinical use. CT-B is an effective adjuvant when used for intranasal immunization of mice.[16] Following intranasal immunization with streptococcal antigen conjugated to CT-B, specific antibodies were found in serum, saliva, tracheal wash, gut wash and vaginal wash and the mucosal immune responses were stronger in intranasally immunized animals than in intragastrically immunized animals.[16] The suitability of a given antigen for use with CT or CT-B cannot be predicted and must be determined empirically in each animal system.

Replicating Vectors

Live vaccine vectors offer another method of stimulating mucosal immune responses to STDs. Bacterial vectors are especially promising because they can specifically target mucosal surfaces and can express multiple viral subunits. In addition, antibiotic therapy can be used to control the vector should the bacteria exhibit unanticipated virulence in an immunocompromised host. Bacterial vectors that are easily manipulated genetically, and enter the host via mucosal surfaces for limited periods of time, may be capable of inducing both mucosal and systemic protective immunity (reviewed in ref. 3). *Salmonella typhi* is a human enteropathogen that may be useful for stimulating mucosal immunity to STDs. Salmonella is invasive and the bacteria multiply in the lamina propria of the intestine and survive within phagolysosomes of macrophages. The genes that play an important role in allowing the bacteria to survive in macrophages have been identified. The genes pagC and pagD, denoting phosphatase activated gene C and D, are transcriptionally activated once the bacteria enter macrophages.[118] The deletion of pagC seems to abolish the pathogenic effects of *Salmonella typhimurium* in mice.[119] These bacteria may be capable of stimulating a strong CTL response;[120] however, bacterial vectors expressing viral antigens may not be capable of inducing effective antibody responses.

A number of groups have used recombinant DNA technology to produce chimeric viruses that may be used as vaccines. These viruses provide a method to deliver the appropriate antigens to mucosal surfaces and elicit specific immune responses in the desired anatomic location. Several virus vectors (poliovirus, adenovirus, poxviruses, herpes viruses) are in varying stages of development. Oral immunization with recombinant adenovirus expressing HSV glycoprotein B protects mice from lethal challenge with HSV-2.[121] Poliovirus constructs[122-126] seem to be especially promising vectors for the delivery of STD antigens to the mucosal immune system. The most effort to date has been directed toward developing vaccinia virus vectors. There are several potential problems with this approach. Pre-existing immunity, due to vaccination or infection, may limit the ability of viral vectors to infect and induce immunity in an individual. In addition, the use of these recombinant viruses in immunodeficient individuals (newborns, the elderly, AIDS patients, therapeutically immunosuppressed patients) may result in a disseminated and life-threatening infection with the vector.

Microspheres and Liposomes as Mucosal Adjuvants

Another approach to mucosal immunization is to incorporate whole-killed virus or viral proteins into biodegradable microspheres. In order to use these as vehicles for mucosal immunization, polymers are crosslinked into microspheres in the size range of 1-10 microns. Oral immunization with microspheres in this size range results in the uptake of the microspheres by M cells. Subsequently the particles are passed to APCs in Peyer's patches where an immune response is stimulated.[127] Liposomes are another antigen delivery system which has the potential to induce significant mucosal immunity. The formulation of the liposome can determine the nature of the immune response to the incorporated antigen.[128] It is particularly significant that incorporation of peptides into pH-sensitive liposomes results in specific CTL responses in immunized mice.[128-130] Rats orally immunized with *Streptococcus mutans* antigen incorporated into liposomes had strong secretory IgA responses in saliva.[131] By encapsulating BSA into liposomes, mucosal and systemic immune responses in orally immunized mice were significantly enhanced.[132] Mice immunized with liposomes containing mRNA encoding influenza nucleoprotein develop specific CTL responses.[133] Intranasal and oral immunization of mice with liposomes containing *Bordetella pertussis* antigens resulted in an IgA response in lung washes that persisted for 75 days after the last boost.[134]

Immunization by DNA transfection in vivo

Recently, the transfection of plasmid DNA encoding immunogenic proteins into mouse skeletal muscle or tumor in vivo has resulted in protection from lethal disease.[135,136] In both cases, protection correlated with the induction of classical humoral and/or cellular immune responses to the transfected genes' products. Previous studies demonstrated that foreign DNA inoculated into mouse skeletal muscle in vivo could be stably expressed for several months and that the plasmid DNA persisted as circular episomes in otherwise normal muscle fibers.[137] Experiments in nonhuman primates have provided similar results, but the levels of foreign gene expression are significantly lower.[138] Although this method of genetic immunization is in an early stage of development, it has the advantage of immunization with replicating vectors and with readily produced, non-infectious molecular immunogens, that can stimulate both MHC Class I- and II-restricted immune responses at targeted mucosal sites.

CONCLUDING REMARKS

Although the challenges to producing a vaccine capable of preventing transmission of STDs are significant, recent advances in our understanding of mucosal immunity and the success of some vaccines in animal model systems are encouraging. However, the difficulty in maintaining prolonged and effective immune responses in the genital tract must be overcome before an effective STD vaccine can be developed. STD pathogen-specific immunity that results from natrual infection does not prevent recurrent infections and, for some STDs, it may be immunopathologic. Vaccine strategies should be directed to novel routes and methods of antigen presentation to stimulate protective immune responses. One intriguing strategy is to use recombinant-attenuated STD organisms (HSV, HIV, chlamydia) as vectors for the delivery of STD antigens to the genital mucosa. It may also be possible to use chimeras of the normal vaginal bacterial flora (*Lactobacillus sp.*) to expose the genital immune system to STD antigens and in this way a persistent immune response could be generated. Thus organisms well adapted to survival in the genital tract and engineered to express STD antigens could be capable of generating long-lasting protective immunity in the genital mucosa.

REFERENCES

1. Wasserheit JN and Hitchcock PJ. Future directions in sexually transmitted disease research. In: Quinn TC, ed. Sexually Transmitted Diseases. New York. Raven Press,1992: 291-325
2. Ada GL. Prospects for vaccination at mucosal surfaces for the control of sexually transmitted diseases. In: Quinn TC, ed. Sexually Transmitted Diseases. New York. Raven Press,1992: 275-90
3. McGhee JR, Mestecky J, Dertzbaugh MT et al. The mucosal immune system: from fundamental concepts to vaccine development. Vaccine 1992; 10:75-87
4. McGhee JR and Kiyono H. Mucosal immunity to vaccines: current concepts for vaccine development and immune response analysis. In: Ciardi JE, ed. Genetically Engineered Vaccines. New York. Plenum Press,1992: 3-12
5. Czerkinsky C, Svennerholm A-M and Holmgren J. Induction and assessment of immunity at enteromucosal surfaces in humans. Clin. Infect. Dis. 1993; 16 (Suppl 2):S106-16
6. Mestecky J and McGhee JR. New Strategies for Oral Immunization. Curr Top Microbiol Immunol 1989; 146:1-10
7. Brandtzaeg P. Overview of the mucosal immune system. Curr. Top. Microbiol. Immunol. 1989; 146:13-25
8. Miller CJ, McGhee JR and Gardner MB. Mucosal Immunity, HIV transmission and AIDS. Lab. Invest. 1993; 68:129-45
9. Anderson DJ, Wolff H, Zhang W et al. Immunology of the male reproducitve tract: Implications for the heterosexual transmission of human immunodeficiency virus. In: Voeller B, Reinisch JN and Gottlieb M, ed. AIDS and Sex: an integrated biomedical and behavioral approach. New York. Oxford University Press,1990: 311-33
10. Holzmann B and Weissman IL. Integrin molecules involved in lymphocyte homing to Peyer's patches. Immunol. Rev. 1989; 108:45-61

11. Holzmann B and Weissman IL. Peyer's patch-specific homing receptors lymphocyte homing receptors consist of a VLA-4-like alpha chain associated with either of two beta chains, one of which is novel. EMBO J. 1989; 8:1735-41
12. Holzmann B, McIntyre BW and Weissman IL. Identification of a murine Peyer's patch-specific lymphocyte homing receptor as an integrin molecule with an alpha chain homologous to human VLA-4alpha. Cell 1989; 56:37-46
13. Bienenstock J, McDermott M, Befus AD et al. A common mucosal immune system involving the bronchus, breast and bowel. In: McGhee JR, Mestecky J and Babb JL, ed. Secretory Immunity and Infection. New York. Plenum Publishing Corp.,1978: 53-9
14. Bienenstock J, McDermott M and Befus A. A common mucosal immune system. In: Ogra PL and Dayton DH, ed. Immunology of Breast Milk. NY. Raven Press,1979: 91-104
15. Mestecky J. The common mucosal immune system and current strategies for induction of immune responses in external secretions. J. Clin. immunol. 1987; 265-76
16. Wu H-Y and Russell MW. Induction of mucosal immunity by intranasal application of a streptococcal surface protein antigen with the cholera toxin B subunit. Infect. Immun. 1993; 61:314-22
17. Lehner T, Bergmeier LA, Panagiotidi C et al. Induction of mucosal and systemic immunity to a recombinant simian immunodeficiency viral protein. Science 1992; 258:1365-9
18. Nichols RL, Murray ES and Nisson PE. Use of enteric vaccines in protection against chlamydial infections of the genital tract and the eye of guinea pigs. J Infect Dis 1978; 138:742-6
19. Ogra P, Leibovitz E and Zhao-Ri G. Oral immunization and secretory immunity to viruses. Curr. Top. Microbiol. Immunol. 1989; 73-81
20. Dimmock N. Mechanisms of neutralization of animal viruses. J. Gen. Virol. 1984; 1015-22
21. Mazanec MB, Kaetzel CS, Lamm ME et al. Intracellular neutralization of virus by immunoglobulin A antibodies. Proc Natl Acad Sci USA 1992; 89:6901-5
22. Mazanec MB, Nedrud JG, Kaetzel CS et al. A three-tiered view of the role of IgA in mucosal defense. Immunol. Today 1993; 14:430-5
23. Parr MB, Kepple L and Parr EL. Antigen recognition in the female reproductive tract: II. Endocytosis of horseradish peroxidase by Langerhans cells in murine vaginal epithelium. Biol. Reprod. 1991; 45:261-5
24. Hoefsmit ECM, Duijvestijn AM and Kamperdijk EWA. Relation between Langerhans cells, Veiled cells, and Interdigitating cells. Immunobiology 1982; 161:255-65
25. Kraal G, Breel M, Janse M et al. Langerhans cells, vieled cells and interdigitating cells in the mouse recognized by a monoclonal antibody. J. Exp. Med. 1986; 981-97
26. Kripke M, Munn C, Jeevan A et al. Evidence that cutaneous antigen-presenting cells migrate to regional lymph nodes during contact sensitization. J. Immunol. 1990; 2833-7
27. Silberberg-Sinakin I, Thorbecke GJ, Baer RL et al. Antigen-bearing Langerhans cells in skin, dermal lymphatics and in lymph nodes. Cell. Immunol. 1976; 25:137-51

28. Merriman H, Woods S, Winter C et al. Secretory IgA antibody in cervicovaginal secretions from women with genital infection due to herpes simplex virus. J Infect Dis 1984; 149:505-10
29. Ogra P and Ogra S. Local antibody response to polio vaccine in the human female genital tract. J. Immunol. 1973; 110:1307-11
30. Waldman RH, Cruz JM and Rowe DS. Immunoglobulin levels and antibody to *Candida albicans* in human cervicovaginal secretions. Cin. Exp. Immunol. 1972; 10:427-34
31. Parr EL and Parr MB. Immunization for secretory immunity in the female reproductive tract. Vaccine Res. 1992; 1:221-5
32. Yang SL and Schumacher GFB. Immune response after vaginal application of antigens in the rhesus monkey. Fert. Steril. 1979; 32:588-98
33. Thapar MA, Parr EL and Parr MB. The effect of adjuvants on antibody titers in mouse vaginal fluid after intravaginal immunization. J. Reprod. Immunol. 1990; 17:207-16
34. Bronson RA. Sperm antibodies. Immunol. Allergy Clin. North Am. 1990; 10:165-84
35. Miller CJ, McChesney M and Moore PF. Langerhans cells, macrophages and lymphocyte subsets in the cervix and vagina of rhesus macaques. Lab. Invest. 1992; 67:628-34
36. Edwards JNT and Morris HB. Langerhans cells and lymphocyte subsets in the female genital tract. Br. J. Obstet. Gynecol. 1985; 92:974-82
37. Bjercke S, Scott H, Braathen LR et al. HLA-DR-expressing Langerhans-like cells in vaginal and cervical epithelium. Acta Obstet Gynecol Scand 1983; 62:585-9
38. Hackemann M, Grubb C and Hill KR. The ultrastructure of normal squamous epithelium of the human cervix uteri. J Ultrastruct Res 1968; 22:443-57
39. Morris HHB, Gatter KC, Stein H et al. Langerhans cells in human cervical epithelium: an immunohistologic study. Br. J. Obstet. Gynecol. 1983; 90:400-11
40. Younes MS, Robertson EM and Bencosme SA. Electron microscope observations on Langerhans cells in the cervix. Am. J. Obstet. Gynecol. 1968; 102:397-403
41. Wira C and Sandoe C. Sex steroid hormone regulation of IgA and IgG in rat uterine secretions. Nature 1977; 534-6
42. Tjokronegoro A and Sirisinha S. Quantitative analysis of immunoglobulins and albumin in secretion of female reproductive tract. Fertil. Steril. 1975; 413-7
43. Kutteh WH, Kutteh C, Blackwell RE et al. Secretory immune system of the female reproductive tract. II. Local immune system in normal and infected fallopian tube. Fertil. Steril. 1990; 51-5
44. Jalanti R and Isliker H. Immunoglobulins in human cervico-vaginal secretions. Int. Arch. Aller. Appl. Immunol. 1977; 402-9
45. Schumacher GFB and Yang SL. Cyclic changes of immunoglobulins and specific antibodies in human and rhesus monkey cervical mucus. In: Insler V and Bettendorf G, ed. The Uterine Cervix in Reproduction. Stuttgart. Georg Thieme Verlag,1977: 187-203
46. Parr E and Parr M. A comparison of antibody titers in mouse uterine fluid after immunization by several routes, and the effect of the uterus on antibody titers in vaginal fluid. J. Reprod. Fertil. 1990; 89:619-25
47. Kutteh WH, Hatch KD, Blackwell RE et al. Secretory immune system of the female reproductive tract: I. Immunoglobulin and secretory component containing cells. Obstet. Gynecol. 1988; 71:56-60

48. Rebello R, Green FHY and Fox H. A study of the secretory immune system of the female reproductive tract. Br. J. Obstet. Gynecol. 1975; 82:812-6
49. Chipperfield EJ and Evans BA. The influence of local infection on immunoglobulin formation in the human endocervix. Clin Exp Immunol 1972; 11:219-33
50. Cameron DW, Simonsen JN, D'Costa LJ et al. Female to male transmission of human immunodeficiency virus type 1: risk factors for seroconversion in men [see comments]. Lancet 1989; 2:403-7
51. Simonsen JN, Cameron DW, Gakinya MN et al. Human immunodeficiency virus infection among men with sexually transmitted diseases. Experience from a center in Africa. N Engl J Med 1988; 319:274-8
52. Miller CJ, Vogel P, Alexander NJ et al. Pathology and localization of SIV in the reproductive tract of chronically infected male rhesus macaques. Lab. Invest. in press
53. Miller CJ, Alexander NJ, Sutjipto S et al. Effect of virus dose and nonoxynol-9 on the genital transmission of SIV in rhesus macaques. J Med Primatol 1990; 19:401-9
54. Hook EWI and Holmes KK. Gonococcal infections. Ann Intern Med 1985; 102:229-43
55. Baker CC, Phelps WC, Lindgren V et al. Structural and transcriptional analysis of human papillomavirus type 16 sequences in cervical carcinoma cell lines. J Virol 1987; 61:962-71
56. Durst M, Gissmann L, Ikenberg H et al. A papillomavirus DNA from a cervical carcinoma and its prevalence in cancer biopsy samples from different geographic regions. Proc Natl Acad Sci U S A 1983; 80:3812-5
57. Pater MM, Dunne J, Hogan G et al. Human papillomavirus types 16 and 18 sequences in early cervical neoplasia. Virology 1986; 155:13-8
58. Schwarz E, Freese UK, Gissmann L et al. Structure and transcription of human papillomavirus sequences in cervical carcinoma cells. Nature 1985; 314:111-4
59. Taylor HR, Johnson SL, Prendergast RA et al. An animal model of trachoma II. The importance of repeated reinfection. Invest Ophthalmol Vis Sci 1982; 23:507-15
60. Monnickendam MA, Darougar S, Treharne JD et al. Development of chronic conjunctivitis with scarring and pannus, resembling trachoma, in guinea-pigs. Br J Ophthalmol 1980; 64:284-90
61. Patton DL. Immunopathology and histopathology of experimental chlamydial salpingitis. Rev Infect Dis 1985; 7:746-53
62. Patton DL and Kuo CC. Histopathology of Chlamydia trachomatis salpingitis after primary and repeated reinfections in the monkey subcutaneous pocket model. J Reprod Fertil 1989; 85:647-56
63. Quinn TC, Taylor HR and Schachter J. Experimental proctitis due to rectal infection with Chlamydia trachomatis in nonhuman primates. J Infect Dis 1986; 154:833-41
64. Tuffrey M, Alexander F and Taylor RD. Severity of salpingitis in mice after primary and repeated inoculation with a human strain of Chlamydia trachomatis. J Exp Pathol (Oxford) 1990; 71:403-10
65. Corey L. Genital Herpes. In: Holmes KK, Mardh PA, Sparling PF et al. , ed. Sexually Transmitted Diseases. New York. McGraw-Hill,1990: 391-413

66. Lukehart SA. Immunology and pathogenesis of syphilis. In: Quinn TC, ed. Sexually transmitted diseases. New York. Raven Press,1992: 141-63
67. Tosca A, Lehou J, Hatjivasiliou M et al. Infiltrate of syphilitic lesions before and after treatment. Genitourin Med 1988; 64:289-93
68. Sabin AB. HIV vaccination dilemma [letter]. Nature 1993; 362:212
69. Ison CA, Hadfield SG, Bellinger CM et al. The specificity of serum and local antibodies in female gonorrhoea. Clin Exp Immunol 1986; 65:198-205
70. Lammel CJ, Sweet RL, Rice PA et al. Antibody-antigen specificity in the immune response to infection with Neisseria gonorrhoeae. J Infect Dis 1985; 152:990-1001
71. Cooper MD and Moticka EJ. Cellular immune responses during gonococcal and meningococcal infections. Clin Microbiol Rev 1989; S29-34
72. Harkness AH. The pathology of gonorrhea. Br. J. Vener. Dis. 1948; 24:137-47
73. Brunham RC, Kuo CC, Cles L et al. Correlation of host immune response with quantitative recovery of Chlamydia trachomatis from the human endocervix. Infect Immun 1983; 39:1491-4
74. Moulder JW. Interaction of chlamydiae and host cells in vitro. Microbiol Rev 1991; 55:143-90
75. Morrison RP, Manning DS and Caldwell HD. Immunology of Chlamydia trachomatis infections: immunoprotective and immunopathogenetic responses. In: Quinn TC, ed. Sexually Transmitted Diseases. New York. Raven Press,1992: 57-84
76. Lukehart SA, Baker ZS, Lloyd RM et al. Characterization of lymphocyte responsiveness in early experimental syphilis. II. Nature of cellular infiltration and Treponema pallidum distribution in testicular lesions. J Immunol 1980; 124:461-7
77. Zhou JA, McIndoe A, Davies H et al. The induction of cytotoxic T-lymphocyte precursor cells by recombinant vaccinia virus expressing human papillomavirus type 16 L1. Virology 1991; 181:203-10
78. Kohl S. Human immune response to herpes simplex virus. J Infect Dis 1982; 146:292
79. Kohl S, Adam E, Matson DO et al. Kinetics of human antibody responses to primary genital herpes simplex virus infection. Intervirology 1982; 18:164-8
80. Gronroos M, Honkonen E, Terho P et al. Cervical and serum IgA and serum IgG antibodies to Chlamydia trachomatis and herpes simplex virus in threatened abortion: a prospective study. Br J Obstet Gynaecol 1983; 90:167-70
81. Coughlan BM and Skinner GR. Antibody activity to type 1 and type 2 herpes simplex virus in human cervical mucus. Br J Obstet Gynaecol 1977; 84:622-9
82. Murphy JF, Murphy DF, Barker S et al. Neutralising antibody against type 1 and type 2 herpes simplex virus in cervical mucus of women with cervical intra-epithelial neoplasia. Med Microbiol Immunol (Berl) 1985; 174:73-80
83. Persson E, Eneroth P and Jeansson S. Secretory IgA against herpes simplex virus in cervical secretions. Genitourin Med 1988; 64:373-7
84. Koutsky LA, Ashley RL, Holmes KK et al. The frequency of unrecognized type 2 herpes simplex virus infection among women. Implications for the control of genital herpes. Sex Transm Dis 1990; 17:90-4
85. Breinig MK, Kingsley LA, Armstrong JA et al. Epidemiology of genital herpes in Pittsburgh: serologic, sexual, and racial correlates of apparent and inapparent herpes simplex infections. J Infect Dis 1990; 162:299-305

86. Nahmias AJ, Lee FK and Beckman NS. Sero-epidemiological and -sociological patterns of herpes simplex virus infection in the world. Scand J Infect Dis Suppl 1990; 69:19-36
87. Mertz GJ, Ashley R, Burke RL et al. Double-blind, placebo-controlled trial of a herpes simplex virus type 2 glycoprotein vaccine in persons at high risk for genital herpes infection. J Infect Dis 1990; 161:653-60
88. Reeves WC, Corey L, Adams HG et al. Risk of recurrence after first episodes of genital herpes. Relation to HSV type and antibody response. N Engl J Med 1981; 305:315-9
89. Archibald DW, Witt DJ, Craven DE et al. Antibodies to human immunodeficiency virus in cervical secretions from women at risk for AIDS. J. Infect. Dis. 1987; 156:240-1
90. Belec L, Georges A, Steenman G et al. Antibodies to human immunodeficiency virus in vaginal secretions of heterosexual women. J. Infect. Dis. 1989; 385-91
91. Lu XS, Belec L and Pillot J. Anti-gp 160 IgG and IgA antibodies associated with a large increase in total IgG in cervicovaginal secretions from human immunodeficiency virus type 1-infected women. J. Infect. Dis. 1993; 167:1189-92
92. Murphy BR and Chanock RM. Immunization against viruses. In: Fields BN and Knipe DM, ed. Virology. New York. Raven Press,1990: 469-502
93. Murphy BR, Sotnikov AV, Lawrence LA et al. Enhanced pulmonary histopathology is observed in cotton rats immunized with formalin-inactivated respiratory syncitial virus (RSV) or purified F glycoprotein and challenged with RSV 3-6 months after immunization. Vaccine 1990; 8:497-502
94. Murphy BR, Prince GA, Lawrence LA et al. Detection of respiratory syncytial virus (RSV) infected cells by in-situ hybridization in the lungs of cotton rats immunized with formalin-inactivated virus or RSV F and G glycoprotein subunit vaccine and challenged with RSV. Virus Res. 1990; 16:153-62
95. Alexander NJ, Fulgham DL and Goldberg E. Contraceptive vaccine development: secretory immune response in mice and monkeys. Vacc. Res. 1992; 1:331-45
96. Clerici M and Shearer GM. A Th1-Th2 switch is a critical step in the etiology of HIV infection. Immunol. Today 1993; 14:107-11
97. Bretscher PA, Wei G, Menon JN et al. Establishment of stable, cell-mediated immunity that makes "susceptible" mice resistant to Leishmania major. Science 1992; 257:539-42
98. McGhee J, Mestecky J, Elson C et al. Regulation of IgA synthesis and immune response by T cells and interleukins. J. Clin. Immunol. 1989; 175-99
99. Stanberry LR, Myers MG, Stephanopoulos DE et al. Preinfection prophylaxis with herpes simplex virus glycoprotein immunogens: factors influencing efficacy. J Gen Virol 1989; 70:3177-85
100. McDermott MR, Smiley JR, Leslie P et al. Immunity in the female genital tract after intravaginal vaccination of mice with an attenuated strain of Herpes Simplex Virus Type 2. J. Virol. 1984; 51:747-53
101. McDermott MR, Brais PLJ, Goettsche GC et al. Expression of immunity to intravaginal herpes simplex virus type 2 in the genital tract and associated lymph nodes. Arch Virol 1987; 93:51-68
102. McDermott MR, Goldsmith CH, Rosenthal KL et al. T-lymphocytes in Genital lymph nodes protect mice from intravaginal infection with Herpes Simplex Virus Type 2. J. Infect. Dis. 1989; 159:460-6

103. Burke RL. Current developments in herpes simplex virus vaccines. Semin. Virol. 1993; 4:187-97
104. Campo MS. Vaccination against papillomavirus. Cancer Cells 1991; 3:421-6
105. Campo MC, Grindlay GJ, O'Neil BW et al. Prophylactic and therapeutic vaccination against a mucosal papillomavirus. J Gen Virol 1993; 945-53
106. Rose RC, Bonnez W, Reichman RC et al. Expression of human papillomavirus type 11 L1 protein in insect cells: in vivo and in vitro assembly of viruslike particles. J Virol 1993; 67:1936-44
107. Hines JF, Ghim SJ, Christensen ND et al. HPV L1 proteins expressed in COS cells display type-specific and neutralizing epitopes. 12th International Papillomavirus Conference. Baltimore, MD. 1993 (abstr.)
108. Miller JN. Immunity in experimental syphilis. VI. Successful vaccination of rabbits with Treponema pallidum, Nichols strain, attenuated by -irradiation. J Immunol 1973; 110:1206-15
109. Gardner MB and Hu SL. SIV vaccines, 1991- a year in review. AIDS 1991; 5 (suppl 2):S115-27
110. Marthas M, Sutjipto S, Miller C et al. Efficacy of live-attenuated and whole-inactivated simian immunodeficiency virus vaccines against intravenous and intravaginal challenge. In: Brown F, Chanock rM, Ginsberg HS et al. , ed. Vaccines 1992. Cold Spring Harbor Laboratory Press,1992: 117-22
111. Marx PA, Compans RW, Gettie A et al. Protection against vaginal SIV transmission with microencapsulated vaccine. Science 1993; 260:1323-7
112. Dertzbaugh M and Elson CO. Cholera toxin as a mucosal adjuvant. In: Spriggs DR and Koff WC, ed. Topics in adjuvant research. Boca Raton. CRC Press,1991: 119-31
113. Elson CO and Ealding W. Cholera toxin feeding did not induce oral tolerance in mice and abrogated oral tolerance to an unrelated protein antigen. J Immunol 1984; 133:2892-8
114. Lycke N and Holmgren J. Strong adjuvant properties of cholera toxin on gut mucosal immune responses to orally presented antigens. Immunology 1986; 59:301-8
115. Lycke N and Holmgren J. Long-term cholera antitoxin memory in the gut can be triggered to antibody formation associated with protection within hours of an oral challenge immunization. Scand J Immunol 1987; 25:407-12
116. Lewis DJ, Novotny P, Dougan G et al. The early cellular and humoral immune response to primary and booster oral immunization with cholera toxin B subunit. Eur J Immunol 1991; 21:2087-94
117. Czerkinsky C, Prince SJ, Michalek SM et al. IgA antibody-producing cells in peripheral blood after antigen ingestion: evidence for a common mucosal immune system in humans. Proc Natl Acad Sci U S A 1987; 84:2449-53
118. Alpuche-Aranda C, Swanson J, Loomis W et al. Salmonella typhimurium activates virulence gene transcription within acidified macrophage phagosomes. Proc. Natl. Acad. Sci. (USA) 1992; 89:10079-83
119. Loomis W, Calderwood S and Miller S. Salmonella vaccine construction using a suicide vector that inserts heterologous antigen within a unique virulence locus. Infect. Immun. in press.
120. Flynn JL, Weiss WR, Norris KA et al. Generation of a cytotoxic T-lymphocyte response using a Salmonella antigen-delivery system. Mol. Microbiol. 1990; 4:2111-18

121. McDermott MR, Graham FL, Hanke T et al. Protection of mice against lethal challenge with herpes simplex virus by vaccination with an adenovirus vector expressing HSV glycoprotein B. Virology 1989; 169:244-7
122. Burke KL, Almond JW and Evans DJ. Antigen chimeras of poliovirus. Prog Med Virol 1991; 38:56-68
123. Burke KL, Evans DJ, Jenkins O et al. A cassette vector for the construction of antigen chimaeras of poliovirus. J Gen Virol 1989; 2475-9
124. Evans DJ and Almond JW. Design, construction, and characterization of poliovirus antigen chimeras. Methods Enzymol 1991; 203:386-400
125. Jenkins O, Cason J, Burke KL et al. An antigen chimera of poliovirus induces antibodies against human papillomavirus type 16. J Virol 1990; 64:1201-6
126. Vella C, Minor PD, Weller IV et al. Recognition of poliovirus/HIV chimaeras by antisera from individuals with HIV infection. Aids 1991; 5:425-30
127. Eldridge JH, Gilley RM, Staas JK et al. Biodegradable microspheres: vaccine delivery system for oral immunization. Curr. Top. Microbiol. Immunol. 1989; 146:59-66
128. Nair S, Zhou F, Reddy R et al. Soluble proteins delivered to dendritic cells via pH-sensitive liposomes induce primary cytotoxic T lymphocyte responses in vitro. J Exp Med 1992; 175:609-12
129. Reddy R, Nair S, Brynestad K et al. Liposomes as antigen delivery systems in viral immunity. Semin Immunol 1992; 4:91-6
130. Reddy R, Zhou F, Nair S et al. In vivo cytotoxic T lymphocyte induction with soluble proteins administered in liposomes. J Immunol 1992; 148:1585-9
131. Michalek SM, Childers NK, Katz J et al. Liposomes as oral adjuvants. Curr. Top. Microbiol. Immunol. 1989; 146:51-8.
132. Fujii Y, Aramaki Y, Hara T et al. Enhancement of systemic and mucosal immune responses following oral administration of liposomes. Immunol. Lett. 1993; 36:65-9
133. Martinon F, Krishnan S, Lenzen G et al. Induction of virus-specific cytotoxic T lymphocytes in vivo by liposome-entrapped mRNA. Eur. J. Immunol. 1993; 23:1719-22
134. Brownlie RM, Brahmbhatt HN, White DC et al. Stimulation of secretory antibodies against Bordetella pertussis antigens in the lungs of mice after oral or intranasal administration of liposome-incorporated cell-surface antigens. Microb. Pathog. 1993; 14:149-60
135. Plautz GE, Yang ZY, Wu BY et al. Immunotherapy of malignancy by in vivo gene transfer into tumors. Proc. Natl. Acad. Sci. U.S.A. 1993; 90:4645-9
136. Ulmer JB, Donnely JJ, Parker SE et al. Heterologous protection against influenza by injection of DNA encoding a viral protein. Science 1993; 259:1745-9
137. Wolff JA, Malone RW, Williams P et al. Direct gene transfer into mouse muscle in vivo. Science 1990.; 247:1465-8
138. Jiao S, Williams P, Berg RK et al. Direct gene transfer into nonhuman primate myofibers in vivo. Hum Gene Therapy 1992; 3:21-33

INDEX

Items in italics denote figures (f) or tables (t).

H

I

J

K

L